/

RECOVERY-ORIENTED COGNITIVE THERAPY FOR SERIOUS MENTAL HEALTH CONDITIONS

Also from Aaron T. Beck and Colleagues

FOR PROFESSIONALS

Cognitive Therapy for Adolescents in School Settings
Torrey A. Creed, Jarrod Reisweber, and Aaron T. Beck

*Cognitive Therapy of Anxiety Disorders:
Science and Practice*
David A. Clark and Aaron T. Beck

Cognitive Therapy of Depression
Aaron T. Beck, A. John Rush, Brian F. Shaw,
and Gary Emery

Cognitive Therapy of Personality Disorders: Third Edition
Edited by Aaron T. Beck, Denise D. Davis,
and Arthur Freeman

Cognitive Therapy of Substance Abuse
Aaron T. Beck, Fred D. Wright, Cory F. Newman,
and Bruce S. Liese

Group Cognitive Therapy for Addictions
Amy Wenzel, Bruce S. Liese, Aaron T. Beck,
and Dara G. Friedman-Wheeler

The Integrative Power of Cognitive Therapy
Brad A. Alford and Aaron T. Beck

Schizophrenia: Cognitive Theory, Research, and Therapy
Aaron T. Beck, Neil A. Rector, Neal Stolar, and Paul Grant

FOR GENERAL READERS

*The Anxiety and Worry Workbook:
The Cognitive Behavioral Solution*
David A. Clark and Aaron T. Beck

Recovery-Oriented Cognitive Therapy for Serious Mental Health Conditions

Aaron T. Beck
Paul Grant
Ellen Inverso
Aaron P. Brinen
Dimitri Perivoliotis

THE GUILFORD PRESS
New York   London

Copyright © 2021 The Guilford Press
A Division of Guilford Publications, Inc.
370 Seventh Avenue, Suite 1200, New York, NY 10001
www.guilford.com

All rights reserved

Except as noted, no part of this book may be reproduced, translated, stored in a retrieval system, or transmitted, in any form or by any means, electronic, mechanical, photocopying, microfilming, recording, or otherwise, without written permission from the publisher.

Printed in the United States of America

This book is printed on acid-free paper.

Last digit is print number: 9   8   7   6   5   4   3   2   1

LIMITED DUPLICATION LICENSE

These materials are intended for use only by qualified mental health professionals.

The publisher grants to individual purchasers of this book nonassignable permission to reproduce all materials for which photocopying permission is specifically granted in a footnote. This license is limited to you, the individual purchaser, for personal use or use with clients. This license does not grant the right to reproduce these materials for resale, redistribution, electronic display, or any other purposes (including but not limited to books, pamphlets, articles, video or audio recordings, blogs, file-sharing sites, Internet or intranet sites, and handouts or slides for lectures, workshops, or webinars, whether or not a fee is charged). Permission to reproduce these materials for these and any other purposes must be obtained in writing from the Permissions Department of Guilford Publications.

The authors have checked with sources believed to be reliable in their effort to provide information that is complete and generally in accord with the standards of practice that are accepted at the time of publication. However, in view of the possibility of human error or changes in behavioral, mental health, or medical sciences, neither the authors, nor the editors and publisher, nor any other party who has been involved in the preparation or publication of this work warrants that the information contained herein is in every respect accurate or complete, and they are not responsible for any errors or omissions or the results obtained from the use of such information. Readers are encouraged to confirm the information contained in this book with other sources.

Library of Congress Cataloging-in-Publication Data

Names: Beck, Aaron T., author.
Title: Recovery-oriented cognitive therapy for serious mental health conditions / Aaron T. Beck, Paul Grant, Ellen Inverso, Aaron P. Brinen, Dimitri Perivoliotis.
Description: New York : The Guilford Press, [2021] | Includes bibliographical references and index. |
Identifiers: LCCN 2020024544 | ISBN 9781462545209 (cloth ; alk. paper) |
ISBN 9781462545193 (paperback ; alk. paper)
Subjects: LCSH: Mental health—Treatment. | Cognitive therapy.
Classification: LCC RA790 .B424 2020 | DDC 616.89/1425—dc23
LC record available at *https://lccn.loc.gov/2020024544*

About the Authors

Aaron T. Beck, MD, is the founder of cognitive therapy, University Professor Emeritus of Psychiatry at the University of Pennsylvania, and President Emeritus of the Beck Institute for Cognitive Behavior Therapy. He is a recipient of awards including the Albert Lasker Clinical Medical Research Award, the Lifetime Achievement Award from the American Psychological Association, the Distinguished Service Award from the American Psychiatric Association, the James McKeen Cattell Fellow Award in Applied Psychology from the Association for Psychological Science, and the Sarnat International Prize in Mental Health and Gustav O. Lienhard Award from the Institute of Medicine. Dr. Beck is author or editor of numerous books for professionals and the general public.

Paul Grant, PhD, is Director of Research, Innovation, and Practice at the Beck Institute Center for Recovery-Oriented Cognitive Therapy. With Aaron T. Beck, he originated recovery-oriented cognitive therapy (CT-R) and conducted foundational research to validate it. He is a recipient of awards from the National Alliance on Mental Illness, the University of Medicine and Dentistry of New Jersey, and the Association for Behavioral and Cognitive Therapies. Dr. Grant developed group, family, and milieu CT-R approaches, and directs large projects implementing CT-R nationally and internationally. He has developed innovative implementation tools and is involved in researching positive beliefs and teamwide culture change as mediators of successful CT-R outcomes.

Ellen Inverso, PsyD, is Director of Clinical Training and Implementation at the Beck Institute Center for Recovery-Oriented Cognitive Therapy. A codeveloper of CT-R, she has created transformative CT-R programming for psychiatric inpatient units, programmatic residences, schools, and community teams, with a special focus on adolescents and young adults, individuals engaging in extreme forms of self-injury, individuals considering transitions into the community following extended periods of institutionalization, and families. Dr. Inverso supervises early career professionals in CT-R, guides her seasoned colleagues to add the approach to their armamentaria, and has coauthored curricula for training peer specialists and expert trainers in CT-R.

Aaron P. Brinen, PsyD, is Assistant Professor of Clinical Psychiatry and Behavioral Sciences at Vanderbilt University Medical Center, where he provides training in CT-R, serves individuals with psychosis, and collaborates on research. Previously, he directed Drexel University's center for the dissemination, development, study, and practice of CT-R. A codeveloper of CT-R, Dr. Brinen worked to formalize the treatment and adapt it for individual and group therapy settings, as well as in team-based psychiatric care and during inpatient treatment. He trains psychiatry residents in CT-R and has been active in training community therapists from around the world. Dr. Brinen also has a small clinical psychology practice specializing in cognitive-behavioral therapy for individuals with schizophrenia, posttraumatic stress disorder, and other disorders.

Dimitri Perivoliotis, PhD, is a psychologist at the VA San Diego Healthcare System and Associate Clinical Professor in the Department of Psychiatry at the University of California, San Diego (UCSD). At the VA, he is the coordinator of the Center of Recovery Education. He is also Training Director of the VA San Diego/UCSD Interprofessional Fellowship in Psychosocial Rehabilitation and Recovery Oriented Services. In these settings, Dr. Perivoliotis conducts individual and group cognitive-behavioral therapy for people with psychosis and co-occurring conditions, such as posttraumatic stress disorder, and provides supervision, training, and consultation to psychology, psychiatry, and social work trainees. He is a codeveloper of CT-R.

Preface

These are exciting times for the treatment of serious mental health conditions. The last two decades have seen a steady growth in effective approaches. Standout therapies—moral therapy, occupational therapy, recreational therapy, creative arts therapy, clubhouse model—have been joined by newer approaches—social skills, supportive employment, supportive housing, cognitive remediation, cognitive-behavioral therapy—all of which have accrued their own evidence base (Jay, 2016; Lieberman, Stroup, Perkins, & Dixon, 2020).

This book represents a leap forward in the approach to these formidable conditions. The know-how contained within this book is the result of 20 years of focused effort. Thousands of people have contributed to our thinking, the most important being those given a diagnosis.

It all began when two of us—Grant and Beck—initiated a side project to advance treatment for individuals given a diagnosis of schizophrenia whom community providers and family members identified as being people they wanted to help more effectively. This side project has become a passion and our mission. Conversations with providers and individuals with lived experience turned to observations of inpatient units, community teams, individual and group therapy sessions, waiting rooms, and family meetings, which turned to research studies.

These studies confirmed our theory that beliefs help us understand how people with serious mental health conditions might get stuck but also how they do well. We developed a powerful and empowering treatment approach and conducted clinical and implementation studies to show that our approach frees people to live a better life, a desired life, a wonderful life.

We know that individuals who find themselves in difficult circumstances are often stronger than they realize. They have potential they may not believe they have. We delight in being able to see them exceed all expectations. To recover. To thrive. To flourish. To enjoy life. To make the world a better place. To find their mission.

While we remain optimistic about the rich possibility residing within every person, we are not Pollyannas. The challenges can seem insurmountable, both to those experiencing them and to those who want to collaborate to make life better.

> He has a blanket over his head. She won't talk. He talks to himself all day. She comes out of her room swinging. He swallows objects. She talks of being God.

How do you find the person who may be obscured in these vexing challenges? This book will show you how.

The work can be hard and trying at times but can also be supremely rewarding. We have shared tears with countless mental health providers and families when the breakthrough comes. And the breakthrough can be many things.

> Making the first friend in 20 years. Dating after 40 years in an institution. Volunteering to help kids. Starting a fashion club in the community. Becoming active in the local church.

If you want to create, sustain, and build on breakthroughs—this book will show you how.

Life is never linear. There are ups and downs for all of us. Setbacks can seem especially crushing for someone who is just beginning—often after decades—to get the life of their choosing.

> Can they tap into their inner strength to keep trying? Can they cultivate resiliency to participate more and help others? Can they see their flourishing is getting stronger when things do not work out?

If you want to empower people to achieve their purpose in the face of life's challenges, this book will show you how.

You may work in corrections, a state hospital (civil or forensic), a long-term hospital, an acute care hospital, a programmatic residence, a community team (assertive community treatment, coordinated specialty care, mobile crisis), a community mental health center, private practice, or a military setting. The approach we detail in this book has seen success in all of these locations.

Your role in care may be as a case manager, creative arts therapist, direct care staff, drug and alcohol specialist, nurse, occupational therapist, peer provider or specialist, psychiatric rehabilitation specialist, psychiatrist, psychologist, social worker, or vocational specialist. Our approach has been useful to practitioners from all of these disciplines.

You will find in the contents of this book a synthesis of many seemingly eclectic elements. The humanistic tradition of Carl Rogers (1951) and Abraham Maslow (1954) is here. The behavioral tradition of B. F. Skinner (Liberman, 2008) and Joseph Wolpe (1990) is here. The psychodynamic tradition of Silvano Arieti (1974) and others is here. The psychiatric rehabilitation tradition of William Anthony (1980) and colleagues is present.

The cognitive model (Beck, 1963) and theory of modes (Beck, 1996) form the theoretical map that links everything together. The targets we are going for are defined by the recovery movement's emphasis on promoting self-defined hope, empowerment, and purpose (Davidson et al., 2008). We call the approach *recovery-oriented cognitive therapy* (CT-R).

You will be able to incorporate the knowledge and proficiency you already possess to make for powerful outcomes. Figure 1 represents the way in which strengths of other therapeutic approaches overlap with CT-R.

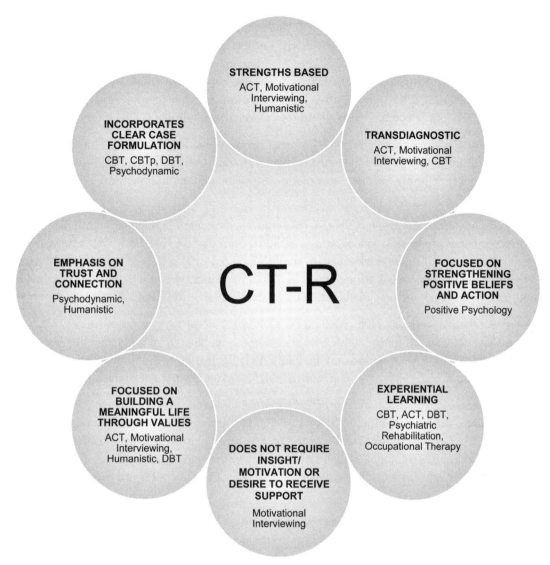

FIGURE 1. Overlap of CT-R with other approaches. CBT, cognitive-behavioral therapy; CBTp, cognitive-behavioral therapy for psychosis; DBT, dialectical behavior therapy; ACT, acceptance and commitment therapy.

The focus in the chapters to come is on how to do things. CT-R is grounded in theory and research. However, the purpose of this book is to aid you in learning and doing.

There are several additional features of CT-R that we think make it worth your time to learn about this therapeutic approach:

- *A focus on the positive.* Much of what you will find in this book aims to foster positive emotions, beliefs, and action. We do not accentuate the positive just because we are nice people. We focus on the positive because it works clinically. It turns out to be a fruitful way to meet people where they are and collaborate with them on building their best life and their best self (Grant & Inverso, in press; Grant, Perivoliotis, Luther, Bredemeier, & Beck, 2018). For people living with serious mental health conditions, there are myriad reasons to avoid seeking help and to not trust promises from clinical contacts who have repeatedly disappointed them (Dixon, Holoshitz, & Nossel, 2016). The positive focus we embrace can help you bridge that divide of mistrust; it serves as a connective and sustaining force, the vitality of CT-R.

- *An action orientation.* You will find that action pervades this book. From how to get started to building up a desired life to developing resilience to flourishing. Purpose is lived. But action is more than just being busy; we use it in a strategic manner to produce dramatic positive change.

- *Empowerment through beliefs.* Action enjoys a dynamic interchange with beliefs; positive experiences are terrific sources to strengthen a person's adaptive view of themselves, others, and the future. Empowerment lies in strengthened personal beliefs of being a good person, a helping person, one who is strong and able to handle things when the going gets tough. The book is replete with guidance to elicit this life-sustaining empowerment.

- *Innovative approaches to challenges.* Delusions, negative symptoms, disorganization, aggressive behavior, self-injury, substance use—using a combination of understanding, our positive orientation, and know-how, we present unique and effective ways to empower individuals with regard to each of these challenges. This is always in the service of what a person really wants in life.

- *Applicability to the complexity of real people.* People experience a diversity of challenges. Our approach to understanding and empowering is grounded in the theory and strategy of Beck's (2019b) cognitive model that, over the past 60 years, has been successfully validated for nearly every problem we might encounter in working with someone. You will see that nobody is too complex, nobody too severely challenged. Everyone can progress toward their desired life.

- *Focus on the whole person.* By including positive actions and beliefs alongside specific challenges, case formulation broadens into a mapping of recovery and resiliency. We do not consider a problem or challenge in isolation from a person's positive interests, aspirations, and assets. We have created a form for guiding the focus on the whole person—the Recovery Map. You will find the Recovery Map in every chapter. It helps to organize your thinking and can aid in the coordination of a multidisciplinary team, as well as continuity across levels of care.

This book can help you develop a spirited savvy in CT-R over the course of 15 chapters, which we have organized into three parts:

Part I—CT-R Model of Transformation and Empowerment. The first six chapters introduce you to CT-R—the basic model and how it works.

Part II—Empowerment for Common Challenges. Building on the basics, the five chapters in Part II extend understanding, strategy, and intervention to the challenges that have historically gotten the person stuck: negative symptoms, delusions, hallucinations, communication challenges, trauma, self-injury, aggressive behavior, and substance use.

Part III—CT-R Contexts. The final four chapters delve deeper into specific settings and applications—individual therapy, therapeutic milieu, group therapy, and families.

Preface   xi

LANGUAGE MATTERS

Throughout this book we have taken care to balance language that is sensitive to people's lived experience while also being accurate. The history of psychiatry is full of terms that carry negative baggage and can limit collaborative success. Some expressions are misleading, some are simply false, some are unnecessarily upsetting, and some can foster stigma.

Our aim is to communicate in a way that is destigmatizing and nonjudgmental, recognizing that we undoubtedly have some room for improvement. In this vein, we have adjusted our language in many ways away from that of traditional psychopathological texts. We have gained valuable perspective from all of our collaborators, especially those with lived experience, on the impact of words, and we imagine that this will continue to develop over time.

In this book, we refer to those whom you are collaborating with, who are receiving care, as *individuals*. These individuals have been *given a diagnosis* and they tend to experience *serious mental health challenges*. It is out of this attempt at balance that we have titled this book *Recovery-Oriented Cognitive Therapy for Serious Mental Health Conditions*. We use the pronouns *they* and *them* to refer to any specific individual in the singular. Case examples discussed in this book are loosely based on actual cases and do not depict any specific person or contain any protected health information. Appendix A defines some of the common terms we use in this volume.

This book was coming to press precisely as the COVID-19 pandemic had a significant impact on the culture. We follow former Surgeon General Vivek Murthy's (2020) observation that the prescription to fight the spread of the virus is not *social* distancing but *physical* distancing. CT-R is an action-oriented approach that emphasizes connection. This connection can be achieved via telehealth and over the phone. Very successful social connection through CT-R is possible while physical distancing. As a result of this success, we have included text on telehealth in Chapters 3 and 12, as well as two online tip sheets that give useful advice for how to succeed in doing action-oriented CT-R when communicating via remote means.

ACKNOWLEDGMENTS

We extend a tremendous amount of gratitude and appreciation for all those who have supported us and have been involved in the completion of this book. We would especially like to acknowledge those who have contributed to essential elements of the text: Elisa Payne, PhD, for many of the ideas in the "Families as Facilitators of Empowerment" chapter; Joseph Keifer, PsyD, BSN, RN, for developing the Recovery Map How-To Guide; Jenna Feldman, PsyD, for construction of the adaptive mode and aspirations decision trees; Nina Bertolami for organization, formatting, and resource supports, and extensive reading and revision at each stage; Marguerite Cruz for organization and graphic design assistance; Shelby Arnold, PhD, Amber Margetich, PsyD, and Adam Rifkin, LPC, for the creation of several appendices and graphic representations of CT-R; Francesca Lewis-Hatheway, PsyD, for significant improvements and practical examples pertaining to aspirations and development of several appendices; and Sarah Fleming and Ivy McDaniels for the creative improvements to appendices, handouts, and graphics. We are grateful to all who provided feedback on earlier versions of the manuscript.

We would also like to thank Judith Beck, PhD (whose book *Cognitive Behavior Therapy: Basics and Beyond* is now in its third edition), for strategy and guidance; Arthur Evans, PhD, for challenging us to truly bring recovery to all; and our many community and hospital partners who have taught us so much.

This book is dedicated to the incredible individuals with lived experience who teach us and help us do better every day—who trust us with their hopes and dreams and partner with us in their pursuit of the life they want!

Contents

I. CT-R Model of Transformation and Empowerment — 1

1. Introduction to Recovery-Oriented Cognitive Therapy — 3
2. Mapping Recovery: Developing a Plan for Transformative Action — 17
3. Accessing and Energizing the Adaptive Mode — 29
4. Developing the Adaptive Mode: Aspirations — 58
5. Actualizing the Adaptive Mode: Positive Action — 79
6. Strengthening the Adaptive Mode — 88

II. Empowerment for Common Challenges — 103

7. Empowering When Negative Symptoms Are the Challenge — 105
8. Empowering When Delusions Are the Challenge — 116
9. Empowering When Hallucinations Are the Challenge — 133
10. Empowering When Communication Is the Challenge — 143
11. Empowering When Trauma, Self-Injury, Aggressive Behavior, or Substance Use Is the Challenge — 155

III. CT-R Contexts — 177

12. Individual CT-R for the Sole Provider — 179

13. The CT-R Inpatient Service — 193

14. CT-R Group Therapy — 211

15. Families as Facilitators of Empowerment — 222

APPENDICES — 231

A. CT-R Terminology — 233

B. Blank Recovery Map — 234

C. Recovery Map How-To Guide — 235

D. Suggestions for Activities to Access the Adaptive Mode — 237

E. Blank Activity Schedule — 238

F. Blank Chart for Breaking Aspirations into Steps — 239

G. Interventions for Individuals Experiencing Negative Symptoms — 240

H. CT-R Benchmarks — 241

Resources — 257

References — 259

Index — 265

Purchasers of this book can download and print copies of the reproducible appendices, and access online-only tip sheets on CT-R strategies during social distancing, at *www.guilford.com/beck15-materials* for personal use or use with clients (see copyright page for details).

PART I
CT-R MODEL OF TRANSFORMATION AND EMPOWERMENT

Part I takes you through each of the stages of recovery-oriented cognitive therapy (CT-R), beginning with the development of a CT-R formulation. The diagram below shows you the core features of CT-R and matches the flow of the subsequent chapters:

THE CORE FEATURES OF CT-R

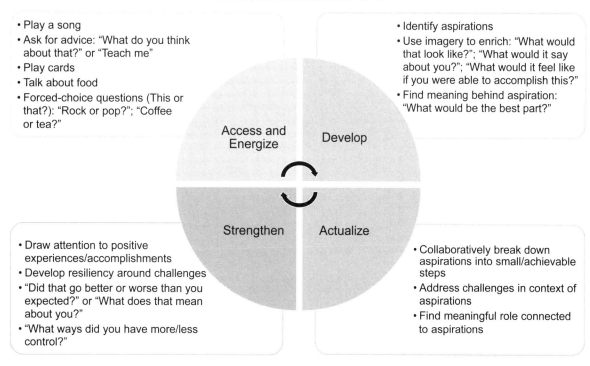

- Play a song
- Ask for advice: "What do you think about that?" or "Teach me"
- Play cards
- Talk about food
- Forced-choice questions (This or that?): "Rock or pop?"; "Coffee or tea?"

- Identify aspirations
- Use imagery to enrich: "What would that look like?"; "What would it say about you?"; "What would it feel like if you were able to accomplish this?"
- Find meaning behind aspiration: "What would be the best part?"

- Draw attention to positive experiences/accomplishments
- Develop resiliency around challenges
- "Did that go better or worse than you expected?" or "What does that mean about you?"
- "What ways did you have more/less control?"

- Collaboratively break down aspirations into small/achievable steps
- Address challenges in context of aspirations
- Find meaningful role connected to aspirations

CHAPTER 1.	Introduction to Recovery-Oriented Cognitive Therapy	3
	How you become familiar with the basic ideas and evidence base	
CHAPTER 2.	Mapping Recovery: Developing a Plan for Transformative Action	17
	How you organize and conceptualize a person's positive and negative experiences	
CHAPTER 3.	Accessing and Energizing the Adaptive Mode	29
	How you get started and build connection and trust	
CHAPTER 4.	Developing the Adaptive Mode: Aspirations	58
	How you discover and enrich aspirations that foster hope	
CHAPTER 5.	Actualizing the Adaptive Mode: Positive Action	79
	How you turn aspirations into action that grows purpose	
CHAPTER 6.	Strengthening the Adaptive Mode	88
	How you impact beliefs and empower throughout each stage	

CHAPTER 1
Introduction to Recovery-Oriented Cognitive Therapy

Michael, a resident of a state hospital for several decades, spent most of his time sitting and staring at the wall. When you did see him walking about, he was usually muttering to himself about having billions of dollars and thousands of wives. He was almost always alone.

Change started with an engaging conversation. A member of the treatment team approached Michael. Noting his football cap, she asked him whether he was a fan, and then where in town he was from. Michael soon shared a few of his interests: music, fishing, and motorcycles. They agreed to talk again.

Over the next few conversations Michael talked about dating and getting back on a motorcycle. The team member said that people often got together in a club to talk about the things they like, and what they wanted outside of the hospital. If he joined, he could teach others about motorcycles and good fishing spots in the city.

Michael did join the club. From the start, he demonstrated tremendous knowledge and love for music of the 1960s, plus a beautiful singing voice. He began to connect with people, dancing to the music and telling others about various singing groups. Those conversations led naturally to others about food and where the club members could eat and listen to music in the community outside of the hospital walls.

Eventually, Michael started to talk more about his desire to have a girlfriend. He sang songs in the club that he would sing to her. He began thinking about what it would mean to have a girlfriend. He wanted to take her out, be a loving and supportive boyfriend, and show her around the town. This would probably be easier if he were not in the hospital. For the first time in decades, Michael contemplated accepting a community housing offer. Ultimately, after a visit, he moved from the hospital into a transitional group home.

At the residence, Michael also discovered a talent for art, and began giving his drawings to other residents as gifts. He talked about his giving as a step toward making and keeping friends and a nice thing to do for a girlfriend. With his case team, Michael and other members visited neighborhood places where they shared food, listened to music, even went to church.

The church invited him to help in the food pantry. Soon Michael asked to join the cooking team in his residence. He recruited a friend from the house to join him in the pantry. Little by little, Michael developed a social network beyond his team. Eventually, he went to a less restrictive residence and began going out more and more on his own in the community. Michael became a familiar face in certain coffee shops. He struck up conversations with other regulars and eventually began dating someone he met at the coffee shop. He also got a job at a nearby diner.

Michael's life transformed dramatically. Decades of relative inactivity and disconnection gave way to an expanding life that realized his desire for meaningful relationships and a daily experience of purpose. The dreams, actions, and success were—and are—his. The guide to this new life: recovery-oriented cognitive therapy (CT-R).

The CT-R approach emphasizes meeting people where they are as the starting point. The team member knew to look for Michael's adaptive personality, finding it in sports and motorcycles. Trust and connection through action help to build momentum. The team first discussed Michael's interests and later offered him the opportunity to join the club. In this way, an interpersonal role for him evolved. The team also knew to draw Michael's attention to his successes and begin to think about his future. Hope came, evidenced by his voicing his wish for a romantic partner, and then action—taking steps to get out of the hospital and participate more fully in the community. The community team met with Michael and the hospital team, picking up the program and continuing his success and emerging autonomy—creating art, giving it away, developing friendships, starting to date, and getting a job.

CT-R reliably produces the right kind of interactions between service partners like yourself and individuals. This book is a how-to guide for partnering with individuals like Michael that enables them to move from languishing to flourishing.

In this chapter, we present the fundamentals of CT-R that lay the foundation for our subsequent work. The basic CT-R model involves the concept of recovery, the cognitive model, and the idea of modes. We introduce recovery mapping and the parts of CT-R. At the end of the chapter, we consider the evidence base for the approach.

RECOVERY—FROM POLITICAL MOVEMENT TO STANDARD OF TREATMENT

Mental health care has changed profoundly since the early 1960s in terms of the location—institution to community—and nature of care—from custodial to empowering (Broadway & Covington, 2018; Lutterman, Shaw, Fisher, & Manderscheid, 2017; Pinals & Fuller, 2017). The modern approach to recovery began as a political movement among individuals who were mostly in state hospitals advocating for themselves and others to receive better (or in some cases, any) treatment (Chamberlin, 1990). Their inspiration was the civil rights movement (Davidson, Rakfeldt, & Strauss, 2011).

A watershed year in turning recovery ideology into practice was 1999, with the publication of the Surgeon General's Report on Mental Health, and the U.S. Supreme Court's decision in *Olmstead v. L. C.* In that decision, mental health was equated with physical health. Effective treatments existed, and the court confirmed that people have the right to receive these treatments and pursue life in the community rather than within institutions: "The notion of recovery reflects a renewed optimism about the outcomes of mental illness, including that achieved through an individual's own self-care efforts, and the opportunities open to persons with mental illness to participate to the full extent of their interests in the community of their choice" (Satcher, 2000, p. 94).

Further steps were advanced in the final report of President George W. Bush's New Freedom Commission on Mental Health (2003), which endorsed a need to completely embrace recovery in mental health care, focusing on full community participation for everyone. In 2005, the Substance Abuse and Mental Health Services Administration (SAMHSA) issued a federal action agenda to carry out the aims of the New Freedom Commission. This document called for a revolution in the organization and delivery of mental health services.

RECOVERY—WHAT IT IS LIKE FROM THE INSIDE

The concept of recovery is admirable and broadly appealing. How to realize it in a person's life can be challenging. Two questions leap to mind: What is recovery-oriented care? and How do you do it?

Individuals who have received psychiatric treatment for serious mental health conditions offer a way forward. One such person created Figures 1.1 and 1.2 to distinguish bad from good approaches, respectively, that providers can take toward treatment. In Figure 1.1, psychiatric diagnosis and treatment is the largest circle, with all of the other factors in life being given lesser importance. In this approach, the provider prioritizes dealing with psychiatric issues, perhaps with the assumption that these must resolve prior to addressing the others.

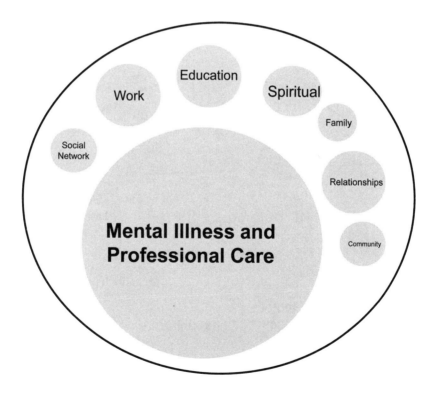

FIGURE 1.1. A less appealing focus of treatment.

As disengagement from treatment predicts a poor quality of life, institutionalization, homelessness, and greater disability for individuals given serious mental health diagnoses (Kreyenbuhl, Nossel, & Dixon, 2009), this first circle suggests why some might choose not to engage or to drop out.

Figure 1.2 contains the more appealing focus. Here aspects of life, such as going to school, dating, making friends, having a meaningful role, and working are much larger circles, with psychiatric treatment being a smaller circle. Providers delivering desirable treatment prioritize life and participation, and place psychiatric treatment within that context. Focusing treatment more squarely on recovery can broaden its appeal and potentially impact people who may not otherwise participate (Dixon, Holoshitz, & Nossel, 2016).

A recovery-oriented approach to treatment should emphasize the pursuit of an individualized sense of purpose (having a job, volunteering, helping your family) and meaningful relationships (friends, collegial, dating), as well as interests and hobbies. Individuals should have the opportunity to discover their inner power to help themselves or seek help when stress or problems arise. Everyone's life has challenges; treatment should promote resilience in regard to problems in the context of a person's fuller life.

> **Recovery means recovery of the individual's:**
>
> ✓ Interests
> ✓ Capabilities
> ✓ Aspirations
> ✓ Ability to problem-solve
> ✓ Ability to communicate effectively
> ✓ Resilience in the face of stress

In CT-R, recovery is defined broadly, in terms of people connecting—or reconnecting—with other people and with values that drive the life they want to be living. There are certain basic human needs that seem to underlie individuals' hopes and aspiration and lead to wellness and expression of their best self—connection, trust, hope, purpose, and empowerment (Harding, 2019).

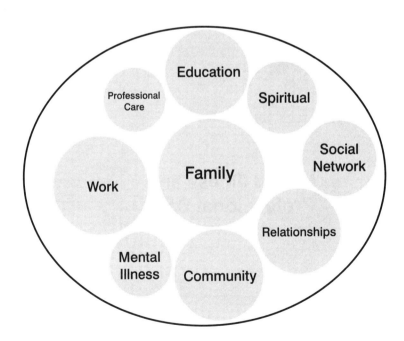

FIGURE 1.2. A more appealing focus of treatment.

THE COGNITIVE MODEL

Now that we have a better sense of what care should look like, how do you realize recovery? The cognitive model is useful in this regard (Beck, 1963). This model helps us understand how people flourish, as well as how they get stuck, in terms of beliefs they hold—about themselves, about other people, and about their future.

We can think of the person's best self, the person they want to be and experience more often (Callard, 2018). This self gets expressed in positive beliefs: "I am a good person," "I am a helping person," "I can be successful," "Others value me," "I belong to the group," "I am loved," "I have a future full of possibility to make a difference." With CT-R we identify this self, help the person live it every day, and strengthen the underlying beliefs.

ADAPTIVE MODE AND NOTICING AT-THEIR-BEST MOMENTS

We all speak of being in "work mode," "vacation mode," "survival mode." A *mode* is a manner of acting or doing that involves beliefs, attitudes, emotion, motivation, and behavior (Beck, 1996; Beck, Finkel, & Beck, 2020). We all have times when we are at our best, as do the individuals we work with. These *at-their-best* moments are an experience of one's best self and might occur during music group, at a birthday party, during a sporting event, or when describing a recipe. What do we see during these times? The person is warm, funny, connected, alert, knowledgeable. We refer to this way of being as the *adaptive mode*.

At-their-best moments occur when the individual connects with at least one other person and participates in a mutually beneficial activity. We can tell that these individuals are in the adaptive mode by their expression and behavior. They become animated, less pressured, and have a good time. Positive beliefs become more available, such as "I can have a good time," "I can be effective," and "I can be friends with other people." These positive beliefs are accompanied by energy, motivation, and good mood that free up latent capabilities and behaviors.

Treatment that focuses on the adaptive mode looks like that prescribed in Figure 1.2. It meaningfully involves other people, as well as a person's own strengths and talents, dreams and ambitions.

The adaptive mode is not exclusive to people given a diagnosis of a serious mental health condition; it is a general feature of being human. In CT-R, recovery means recovery of the adaptive mode: recovery of the individual's interests, values, capabilities, and aspirations, as well as their ability to problem-solve, think flexibly, communicate effectively, and be resilient in the face of stress. Recovery means flourishing in a desired life.

CHALLENGES AND THE STUCK QUALITY OF THE "PATIENT" MODE

Individuals may not get to experience their best self or adaptive personality that often. This may be a large part of why they are in care. Days may be dominated by the experience of low motivation, lack of pleasure, hallucinations, delusions, aggressive behavior, disorganization, or self-injury. These experiences are frequently fluctuating and time limited, yet can pose a significant challenge to daily living (Mote, Grant, & Silverstein, 2018).

The cognitive model (Beck, 1963) is also useful for our understanding of challenges. When in this "patient" mode, individuals see themselves as weak, incompetent, incapable; they see others as threatening, rejecting; and they see their future as uncertain and forbidding (Beck, Himelstein, & Grant, 2019). These beliefs have gravity. They seem like facts. It becomes hard to access motivation, easy to be consumed by hallucinations and delusions—and above all to be held back from the life of one's choosing. The negative beliefs coalesce into a negative sense of self that can have a strong pull on a person—the essence of being stuck.

PUTTING IT ALL TOGETHER

The whole focus of the CT-R approach is to locate the adaptive mode in the individual. Because the mode tends to be dormant, we need to energize it and then help the person develop, actualize, and strengthen it. Accessing the adaptive mode generally involves activities that do not look like traditional talk therapy.

What really works for people is the pursuit of some purpose that brings them a tremendous amount of meaning (Frankl, 1946). It's not about being busy or convincing yourself that things are okay; it's about making a difference. At the heart of CT-R is collaborating with individuals so they might develop and realize their mission in life.

CT-R helps individuals to locate their best self, develop it, and live their purpose every day. It focuses on what matters to individuals and places psychiatric problems in the context of the lives they want to live. It meets them where they are, even if they have low access to motivation and minimal interest in treatment or trust of service providers.

Figure 1.3 illustrates the essential components of CT-R. The adaptive mode is the focus of each part: accessing and energizing it, developing it, actualizing it, and strengthening it. The arrow itself is an image of progress. And the rectangles show how each of the components will

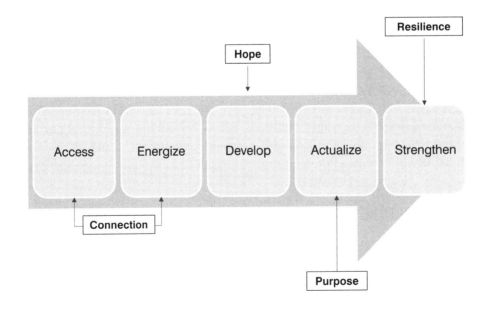

FIGURE 1.3. The CT-R arrow.

help you bring about the key aspects of recovery and wellness: connection, hope, purpose, and resilience. The CT-R arrow will be our guide throughout the first part of this book.

Introducing Recovery Mapping and the Recovery Map

CT-R requires a focus that expands beyond challenges to include interests, aspirations, and positive beliefs. We use the term "recovery mapping" to refer to the process of collecting information about all of these, develop an understanding in terms of beliefs, and planning treatment. The Recovery Map (see Appendix B) is a one-page living document that you can use individually or with your team. It guides the development of your CT-R understanding. It helps you plan strategies and interventions—with concrete targets for change—that collaboratively promote a meaningful life. The Recovery Map keeps you focused on beliefs at each step of treatment and helps ensure that problems are kept in the context of the whole person, especially their interests, aspirations, and meanings. In Chapter 2, you develop your recovery mapping skills.

The following describes the parts of the CT-R approach, including how the Recovery Map comes into play at each step.

Accessing and Energizing the Adaptive Mode through Connection

A significant number of people given a diagnosis do not say they want treatment, a diagnosis, or help. They may be discouraged, feeling that whatever they're doing is as good as it gets. They might not be trusting of mental health professionals.

Because of these concerns, you have to meet them where they are. This is a matter of finding and accessing their adaptive mode. We do this through human connection over shared interests and activities that excite the person. Accessing the adaptive mode requires an understanding of why a person might not initially want to engage with you. It also entails persistence to keep trying interests and activities until one of them generates a response. You can recognize when individuals are at-their-best and help to make these experiences happen more often.

But accessing the adaptive mode is not enough. We need to help the individual energize it. The aim is for the adaptive mode to occur more frequently and predictably. You can repeatedly develop the connection through shared interests that involve the individual helping you in some way. Energizing the adaptive mode requires repeated activity, based on the person's interests, that increases energy over time and lead to easier access of the adaptive mode. Ultimately, the individual can begin to project a future. The first row of the Recovery Map (see Appendix B) tracks accessing and energizing the adaptive mode.

As your relationship and doing activities together—either individually or as a team—is central to accessing and energizing efforts, this part of CT-R embodies human connection, which is an important feature of recovery and wellness. Chapter 3 enhances your skill at accessing and energizing the adaptive mode.

Developing the Adaptive Mode by Eliciting and Enriching Aspirations

When individuals become more connected to other people, develop trust, get more energy, and gain more access to motivation, it is time to focus on the life the person really wants to have. Specific features of that life could include owning a home, getting a romantic partner, starting a family, becoming a nurse, starting a business, or helping animals or the less fortunate. We use the term "aspirations" to refer to what people really want in their lives. Critical to CT-R is identifying aspirations that are big, meaningful, motivating desires.

It is particularly important to elicit meaning, which almost always involves helping other people, making a difference in the world socially, contributing in a significant way to family, or giving to others who are struggling. The meanings of aspirations are targets for everyday action. You can help enrich aspirations through the development of a recovery image that helps empower the person when stressful experiences occur. Individuals experience a palpable sense of hope when developing their adaptive mode. Hope is key to successful recovery and sustained wellness.

The second row of the Recovery Map (see Appendix B) is the place to record aspirations and the meanings driving them. Chapter 4 helps you develop skill in eliciting and enriching aspirations.

Actualizing the Adaptive Mode with Positive Action

It is not enough to just dream—recovery and flourishing are about realizing dreams. Aspirations help us to know what matters most to the person. Once we know the meaning of a person's aspiration, we need to get that into their life to actualize it every day. Individuals create their own desired life through positive, daily action that realizes their valued meanings. Such actions can be taking a step toward reaching the aspired-to goal or engaging in an activity that has the same underlying meaning—for example, helping people. Each success in these kinds of daily activities can strengthen positive beliefs and weaken negative ones. You can introduce flexible schedules to help the person structure their desired life.

Skipping over the third row for now (which we come back to when discussing challenges), the fourth row of the Recovery Map captures your action steps in CT-R as well as targets for positive change. This is where you enter positive action that lets individuals have a daily sense of purpose through experiencing the meaning of their aspirations. Purpose is another critical aspect of recovery and wellness (Harding, 2019). Chapter 5 helps you develop skill with positive action.

Strengthening the Adaptive Mode by Drawing Conclusions and Empowering Resilience

The fifth box in the CT-R arrow (see Figure 1.3) features strengthening the adaptive mode. CT-R is an experiential process, and each of the four boxes to the left require a process of drawing conclusions during the experiences. Succeeding interpersonally, making a difference with other people, getting a desired life—these are all opportunities to strengthen positive beliefs about self, others, and the future. Individuals are capable, lovable, can enjoy things, can connect, and are caring. Other people appreciate them, care, and want to know them. They can make a difference in the future.

The box appears at the right-hand side near the tip of the arrow in Figure 1.3 to illustrate the importance of drawing conclusions to progress with CT-R. This collaborative process helps the person get the most out of experiences that reveal their potential in action. You can focus attention on these positive meanings and draw conclusions with straightforward, custom-tailored questions. The fourth row of the Recovery Map also captures these meanings. Individuals develop resilience and empowerment through this process. Chapters 3–5, and especially 6, show you how.

Challenges, Resilience, and Empowerment

Everyone's life has stress in it. As you help the person begin to live the life they want, stressors and challenges will likely crop up. When life is more difficult, challenges can emerge, such as negative symptoms, hallucinations, delusions, aggression, and self-injury.

Resiliency is about discovering and developing a sense of empowerment with regard to these stressors. It involves the person knowing they can get beyond them. Stress may raise the desire to isolate, listen to voices, focus on delusions, increase aggressive urges—but one can learn how to refocus away from such desires and toward the activities that matter most. As specific challenges come up, CT-R emphasizes understanding them and promoting strategies for empowerment. The third row of the Recovery Map captures the challenges and the beliefs that underlie them.

Resilience enables a person to continue pursuing goals and aspirations despite challenges that arise. One of the greatest discoveries we can help an individual make is that when things don't work out, it's not a catastrophe; all hope is not lost. Developing resilient beliefs of this sort is another essential part of CT-R that propels and sustains individuals as they pursue the life they want to live. Chapters 7–11 show you how.

BOX 1.1. CT-R Is Good Medicine

Epidemiologists have discovered that individuals who are given a diagnosis of schizophrenia and other serious mental health conditions live, on average, 20 fewer years than the average person, early death being most likely caused from a physical illness (e.g., digestive and endocrine diseases, infectious diseases, respiratory diseases, heart condition, metabolic imbalance) rather than directly from a mental health feature, such as suicide (Lee et al., 2018; Saha, Chant, & McGrath, 2007).

At the same time, a revolution in the field of public health over the past 30 years has identified social factors—disconnection, lack of purpose, lack of hope, disempowerment—linked to poorer physical health outcomes and lower life expectancy independent of the presence of a mental condition (Harding, 2019; Murthy, 2020).

This makes CT-R good medicine, as the focus is on social connections, meaningful aspirations, purpose-infused action, and sustaining empowerment. The cognitive model becomes a mediator of wellness—developing and living one's best self can lead to a richer and longer life.

Evidence that this formula for wellness works comes from a study of 50 high-achieving individuals who were given a diagnosis of schizophrenia. Common factors the group cited in their success were having valuable relationships, personally meaningful action every day, and a way to manage stress (Cohen et al., 2017).

STRUCTURE OF A CT-R INTERACTION

Whether you are working with an individual in one-to-one therapy, in group therapy, on a milieu, or in the community, any interaction can be a CT-R interaction. The key components include (1) opening by tapping into the individual's adaptive mode, (2) establishing a collaborative target for your time together, (3) developing or reviewing an individual's aspirations and their meaning, (4) addressing challenges or taking steps in the context of aspirations, and (5) collaboratively developing an action plan that helps translate whatever you did together into the individual's daily life (see Figure 1.4).

Starting any interaction with access to the adaptive mode brings energy, focus, and connection. It communicates that you are invested in the individual as a whole person, not just in the challenges, and it provides enough momentum to progress through the rest of the steps.

Next, a meaningful bridge, similar to traditional cognitive therapy (Beck, 2020), gives you the opportunity to check in on any activities or aspiration steps the individual took since your last interaction. It also gives you the opportunity to reestablish the mission you and the individual are on together. In some circumstances, this will revolve around achieving aspirations and their meaning. In other circumstances, it will be about readiness to transition to a less restrictive level of care, while for others it could be about turning dreams into action. The mission should be developed together.

Aspirations provide the driving force for any CT-R interaction and should be regularly developed, enriched, and referenced. Aspirations are "why to try things out." Strategizing helps identify "what to try." Challenges are addressed when they impact progress toward the aspirations. Finally, an action plan puts aspirations into practice. It is what the person takes away from the interaction. Would it be worth it for the person to do more outside of time with you? What can they do the rest of the day or week to keep the momentum going?

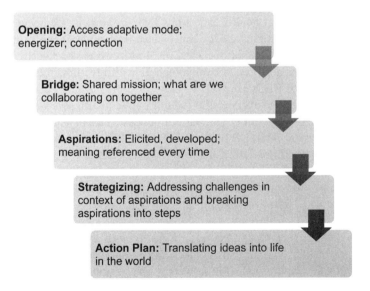

FIGURE 1.4. The structure of a CT-R interaction.

HOW DO WE KNOW THAT CT-R WORKS?

CT-R is an evidence-based practice. Research studies support the cognitive model as a good guide for how people with serious mental health conditions thrive and how they get stuck (Beck, Himelstein, & Grant, 2019; Beck, Rector, Stolar, & Grant, 2009; Grant & Best, 2019). A randomized controlled trial supports the effectiveness of CT-R to promote living better lives of their choosing (Grant, Huh, Perivoliotis, Stolar, & Beck, 2012). Program evaluation outcomes show that CT-R makes an impact across levels of care where individuals find themselves, and across disciplines of care providers they might be working with (Grant, 2019a).

Evidence Supporting Positive Beliefs in Helping People Do Better

The power of positive beliefs to promote recovery can be seen in a study where we simulated the therapeutic process of CT-R by collaborating with individuals to succeed at a task. Success was best predicted by the person's increase in positive beliefs about themselves and others, as well as an increase in their experience of positive emotion (Grant, Perivoliotis, Luther, Bredemeier, & Beck, 2018). In a related study, we found that people with serious mental health challenges who had higher levels of positive beliefs were participating more in the community 6 months later. They were also experiencing less disruption from negative symptoms, hallucinations, and delusions (Grant & Best, 2019).

Evidence Supporting the Role of Negative Beliefs in People Getting Stuck

When we asked a person why they no longer did the things they used to enjoy (such as basketball or cooking), they said things like "Why try, I'm only going to fail." We labeled these kinds of statements "defeatist beliefs," because the person is protected from failure by being inactive.

We conducted a study (Grant & Beck, 2009a) showing that defeatist beliefs were related to negative symptoms and performance on tests of memory, attention, and problem solving—factors that predict living a less full life. Our original finding has now been reproduced many times, both in the United States and in other countries (Campellone, Sanchez, & Kring, 2016).

People who are given a diagnosis experience defeatist beliefs more in their daily life, and these beliefs are related to being less likely to leave their house, and less likely to physically move (Ruiz et al., 2019). If they feel rejected and not a part of any social group, they are much more likely to endorse defeatist beliefs (Reddy, Reavis, Polon, Morales, & Green, 2017). And, on the flip side, when defeatist beliefs become less strong, people given a diagnosis have more success at work, and also more success socially (Mervis et al., 2016).

Defeatist beliefs are a general factor impacting negative symptoms and impeding individuals' pursuit of the meaningful life they would otherwise want. The disruptive power of the beliefs emerges in adolescence (Clay et al., 2019; Perivoliotis, Morrison, Grant, French, & Beck, 2009), cutting the person off from being a part of something bigger with other people (Fuligni, 2019) and leading to isolation and disability.

Our interviews also uncovered asocial beliefs, preferences to be alone rather than with other people (Grant & Beck, 2010)—for example, "People sometimes think I am shy when I

> **BOX 1.2. The Meaning of Difficulties with Attention, Memory, and Problem Solving**
>
> Poor performance on tests of memory and attention have been taken to mean that there's something broken about the test-taker's brain (Andreasen, 1984). We don't think this is true. We published a review study that inspires hope for individuals given a diagnosis of schizophrenia and their families and care providers (Beck, Himelstein, Bredemeier, Silverstein, & Grant, 2018).
>
> In the paper, we show that there are many factors that generally contribute to poor performance on tests and tasks independent of a mental health diagnosis: elevated stress, low mood, expectations of failure, low effort, and low access to motivation. These factors also contribute to poor performance for people given a diagnosis of schizophrenia. These factors can all be addressed with psychosocial treatments. The upshot is that individuals are not limited and can succeed; they hold the key to their own potential to contribute (Grant, Best, & Beck, 2019).

really just want to be left alone." These beliefs protect individuals from the pain of social rejection. In one study (Grant & Beck, 2010), we demonstrated that asocial beliefs predicted a future of not doing activities or spending much time with others. Another study looked at defeatist and asocial beliefs, finding both to be linked to less access to motivation and lower community participation (Thomas, Luther, Zullo, Beck, & Grant, 2017).

As we will see, the key to empowerment in CT-R is to start with participation, increase access to motivation, and then strengthen positive beliefs about capability and the value of other people.

Randomized Trial

In our clinical trial, we recruited individuals with elevated negative symptoms and randomly assigned them to continue their standard treatment in the community or to receive weekly CT-R (Grant et al., 2012). Active treatment lasted up to 18 months. To get a feel for how people were doing at the start of the study, if each participant took snapshots of themselves and their surroundings each hour for an entire day, you would see cigarette smoke, the television, mealtimes, a case worker, a psychiatrist visit—not a lot of activity.

At the end of 18 months of treatment, the assessors—who were blind to condition—determined that individuals in standard treatment had not improved. By contrast, people in the CT-R condition showed improved functional outcomes. They had increased motivation, and their hallucinations, delusions, and communication disturbances were reduced. In real-world terms, the change experienced by the typical person in the CT-R condition was from spending all week smoking cigarettes and watching TV, to making a friend, volunteering, starting to go back to school, starting to date—well on the way to the life of their choosing.

After 6 months during which no treatment was delivered, the people in the CT-R condition still had greater functioning, greater motivation, and reduced hallucinations, delusions, and communication disturbances as compared to people in the standard condition (Grant, Bredemeier, & Beck, 2017). Importantly, improvement in positive beliefs over the 24 months of the study best predicted improvement in community involvement and participation (Grant & Best, 2019). Positive beliefs are the royal road to recovery and living a desired life.

A source of hope is that people who received a diagnosis 20, 30, or 40 years before entering the study still showed improvement by 24 months. Recovery extends to all; everyone can start the life they want.

Program Evaluation Outcomes

CT-R has been successfully implemented in large state and municipal systems of care in Pennsylvania, New York, Montana, Vermont, New Jersey, Massachusetts, and Georgia. This has involved diverse settings, such as long- and short-term hospitals, programmatic residences, and forensic settings, and community, specialty care, and integrated health teams. These implementations involved direct care staff, nurses, art therapists, recreational therapists, occupational therapists, social workers, peer specialists, psychologists, and psychiatrists. Successful CT-R has taken the form of individual therapy, group therapy, milieu, and team-based applications.

Outcomes show that CT-R improves care providers' ability to promote recovery and resiliency in individuals who had been stuck. In acute and long-term hospital settings, CT-R has produced a dramatic reduction in the use of instruments of control (Chang, Grant, Luther, & Beck, 2014)—restraints, seclusion, medications to calm—and eliminated mechanical restraints completely. Individuals came out of their rooms more often to participate. Fee-for-service teams report more quality contacts evidenced by an increase in units of service. Hospitalization rates have lessened, jail days have been reduced, and individuals have moved to less restricted levels of care. They report being less lonely, more hopeful, and starting to flourish. They find use for

---

WORDS OF WISDOM

BOX 1.3. Recovery Is a Process of Flourishing

Recovery is not a destination; it is the evolution of a pathway of flourishing. It is successful participation and involvement in the community of one's choosing. In CT-R, recovery is the active fulfillment of one's highly valued aspirations. It involves a series of milestones as one's life space widens. Occasional setbacks provide the opportunity to build resilience and discover inner strength. Some individuals move rapidly along the recovery pathway, whereas others take longer. With CT-R and sufficient time, all individuals can achieve varying degrees of flourishing. Research shows us that *recovery extends to all*. Milestones include but are not limited to:

- Engagement and accessing the adaptive mode.
- Repeated activation of the adaptive mode.
- Preparation of the Recovery Map.
- Selection and enrichment of aspirations.
- Success achieving the meaning of aspirations.
- Resilience experiences and conclusions.
- Empowerment relative to personal challenges.

the skills of everyday living. In one large system, two-thirds of individuals improved on at least one of the four SAMHSA recovery dimensions within 6 months of supervised CT-R (Grant, 2019b).

The cognitive model guides a person-centered, individualized way of understanding how people thrive and how they get stuck. The theory is supported by a diverse set of research studies. The therapy has been validated in a randomized trial and shown to improve outcomes for diverse care providers in diverse settings. Recovery extends to all, and there are concrete and effective procedures for bringing it about. All individuals have an adaptive mode within them, and everyone who works with them can collaborate to promote flourishing. Subsequent chapters show you how to do it.

SUMMARY

- CT-R is a procedure that reliably produces the right kind of interactions between you and individuals with lived experience to promote recovery, resiliency, and empowerment.
- A mode is a manner of acting or doing that involves beliefs and attitudes, emotion, motivation, and behavior. We use the term "adaptive mode" to describe what seems to drive adaptive behavior. We believe the adaptive mode is present, but inactive, when the individual is experiencing challenges. On the other hand, when individuals are drawn into a meaningful, pleasurable activity, the adaptive mode becomes activated.
- The core components of CT-R and the adaptive mode are accessing and energizing the adaptive mode, developing the adaptive mode, actualizing the adaptive mode, and strengthening the adaptive mode.
- The Recovery Map is a one-page, living document that can guide you in developing a CT-R understanding of an individual and in developing strategies and interventions for collaboratively promoting a meaningful life.
- There is a strong evidence base proving the efficacy of CT-R, including a randomized controlled trial, follow-up to that trial, and program evaluation outcomes.
- Positive beliefs are the royal road to sustained recovery and flourishing in the community of one's choosing.

CHAPTER 2
Mapping Recovery
DEVELOPING A PLAN FOR TRANSFORMATIVE ACTION

Jackie has been living in the same locked community residence for the last 25 years. She has been hospitalized several times since moving to this residence—often a result of wandering her town, sometimes walking into traffic, and screaming loudly at what is assumed to be voices. Jackie's treatment team includes the residence's direct care staff and an outpatient case manager, therapist, and psychiatrist.

They describe Jackie's days as empty and bleak. Much of her time is spent in bed. She wears the same clothes from one day to the next. The residential staff report that sometimes Jackie will come to the dayroom when other residents are working on craft projects, but she rarely stays long enough to work on anything with them. When she does stay with the group, it's typically when they are making jewelry. Occasionally a relative visits Jackie, but during those visits Jackie often walks out of the room and begins screaming different phrases or words in a way that is disjointed and difficult to make sense of.

When the staff or her therapist try to talk to Jackie about her day or things she might like to do later, Jackie responds in either the same disorganized way, or by sharing ideas about having the ability to bring people back from the dead and generate multiple body parts.

It has been difficult for Jackie to develop and keep relationships with others.

Jackie's experience presents several striking challenges, but also offers some glimpses into possible interests and desires. All of this provides valuable information on how we may partner with her in her recovery. To collaborate with Jackie effectively, we need to develop a richer understanding of the things she likes, what hopes and dreams she has, and what beliefs or behaviors may make her feel stuck in her pursuit of those dreams.

Mapping recovery is a process of deepening our understanding of the person and developing a plan for transformative action that enhances positive beliefs and empowers the individual. Recovery mapping is a broader approach to what some may have learned as case conceptualization or formulation (Beck, 2020; Beck, Rush, Shaw, & Emery, 1979); it involves an expanded understanding of individuals and their experiences—both positive and challenging—and helps organize this understanding so that interventions are targeted and documentation is clear.

This chapter highlights how you can map recovery, even when you have little information, and features the Recovery Map, a practical tool that can be used to guide treatment.

INTRODUCING THE RECOVERY MAP

The Recovery Map is a one-page document that contains the core features of CT-R, each of which is elaborated on in Chapters 3–6. As shown in Appendix B, there are a total of eight boxes arranged into four rows and two columns. Looking at the rows first, you can see the top row contains two boxes focused on accessing and energizing an individual's adaptive mode. The boxes in the second row concern an individual's aspirations—their hopes or dreams for the future. The boxes in the third row center on challenges that might impact an individual's progress toward their aspirations. The bottom row contains positive action and empowerment plans that are developed based on the content of the top three rows.

If we now look at the Recovery Map columns for the top three rows, the left-hand side contains what we know about the person for accessing and energizing the adaptive mode (row 1), aspirations (row 2), and challenges (row 3). The right-hand column represents the beliefs and meanings associated with each of these.

The columns in the bottom row are a little different. The box on the left contains CT-R strategies and interventions. The right-hand box contains the belief, meaning, or challenge targeted by those strategies and interventions.

BENEFITS OF THE RECOVERY MAP

Sole-practice providers can use the Recovery Map to plan sessions based on clear targets. Multidisciplinary teams can use this form to coordinate their understanding and planning in a unified way. Any provider, regardless of position, has an opportunity to contribute based on their respective role with the individual. Each provider may see individuals at-their-best in different contexts and may also have information about when challenges are more likely to persist.

The Recovery Map supports continuity of care, since it can be passed along and further developed as the person steps into greater independence, ensuring a shared understanding across providers that is oriented around the person's desires. Similarly, if an individual requires a higher level of care, the Recovery Map can provide valuable information that may jumpstart effective recovery-oriented treatment by the receiving provider.

The Recovery Map can be completed outside of sessions and visits and can also be used in direct collaboration with the individual in some circumstances.

HOW TO FILL OUT A RECOVERY MAP

We recommend that you print out or copy the Recovery Map (see Appendix B). You will change your answers over time, as you learn more about the person. Each strategy and corresponding intervention will lead to updates, too. You can start with very little information and soon find your Map is a cornucopia of the person's best self and desires for a fuller life imbued with resilience. Teams often store Recovery Maps in binders or charts for quick access for all of the staff.

Positive Action and Empowerment

Though you will fill out the bottom row of the Map last, it will be good to keep it in mind as you fill in the Map from the top. This row helps you specify your action plan for collaborating with the individual. It can also help you accurately document your interactions with the person in whatever manner your organization requires.

Let's start by clarifying between *strategy, intervention,* and *target.*

A CT-R *strategy* is a broad plan, a statement of the overall mission. It is what you are going for. One strategy might be that you want to learn about a person's interests, or you might want to discover and develop their aspirations. You might wish to collaborate with the individual to build the meaning of the aspiration into everyday life or empower them relative to challenges.

Interventions are the means to accomplishing the broader mission. This is how you are going to do it. Interventions may include listening to music or asking family members for information on interests to achieve the strategy of accessing and energizing the adaptive mode. They could include questions and use of imagery for the strategy of identifying and enriching aspirations. It could be practicing progressive muscle relaxation to empower the person relative to stress.

Targets are what will change as a result of the intervention. These could include:

- Positive beliefs you're hoping to activate and strengthen with your interventions, like the beliefs from the Accessing and Energizing the Adaptive Mode section
- Aspirations you're working toward together
- Meanings to help the person experience and notice through action
- Negative beliefs you're hoping to reduce
- The specific behavior or symptom being targeted by your interventions

The bottom row of the Recovery Map is the place where you translate the upper three rows into your action plan. Strategies and interventions will go in the left box and targets for change in the right box. You will write these in based on what you have entered in the first three rows. We return to the Positive Action and Empowerment section of the Recovery Map after considering the other three sections.

Accessing and Energizing the Adaptive Mode

In the top-left section of the map—the box labeled "Interests/Ways to Engage"—you should note any of the individual's known interests, preferred activities, areas of specific knowledge, or skills. This box is intended to capture all the times an individual is at-their-best. You might learn about this from the person's own descriptions, speaking with a loved one, paperwork from a referring provider, observations on a milieu, or more. If you do not know enough about the person to fill in anything here, discovering interests, excitements, and best-self moments will be your first priority for CT-R.

In the top-right section—the box labeled "Beliefs Activated while in Adaptive Mode"—you should note positive beliefs about the self, others, and the future that the person might experience when at-their-best or engaged in interests. These might be beliefs about being skilled, capable of enjoying things, being helpful, and so on.

It is essential to CT-R that you think in terms of beliefs from the very start. This will likely involve guesswork at the beginning. Over time, you will be able to confirm your guesses. This way you are always focused on important meanings. Beliefs are the glue that provide continuity between positive experiences and are the basis for growing and sustaining a desired life.

To make a guess, ask yourself, "How might I feel or see myself if I were doing that activity?" You can write your guesses into the upper-right box, indicating that it is a hunch that you can update as you proceed in your collaboration with the person.

The most accurate account of what these beliefs are will be given by individuals. The best time to ask is when you are doing the preferred activity together. You can ask, "What's the best part of [fill in activity]?" or perhaps, "How do you feel about yourself when you're doing that?" Place the answer in the upper-right box.

These positive beliefs are important for progress. You will want to help individuals notice and strengthen them. Often you will find that beliefs activated when the person is in the adaptive mode are the opposite of the beliefs that dominate their daily life when in the "patient" mode. Chapter 3 details how to access the adaptive mode and strengthen beliefs that will energize it.

Let's consider the example of Jackie presented earlier. The first section of her Recovery Map might look like Figure 2.1.

At the start, we have little information. What are Jackie's interests, areas of knowledge, or skill? One clue is that there are times when she is a little more active—while others are doing crafts and making jewelry. What beliefs might be activated during those activities? Why might anyone join with others during certain activities rather than during others? These are just some of the questions you can consider when making guesses about the beliefs activated when the person is in a more adaptive mode.

BOX 2.1. The Importance of Guessing in CT-R

Many of the activities central to CT-R are pursuits that individuals have engaged in off and on throughout their life without necessarily getting a sustained benefit. By focusing our thinking on potential beliefs that could be activated during these activities, we are changing this script. The experience of each activity is replete with potential. The meanings and beliefs are our way to realize it. Individuals may not know or cannot say what these benefits will be, since they may have never noticed them before. This is why we start with guessing. Since there is a universal quality to a lot of the activities, thinking about how we would feel and think about ourselves is a good place to start. This better readies us for helping to choose the activity and then drawing conclusions about meaning during it. Soon our guesses are confirmed, and the person's life begins to take on important meanings more of the time—being capable, contributing, feeling appreciated, making a difference.

ACCESSING AND ENERGIZING THE ADAPTIVE MODE	
Interests/Ways to Engage: • Arts and crafts • Jewelry making	**Beliefs Activated While in Adaptive Mode:** • Guess: I am capable or skilled • Guess: It's worth being around and spending time with others when we're doing things I enjoy

FIGURE 2.1. Jackie's Recovery Map: Accessing and energizing the adaptive mode.

Aspirations

The second row of the Recovery Map contains aspirations and their meanings. The box on the left is for the individual's stated goals. These hopes and dreams should be meaningful, long-range, and able to generate experiences that constitute the person's desired life. In many cases, you will not know what the person's aspirations are. This is to be expected.

Make discovering the person's desired life a priority for CT-R. To start, you can make guesses and write them into the Recovery Map, updating when you have a better sense of the person's aspirations.

As you learn what the person is looking for in their life, you can develop the aspiration with imagery, which can further enhance the information captured on the Recovery Map. The process for discovering and enriching aspirations is detailed in Chapter 4.

In the second row on the right is the box for the meaning of the aspiration. You may not be sure what this meaning is, but you can start with guesses. The process is similar to what we saw with beliefs activated by the adaptive mode.

You can ask yourself, "What might be the best part of the aspiration?" and "What might she feel by achieving the aspiration?" You can write answers in the Recovery Map, noting that each is a guess that you can update as you learn more about the person.

Meanings underlying aspirations tend to be the opposite of the negative beliefs the person has about themselves, others, and the future. They reflect a desired self-concept—"I am a helping person, not a hurting person"; "I am a good person"; "I can succeed"; "I can make the world a better place."

When you know a person's aspiration, you can ask, "What might it say about you to accomplish this?" or "What would be the best part?" The meaning you get can be entered into the Recovery Map.

Since some aspirations are far off (e.g., starting a business, getting a nursing degree) or seemingly impossible to achieve (e.g., becoming the supreme world leader), meanings become your prime currency of progress and recovery. The reason: meanings can be experienced every day. For example, the best part about becoming a nurse might be helping people and making the world a better place.

This makes the meaning of the aspirations section of the Recovery Map especially important—it is the heart of what a person is ultimately looking to gain in their life and is central to your collaboration with them.

The aspirations section of Jackie's Recovery Map is particularly tricky, as many of her desires are unknown at this point in CT-R. To start, it might look like the aspirations section in Figure 2.2.

ASPIRATIONS	
Goals: • Not known yet—need to develop further • What might her belief about bringing people back from the dead mean? Is there something desired there? • Jewelry making	**Meaning of Accomplishing Identified Goal:** • Guess: Connection? • Guess: Power or importance? • Guess: Capability?

FIGURE 2.2. Jackie's Recovery Map: Aspirations.

Since the team doesn't know much about Jackie's desires, discovering them becomes a priority. One clue is that Jackie frequently speaks of "bringing back the dead." The team thinks about what it might mean about her if she were able to bring people back. Would it provide connection? Would she be important? Though initially these are guesses, the more the team learns about Jackie's interests and desires, the better refined the Recovery Map becomes—for example, the team can think about how she might achieve these meanings and then begin to try these activities with her.

Challenges

The third row of the Recovery Map contains the challenges section. This provides a snapshot of behaviors and beliefs currently driving the "patient" mode. Challenges are a focus of treatment only when they pose a hindrance to the individual's aspirations. Later we consider negative symptoms (Chapter 7); positive symptoms (Chapters 8 and 9); communication challenges (Chapter 10); and self-injury, aggressive behavior, and substance use (Chapter 11). Descriptions of the challenges are listed on the left side of the third row; beliefs that might underlie the challenges are listed in the box on the right side.

In our experience, you will find the box on the left in this row to be the easiest one to fill out of all eight on the Recovery Map. Most intakes focus on presenting problems. In congregate residential, hospital, and forensic, as well as community team settings, the challenges are frequently noted to justify the need for a higher level of care.

The accompanying beliefs might take a little more work. As we have seen for the previous two rows, a little educated guesswork can go a long way. To make some initial guesses about the negative beliefs that drive the challenges, we can consider questions such as:

- Why might someone engage in this behavior?
- What might they believe about themselves, others, or the future?
- What need might more expansive beliefs (e.g., grand delusions) fulfill?

You can enter the answers you suspect could be right in the beliefs box in the challenges row, again indicating that you are guessing. You will be able to confirm these beliefs over time, updating the Map as you go. To verify beliefs underlying challenges, you can:

- Use summaries and empathic statements to float possible beliefs (e.g., "I'm hearing you say you are being targeted, have I got that right? I imagine that has to be frightening.

I'm wondering whether this makes you feel like you're unsafe or that other people are untrustworthy?").

- Do a chain analysis (see Chapter 6) with individuals to learn about what leads to the challenge and what they are thinking about themselves, others, and the future throughout that pathway.

The beliefs underlying the challenges are important to your understanding, as the activation of these are a primary source of the person not living the life they desire. The more you know the specific beliefs, the better you can navigate your work and ultimately help the person develop resiliency.

Challenges are often the first material you will know about someone, especially early in developing a relationship with them. This was certainly the case with Jackie. The treatment team had only a vague sense of her interests and desires but could clearly identify what behaviors were keeping her stuck. The challenges portion of Jackie's Recovery Map might look like Figure 2.3.

Jackie's team developed initial ideas for possible beliefs based on what Jackie had said in the past. They also made guesses based on their knowledge of common beliefs that underlie certain challenges (see Part II). The team will likely get clarity on which negative beliefs are most relevant to Jackie's experiences as they learn more about her adaptive mode and which positive beliefs run counter to those activated when challenges are present.

Return to Positive Action and Empowerment

Once you have filled in the first three rows of the Recovery Map, you are ready to determine your strategies, interventions, and targets, writing these in the bottom section of the recovery map.

When developing the action plans, the Recovery Map can be used to organize the roles of treatment team members while all are working toward the same recovery targets. This section can inform clinical documentation, as it provides both the treatment objective and the rationale for the interventions. Figure 2.4 shows what this would look like for Jackie.

CHALLENGES	
Current Behaviors/Challenges: • Paying attention to voices to the point of reduced awareness of her environment (e.g., walking into the street) • Isolation • Difficulty with verbal communication (disorganization) • Delusions around bringing people back from the dead and generating body parts	**Beliefs Underlying Challenges:** Guesses: • I have no control • What's the point of doing things with others? I will fail anyway • I can't enjoy the things I used to anymore • People don't like me • People can't understand me • The world is unsafe • I have nothing to offer, I'm incapable • I'm unimportant and have little value

FIGURE 2.3. Jackie's Recovery Map: Challenges.

POSITIVE ACTION AND EMPOWERMENT	

Current Strategies and Interventions:
1. Identify ways to activate the adaptive mode
  • Ask for advice about craft projects
  • Ask for help setting up crafts and other activities
  • Ask Jackie and her family about things she used to enjoy doing
2. Identify and enrich aspirations
  • Create recovery image
	Beliefs/Aspirations/Meanings/Challenge Targeted:
	1a. Beliefs about capability
	  • I am capable and can be connected
	  • The more I do that I enjoy, the better I feel
	  • I can enjoy more than I thought and can still do the things I used to enjoy
	1b. Reduce isolation
	2. Beliefs about the future
	  • Hope and purpose for the future

FIGURE 2.4. Jackie's Recovery Map: Positive action and empowerment.

Accessing, energizing, and developing the adaptive mode are foundational elements of CT-R. For Jackie, not a lot of information is available to get a good sense for what she might really enjoy, want to do more of, or desire for her future. Therefore, the initial positive action strategies are to discover and enrich Jackie's interests and aspirations. Interventions to achieve these strategies are elaborated on in greater detail in Chapters 3 and 4.

The team also has made guesses about beliefs—for example, capability, connection—that could become active when Jackie does activities she enjoys with others. Isolation is an important challenge the team can address through doing preferred activities with Jackie. Because they know the least about Jackie's aspirations for the future, it is important that the team also include identifying aspirations as a critical positive action step.

THE RECOVERY MAP OVER THE COURSE OF TREATMENT

The Recovery Map is a living document that is flexible, captures current understanding, and guides strategy and positive action. You can modify the Map as you learn more about the individual. Many sources can contribute to updating and personalizing the Recovery Map:

BOX 2.2. Recovery Mapping and Documentation

By design, your work in CT-R may not look like traditional treatment. An auditor or person unfamiliar with the approach may not see how what you are doing is bona fide treatment. The Recovery Map is a useful tool for writing progress notes and other documentation that clearly links what you are doing to underlying beliefs and progress toward a desired life. The fourth row is your guide for this—for example: "Strategy during the contact was strengthening the individual's beliefs about being capable to make a difference and matter to others. Helped him lead the group in calling out birthdays and good qualities of each person. Used guided discovery [strategy and interventions from left box] to help individual notice how successful he was and how others appreciated what he did and that this would be worth doing more in the future [beliefs from right box]."

- New information about the individual's experiences or history
- Confirming or refuting some of your guesses
- New guesses for beliefs and meanings
- An intervention that did not work
- New aspirations
- New interests

As challenges to progress arise over the course of treatment, you or your team can collaborate with individuals to address them through positive action, resiliency, and drawing conclusions to strengthen positive beliefs and minimize negative beliefs. If the initial strategy is unsuccessful, develop a new one that may work better, updating the Recovery Map as you go. Jackie's initial full Recovery Map is shown in Figure 2.5.

In Appendix C you will find an abbreviated Recovery Map How-To Guide—a cheat sheet for completing a Recovery Map—that you can use along with the blank Recovery Map form (see Appendix B) for each client. This guide includes reminders of what information goes in each box, as well as questions you might ask yourself or individuals to get accurate information for each section.

ADDITIONAL CONSIDERATIONS

Following the Flow of the Recovery Map from Top to Bottom

Though there may be substantially more information known about one section (typically, the challenges) compared to another, it is important to try to work from the top down when completing the Map. To be most successful you need to identify what activates the individual's adaptive mode and their aspirations for the future. Both provide powerful and empowering directions for treatment and are very important in developing and maintaining connection. It also helps with putting together a more comprehensive representation of a person that does not focus entirely on their challenges.

This is, perhaps, especially true if you are developing a Recovery Map in collaboration with the individual. It is likely they have a lot of experience being asked about challenges, and much less often have had the opportunity to share values and meaningful hopes for the future. Completing the Map in this order more accurately reflects the CT-R process as a whole and can guide the approach. For example, if you find that you don't have any information on the aspirations section, this lets you know that your strategy and interventions (positive action and empowerment section) should be focused on identifying aspirations.

The Recovery Map and Treatment Planning

The Recovery Map incorporates components commonly found in treatment plan documents across a variety of settings: goals for the future, targets for change, and justification for interventions based on beliefs. It is possible that the Map can inform treatment planning and documentation in the formats currently used in programs and organizations or may be a suitable replacement to such forms. This allows the opportunity for a collaborative process that ensures the individual's priorities are central to treatment planning.

Recovery Map
ACCESSING AND ENERGIZING THE ADAPTIVE MODE

Interests/Ways to Engage: • Arts and crafts • Jewelry making	**Beliefs Activated While in Adaptive Mode:** • Guess: I am capable or skilled • Guess: It's worth being around and spending time with others when we're doing things I enjoy

ASPIRATIONS

Goals: • Not known yet—need to develop further • What might her belief about bringing people back from the dead mean? Is there something desired there? • Jewelry making	**Meaning of Accomplishing Identified Goal:** • Guess: Connection? • Guess: Power or importance? • Guess: Capability?

CHALLENGES

Current Behaviors/Challenges: • Paying attention to voices to the point of reduced awareness of her environment (e.g., walking into the street) • Isolation • Difficulty with verbal communication (disorganization) • Delusions around bringing people back from the dead and generating body parts	**Beliefs Underlying Challenges:** Guesses: • I have no control • What's the point of doing things with others? I will fail anyway • I can't enjoy the things I used to anymore • People don't like me • People can't understand me • The world is unsafe • I have nothing to offer, I'm incapable • I'm unimportant and have little value

POSITIVE ACTION AND EMPOWERMENT

Current Strategies and Interventions:
1. Identify ways to activate the adaptive mode
  • Ask for advice about craft projects
  • Ask for help setting up crafts and other activities
  • Ask Jackie and her family about things she used to enjoy doing
2. Identify and enrich aspirations
  • Create recovery image
	Beliefs/Aspirations/Meanings/Challenge Targeted:
	1a. Beliefs about capability
	  • I am capable and can be connected
	  • The more I do that I enjoy, the better I feel
	  • I can enjoy more than I thought and can still do the things I used to enjoy
	1b. Reduce isolation
	2. Beliefs about the future
	  • Hope and purpose for the future

FIGURE 2.5. Jackie's full initial Recovery Map.

Developing Shared Recovery Maps

Many times, individuals are involved with multiple systems. Someone might live in a programmatic residence and also have the support of a community-based team or individual therapist. Some individuals may be in school and have both school- and community-based collaborators. Other individuals may have family members or caregivers who are eager to contribute to the treatment planning process.

In any of these situations, it can be helpful to develop shared Recovery Maps—Maps that can be used in multiple settings, based on insights from each of the sources involved. Everyone involved in an individual's life may have unique experiences that highlight when the person is at-their-best, what they hope for in the future, and what may bring about the challenges. Ultimately, the aim of the shared Recovery Map is to foster both collaboration and consistency.

Shared Maps can be developed in a few different ways: everyone can convene at one time through meetings or conference calls to develop the Map together or each party can work on the map separately, then share with the larger group to create an overall Map.

Deciding When to Use a Recovery Map with Individuals

The Recovery Map is intended to be a tool that reflects a deep, holistic understanding of a person. This is helpful in generating strategies for treatment rooted in beliefs and meaning. There are some situations, however, when using the Recovery Map during an interaction with an individual ends up interfering with the process of treatment.

For some individuals, a provider emphasizing use of a chart or worksheet represents a hierarchical divide between the treater and the treated. It can feel like more of the same old thing. Evidence of this could be if an individual, upon seeing the Map, expresses very grand ideas, such as being the provider's boss, or owning the agency. Similarly, some individuals may express fears or anxiety around what is being recorded. Others may shut down and retreat from the conversation altogether.

In these circumstances, it may be more effective to focus on an activity or conversation that will provide you with the information needed to complete the Map outside of the interaction with the individual. For others, however, working collaboratively on the Recovery Map can be a powerful experience of control over the sharing of their stories and experiences—they are the experts in their life, guiding their own treatment.

Some individuals may be interested in this approach right away. Others may not respond favorably to the Map at the start of treatment, but after making progress may want to complete the tool with you to highlight where they are now and where they want to continue to go, even as they step out of services.

When using the Map with individuals, focus the time on the first two rows (accessing and energizing the adaptive mode and aspirations). Move to challenges only when rich and meaningful aspirations have been identified and elaborated upon. For some, this process can occur by completing one section per interaction; for others, it may take more time.

Limiting the amount of time spent on the Map can help ensure it is not the sole focus of the interaction. Finally, be sure to get feedback from individuals along the way: "How is this going?"; "Does this seem helpful?"; "What are your thoughts on how or why this might be helpful?"

> **WORDS OF WISDOM**
>
> **BOX 2.3. Mapping the Whole Person to Unleash the Power of the Positive**
>
> The cognitive model (Beck, 1963) helps clinicians understand psychiatric challenges in terms of negative beliefs about self, others, and the future. Strategy and selection of interventions target the beliefs to bring about amelioration of distressing behavior and emotion. Case formulation based in beliefs is at the heart of cognitive therapy.
>
> Clinical observation and recent research show that as individuals start to improve, *positive factors* lead the way and become dominant, as the weight of negative beliefs lessens (Grant & Best, 2019; Grant & Inverso, in press). The cognitive triad turns out to be an excellent formula for building one's best self: I am confident, successful, and a good person; others care about me, are great partners and collaborators; and the future is bright with my flourishing.
>
> To better guide our work in CT-R, we expand the notion of case formulation to include these positive attributes in terms of interests and aspirations, which we frame in terms of the adaptive mode. In this way, the challenges are in their place and the whole person is represented.

In the next several chapters, you learn different methods for implementing CT-R following the same format that is used in the Recovery Map. We continue to use Jackie's experience as an example of how the Recovery Map evolves over the course of treatment using these approaches.

SUMMARY

- The purpose of recovery mapping is to organize your understanding of an individual both at-their-best and when challenges are present.
- The Recovery Map is a living document and practical form that supports a clinician or team's collaboration with an individual, promotes continuity of care, enhances communication among all those involved with an individual, and eases documenting of interactions.
- The Map helps you to design effective strategies, interventions, and targets for positive change.
- The Recovery Map can guide treatment by highlighting aspirations and linking them to treatment targets.
- The Recovery Map supports the ultimate realization of an individual's preferred life.

CHAPTER 3
Accessing and Energizing the Adaptive Mode

Jackie spent several consecutive days alone in her room. The staff at her residence wished to find sources of interest that could foster connection to others in the house. The staff knew the one thing Jackie seemed to enjoy was crafting and making jewelry. One afternoon, the staff went to her room and asked for advice about different types of jewelry-making materials: Which color of beads should they buy? They showed Jackie a picture of color choices from a crafting magazine. Jackie gave a recommendation from her bed—pointing to blue and purple beads. The staff thanked her for her help, and said they hoped she'd give them some more ideas in the future.

Over the course of the next several days, the staff would ask Jackie for other suggestions: whether they should use colored string, metal, or plastic for the jewelry; what size beads would be best; and could she think of people who might appreciate receiving jewelry as a gift. When given a choice between materials, Jackie continued to give her recommendations from bed. Each time she made a recommendation, the staff pulled up a picture of the jewelry-making supply on their phones or showed a picture from a magazine to be sure they picked the right one. As the staff showed pictures, Jackie gradually began to sit up and look. The staff noticed that she was very clear in her opinions and that, as time went on, she became less disorganized as she spoke.

After a week or so, when it came to getting advice on who might like to receive the jewelry as a gift, Jackie replied, "People who are alone in a nursing home might." The staff told her they thought that was a great idea and invited her to share this idea with the group: "Come on downstairs to lunch, we can let the other residents know! Everyone really appreciates your ideas—you're very helpful." Jackie came down to join the others and the staff, and she shared her idea. Other residents agreed that Jackie was probably right and asked whether they could start a project to make jewelry for nursing home residents.

The staff and residents made a plan to work on jewelry making throughout the month and to ultimately deliver the jewelry to the nursing home. Jackie joined every time they worked on the jewelry, and the staff noticed that when she did, she was focused, occasionally smiled, and very helpful.

In Jackie's initial presentation (see Chapter 2), the staff knew little about what might excite her, bring her joy, or energize her—her adaptive mode. Her challenges were pretty clear, and it seemed that she spent considerable time in modes of disconnection. Crafting and jewelry making turned out to be the place to start with Jackie, spurring energy, connection, and trust. Drawing attention to these successes, the staff helped Jackie develop a desire for more. In her adaptive mode, Jackie is a capable and contributing person who others appreciate.

This chapter describes how to get started with individuals. You will bridge from the guesses of your initial recovery mapping to action with the person. Accessing the adaptive mode is a personalized process that often requires persistence, trial and error, and creativity. Individuals have many reasons to not trust. Their "patient" mode can be quite strong. You will learn systematic ways to break through, find the adaptive mode, and energize it over time. You will strengthen positive beliefs—about self, others, and the future—all leading to less time spent in the "patient" mode.

HOW TO ACCESS THE ADAPTIVE MODE

Objective: What You Are Going For

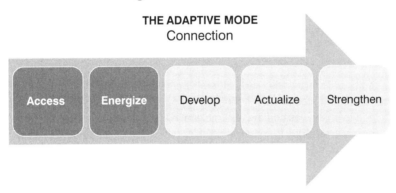

Accessing the adaptive mode is the first step of recovery-oriented cognitive therapy. It involves experiences that increase energy, motivation, access to the cognitive resources, connection with others, and a feeling of control. It also involves drawing the person's attention to these benefits while they are in the adaptive mode. Repeatedly accessing the adaptive mode energizes it, increasing trust and, ultimately, the desire to think about a more hopeful and meaningful future—the aspirations—and to share this vision with others. Accessing the adaptive mode is a process that naturally creates a highly personalized connection, realizing an important recovery dimension.

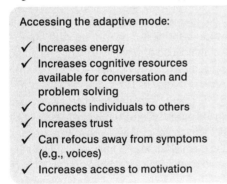

Accessing the adaptive mode:
- ✓ Increases energy
- ✓ Increases cognitive resources available for conversation and problem solving
- ✓ Connects individuals to others
- ✓ Increases trust
- ✓ Can refocus away from symptoms (e.g., voices)
- ✓ Increases access to motivation

Getting Ideas

The first step is to develop ideas about what types of activities excite the person, as well as to think about beliefs that might occur during the activity. While you will still be making reasonable guesses about the beliefs, you can move beyond guessing for the activities. "At-their-best" moments are royal roads to the adaptive mode. You may have had the fortune to observe this with the person, or you might ask others: family, friends, other team members, or providers. For individuals who are more verbal, you may be able to ask them directly.

Identifying At-Their-Best Moments

You may see individuals smiling, laughing, being more talkative or having clearer speech, sharing skills or knowledge, being more spontaneous in conversation or actions, taking more initiative, and so on. These signs tend to happen during social activities, activities that involve sharing talents, when individuals are helping others, or when taking a meaningful action step toward an aspiration. These activities may include listening to music, playing cards with others, gardening, going on a picnic outing, volunteering at the food bank, teaching someone how to fish, or when someone is sharing her grandmother's traditional holiday recipes. The possibilities are endless for what might get someone into the adaptive mode. No matter how long or how significantly individuals have been impacted by challenges, all have these at-their-best moments.

Asking about At-Their-Best Moments

For those who know the person well enough, you might ask, "What is Richard like at his best? What types of things is he doing?" You can also ask about past hobbies or desires that individuals expressed prior to the challenges becoming especially prominent ("What did he like to do before all of this?"). You can also pose similar questions directly to the person (as this can access the adaptive mode for some people; see below).

Clues to Look For

Some people wear interests, literally, on their sleeves. Take note of sports jerseys, hats, and other memorabilia. This could be a sign of allegiance to a favorite team, and a great entry to the adaptive mode. Certain types of shoes or clothes, or specific ways of doing nails or hair, could show interest in fashion, another lead. Room decorations offer another clue—posters of music groups, celebrities, movies, animals, video games.

If You Have No Leads

There may be instances when you have no information about "at-their-best" moments. Table 3.1 can be your guide when this occurs, as it contains the types of activity that we have seen be successful at accessing the adaptive mode. You can keep these activities in mind as you try different activities while looking for the spark that might light up the person's adaptive mode. Our experience is that this search process is very forgiving—you just need one successful activity for it to work. Appendix D provides additional suggestions broken down by targeted beliefs.

Sharpening Your Role in the Activities

Your own enthusiasms and those of some of the individuals may overlap—you like the same thing or things, or, conversely, there may be activities that you know little about or have never

TABLE 3.1. Common Activities for Accessing the Adaptive Mode

Music—current, from the individual's youth, from pop culture, such as theme songs, songs with cultural significance	Pop culture—TV shows, movies, historically significant events, comic books, video games
Sports—local teams, region-specific activities, nationally televised competitions, outdoorsmanship	Food—cooking, family recipes, cultural meals, best things to make when someone is sick, local delicacies, best places to go for certain foods, gardening
Creative pursuits—art, crocheting/knitting, storytelling, photography	Animals—pets (current, past, desired), nature, shelter animals, funny animal videos

pursued. You can take advantage of each of these situations to make your accessing interventions more effective.

Shared Interests

A basic way people connect with one another is through shared interests. These pursuits can be a source for much action and conversing. There are so many possibilities: food, sports, where a person is from, holidays, TV shows, music, vacation spots, and so on. A variation of shared interests occurs when people like opposing sports teams and tease one another. When you find the right activity, doing it together can be effortless and fun. Both of you can be experts or enthusiasts, sharing knowledge, positive emotions, and being a team. In this way, a natural manner of interacting for all people becomes a vehicle for accessing the adaptive mode and developing connection and trust.

Seeking the Individual's Advice

Another basic form of connection involves one person teaching another. There is no better way to show interest and curiosity than to ask a person for advice or to share something they know. Asking for advice places the individual in the expert role and can be very motivating, especially for individuals who are more withdrawn.

There are a few different ways you can ask for advice. You can:

- *Seek help for a problem.* "I'm trying to think of a way to get my next therapy group energized, what music should I play?"
- *Get opinions on possible topics of interest.* "Should I paint my nails red or blue next week?"
- *Seek advice about specific areas of knowledge.* "I notice you have a lot of pictures of dogs, do you have any idea of what are good lapdogs?"
- *Seek advice on how to do something that is a skill of theirs.* "Do you have a good macaroni-and-cheese recipe?"
- *Consider areas that you want to learn more about and see how the individual may be able to help.* "I have been trying to learn how to keep plants alive, any chance you know anything about gardening?"

Being in a helping role energizes the individual by accessing personal skill areas and the desire to care for others. It also establishes a connection between the individual and the person they are helping, demonstrating that both bring something important to the relationship. Sometimes seeking advice helps because it takes the pressure off individuals talking about themselves, and instead shifts the focus onto you. The advice you seek is not on anything exceedingly personal—rather, the purpose is finding opportunities for the person to help, have a role, and connect.

Getting Started

Keep in mind you will be able to clearly observe when someone is in the adaptive mode. You will know when the activity or conversation is going the right way, as the person becomes immediately more animated, relaxed, clear, funny, warm, and connected. What you are going for is this public change in their demeanor.

Each person is different—both in their interests and source of disconnection. Hitting on the right thing will likely take some persistence. You should expect a process of trying an intervention and adjusting your approach based on the response you get back. Fortunately, there are effective things you can do to access the adaptive mode when your initial attempt does not succeed.

To help navigate accessing the adaptive mode, you can follow a decision tree (see Figures 3.1–3.5). This takes into account the sources of disconnection, proposing specific interventions for each one that holds promise to succeed. We take as a starting point the person who responds well to your verbal attempts at access to the adaptive mode. Over time, as you energize the adaptive mode, more and more of your interactions will start with direct verbal access.

But at the start—when you may not have enough trust or other factors may intrude—direct verbal attempts may not work. This could be because the person is particularly withdrawn and isolated, they may be hard to understand, or they could be rejecting and guarded. Another possibility is that the person responds readily to inquiries about being at-their-best, but talks about high-risk activities (e.g., using drugs). The decision tree helps you work with each of these.

The Direct Verbal Approach (See Figure 3.1)

You may well have some ideas about what gets the person excited from observing them or talking with others who have seen them at-their-best. You can lead with these ideas. If you do not know what interests the person, you can also ask what they enjoy doing, what they are interested in, what hobbies they have currently or had growing up, and other open-ended curious questions (using Table 3.1 and Appendix D as a guide).

Some individuals, especially those who have negative beliefs about their abilities to enjoy things (e.g., "I can't enjoy things I used to because I have a diagnosis"), may be unsure about their interests or say that they don't have any. If this comes up, narrow the scope of your question to include specific topics that many people might be interested in, such as asking what type of music they like, or what sports they used to play.

Be attentive for the topic that sparks the most excitement. You want to be prepared to go through a few possibilities until you hit on the right one. The person's excitement will be your guide. Your curiosity will be the oxygen of connection, especially asking about the best part of the interest.

Importantly—you or another team member should turn conversation into action. What can you do together that will activate the person's adaptive mode and produce experiences that can be noticed to strengthen it?

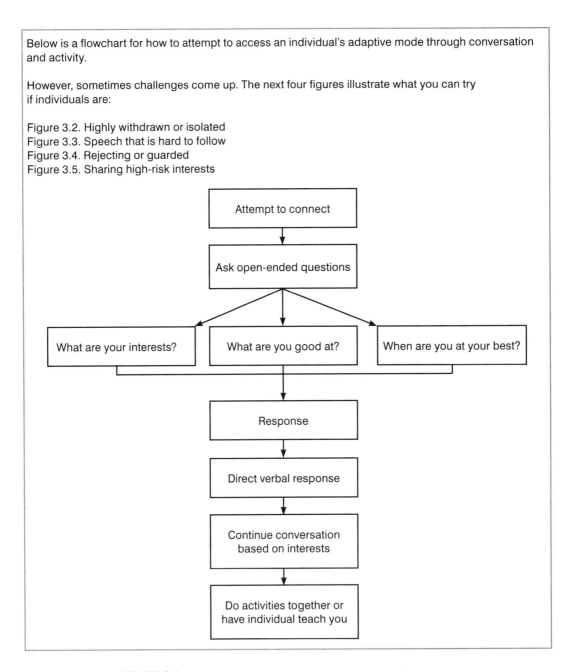

FIGURE 3.1. Accessing the adaptive mode: direct verbal response.

When the Person Is Withdrawn or Isolated (See Figure 3.2)

Some individuals do not have a lot of energy or tolerance for personal questions, even ones that probe positive topics. They may not respond, they may walk away, they might pull covers over their heads. Your strategy here is to make the accessing experience less demanding and easier. Figure 3.2 shows at least three choices you might make, each reducing the energy and effort to respond to your attempts at accessing the adaptive mode.

Narrow the Scope of Questioning and Use Media

As we saw above, simplifying the questions can make things easier. Use questions that provide a couple options and try basic activities. You might try different musical groups (Backstreet Boys or 'NSync?) or food (pancakes or waffles?) or sports (baseball or football?) or activity (yoga or Zumba?).

Media can be especially helpful. It can be effortless to watch a video or listen to a favorite song. Try playing a song on a smartphone or portable music player. Video of a sports highlight, a TikTok video, a humorous animal video, a celebrity chef—all of these can spark the adaptive mode of a person who tends to be more withdrawn.

You want to work up to action. Doing activities that help you in some way can be especially appealing to the person. You can say, "I've been indoors all day. How about we go for a walk? It would help me." You could also bring playing cards and offer the choice: "Blackjack or Go Fish?" and start dealing the cards. It is important to initiate the activity as soon as possible. The longer the delay between proposing the activity and its start, the greater the chance the individual will be drawn back into disconnection or reject the idea. It is also helpful to present the activity matter-of-factly ("Let's go for a walk," or "Do you know this song?" or "Check out this video").

Brief Interactions

Some individuals can find any prolonged interaction intolerable or overwhelming. For them, you can shorten the duration of encounters, relying on single closed-ended questions during each visit—for example, you can say, "Should the group watch *Judge Judy* or *Wheel of Fortune*?" or "Should I make pizza or biscuits and gravy?" The brief duration and concrete focus of the interaction further reduces pressure they might experience. While keeping things short, you can also increase the frequency of your visits. This helps the person become more comfortable with the interaction, shows that you care what they have to say, and that you mean it when you say you will return.

You can use many of the interventions we have already discussed. Ultimately, by introducing media or activities, the person develops trust and you will be able to access their adaptive mode for longer stretches of time. The person teaching you about an area of their interest will be particularly effective in accessing the adaptive mode.

Bring Activity to the Person

There are some individuals who have so little energy that they will not get out of bed or leave the dayroom. To make any interaction possible at all, we need to bring the activity to them. The encounters also need to be brief and frequent at first, following the program of the previous section.

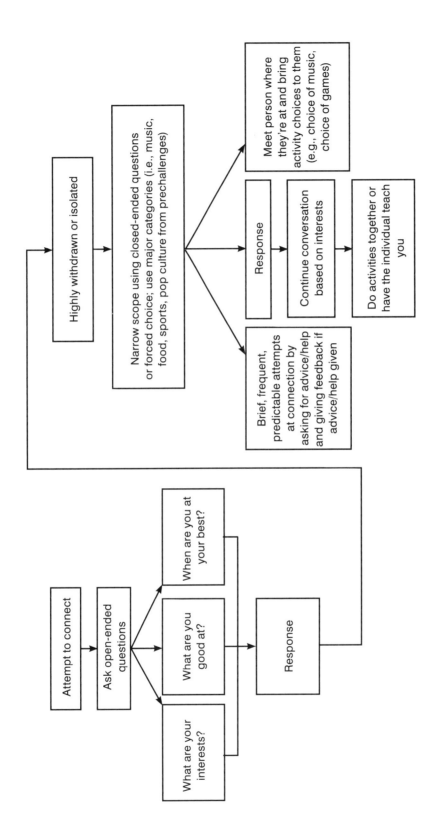

FIGURE 3.2. Accessing the adaptive mode: highly withdrawn or isolated.

This was the approach the team took with Jackie. Attempts at extensive conversation often resulted in increased disorganization and utterances that were hard to follow. Instead, her treatment team made a guess about a possible area of interest through observation of times when she didn't seem to be experiencing as many challenges. In an effort to expand on what the staff in the residence knew about Jackie's interest in jewelry making, they sought her out to get her opinions on different materials and ways of making the jewelry. They initially presented her with short questions that provided just a few options (e.g., plastic vs. metal). Taking this approach had a couple of benefits: answering a choice-based question requires little energy or cognitive resources to come up with a helpful answer. By providing a suggestion, Jackie was able to have a role in an activity without initially getting out of bed or being with the other residents. The staff were able to express appreciation for her helpfulness with every suggestion both in the moment but also after following her advice. Jackie was able to fulfill an *expert role*, shifting some of the dynamic between herself and the staff. Over time, as the staff consistently reached out to her and she was helping more and more from her room, it became easier for Jackie to share her ideas and answer more open-ended questions (e.g., Who might like to receive the handmade jewelry?).

When the Person's Speech Is Hard to Follow (See Figure 3.3)

For various reasons—stress, low energy—some individuals can have a difficult time communicating. You might not initially understand their answer to your query about what they find fun or when they are at-their-best. Not being understood is a key experience of the "patient" mode and is a reason that they can feel they do not belong. To successfully get around this communication challenge and connect successfully with them, you have a couple of choices depending on how much speech is getting in the way.

Reflect What You Heard

Your first move is to show your desire to understand, which can reduce the person's stress related to fear that you might judge them. You can gently interrupt and do your best to summarize back what they said, indicating how important it is for you to understand. Sometimes this intervention releases the pressure enough for you to access the adaptive mode and get moving toward action.

Reduce Verbal Demand

If reflecting does not seem to be effective, try using questioning that can be responded to with less extensive verbalizing. As we say in the previous section, closed-ended questions that offer choices are particularly good. Use of media aids can also be helpful.

Lead with Action

This is where you can use any knowledge of activities where the person seems more at ease (games, singing, exercise, crafts). You can try these out with them and see whether you get the desired effect of accessing the adaptive mode.

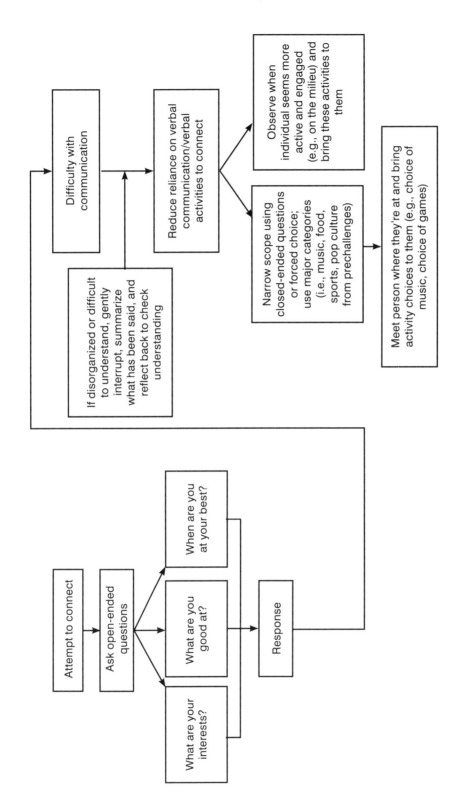

FIGURE 3.3. Accessing the adaptive mode: difficulty with communication.

Meet Them Where They Are

Some people might have low energy and also can be difficult to understand. As we saw in the previous section, we can meet them where they are, bring the activity to them, make it short and predictable, build the interaction over time, and access the adaptive mode more and more.

Jackie also showed speech that her team found difficult to follow. The staff used all of these methods to connect with her and not have Jackie's low energy or speech get in the way of successfully activating her adaptive mode.

When the Person Is Rejecting or Guarded (See Figure 3.4)

Another response you can get when approaching an individual to discover their best self is to be blown off. The person might yell at you colorfully, telling you to go away. They might walk away in irritation, muttering to themselves. They might just say no impassively. These responses show us that the person feels vulnerable. Personal questions could be firing up their heightened sensitivity around control. They might also fear being exposed, devalued, or rejected.

In this instance, the act of trying to access the adaptive mode directly fires up the "patient" mode. To get around this, you can make adjustments to your questioning that explicitly give control back to the person and make the interaction safe and ultimately successful.

Control and Safety

You can turn everything you say into a choice: "Can I talk with you now or later?"; "Is it okay if we talk about you at your best?"; "Do you want to listen to a song?"; "Can I ask a question?"; "Is it okay if I ask again later?"; "Can I come by and see you tomorrow?"

If you treat each exchange as an opportunity for them to have control, you will be less likely to stir up their vulnerability. A careful use of choice-based questions can also put you in a position of offering alternatives while not including the choice of them rejecting you outright ("Can I see you now or later today?").

You can, at the same time, be clear in your intention, which is to connect and find out about them and determine which of these things you might do together—if they agree, of course.

Clear Messaging of Your Interest and Availability

You may still get "no" while you are enhancing the control and safety of your approach. A next move is to be clear that you desire to get to know them better and that you are available to talk when they feel like it. Your message, if genuine and sincere, gives complete control to the person and shows positive intention.

Brief, Frequent, Predictable Interactions

As in the previous sections, keeping things short can take the pressure off and allow the person to warm up to you over time. The person who is feeling vulnerable can come to see that you will keep coming back, possibly countering their belief that you don't really care or will just reject

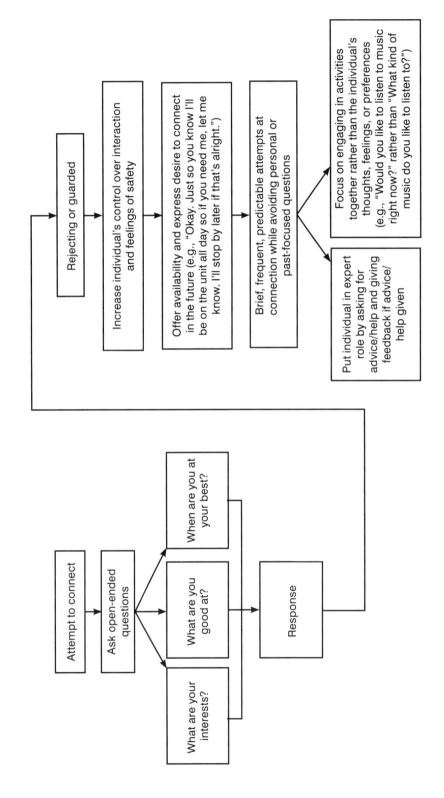

FIGURE 3.4. Accessing the adaptive mode: rejecting or guarded.

them in the end. Each time you are with them you can focus the interaction on asking them a question, playing a song, or looking at a funny video.

Getting Advice

The person is likely hypersensitive to being one down. But, they are, correspondingly, likely to relish being in an expert role. In your brief interactions, you can ask them for advice, noticing (in question form) how helpful they are being, or how much they know. If the advice helps you, you can give them feedback. Each bit of help you get is moving you toward better connection, trust, and longer activation of the adaptive mode together.

Doing Together

As you are able to do more that brings out the person at-their-best, you want to take care to minimize psychological talk. This can touch on vulnerability and reimpose the "patient" mode. Your person is action oriented; focus on what you are doing or going to do rather than preferences, thoughts, and the like.

When the Person Gives High-Risk Responses (See Figure 3.5)

Sometimes individuals give answers that reflect a preference for potentially high-risk activities. In answer to the "when they are at-their-best" question, the person might say, "When I am high," or "When I am prostituting." Here, the decision tree gives you a good procedure to get interests that you can work with.

What's the Best Part?

Your follow-up question can be "What is the best part about that?" In the case of substance use, for example, this could be several possibilities: "I feel accepted," "I feel loved," "I feel so awesome," and so on. You are looking for the meaning or value to the person in the high-risk activity.

Other Ways to Get It

Once you know the function, you can find out whether the person knows of other ways to experience that meaning and feeling. If the answer is yes, then you can discuss these activities and see which ones it might be good to do together or have the person teach you about. We have seen people who have given substance use responses come up with very rich alternatives—for example, they have a big interest in fashion and fitness, a great source for accessing their adaptive mode.

Narrow the Focus

If the person cannot report an alternative way to get the feeling or meaning of their high-risk answer, you can validate that and then try other means to find out what else might excite them. You have a few tacks you can take. You can try a choice approach using the categories of interests

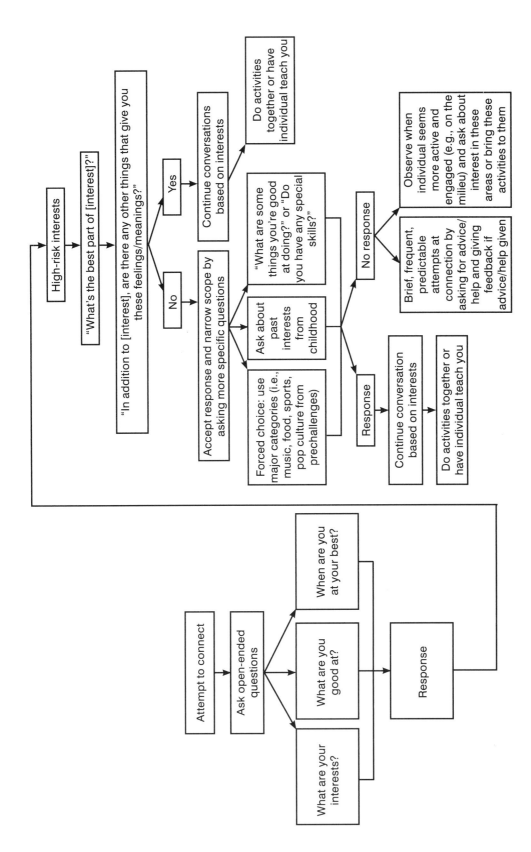

FIGURE 3.5. Accessing the adaptive mode: high-risk interests or response.

(tennis or boxing? *Friends* or *Cheers*?). You can also ask the person what they are particularly good at. A third approach is to ask them if they recall interests from their youth. Any of these might hit something that shows the spark and lets you know you have accessed the adaptive mode.

Brief Interactions

If you still do not have anything after the different types of questioning, you can always move into the least demanding approach: brief, frequent, predictable encounters where you ask for help or try activities that you have seen the person respond to or think they might like.

STRENGTHENING POSITIVE BELIEFS WHEN ACCESSING THE ADAPTIVE MODE

Accessing the adaptive mode brings about apparent behavioral change; it is during these times that the positive beliefs individuals have about themselves are also considerably more accessible. These beliefs are ones that an individual may already possess, though they may not be as strongly held yet as the ones that underlie certain challenges. The beliefs might also be new for the person. See Table 3.2 for a list of some examples of common positive beliefs made accessible in the adaptive mode.

Confirming or Correcting Guesses

When planning to access a person's adaptive mode, you initially conjecture about what beliefs could be activated when they are doing the activity. Once you are doing the activity, you have

TABLE 3.2. Common Positive Beliefs Made Accessible in the Adaptive Mode

About the self
- I am competent.
- I am knowledgeable or skilled.
- I am capable.
- I am helpful.
- I have value.

About others
- Other people care about me.
- Others are interested in what I have to offer.
- It's worthwhile to interact and connect with others.

About the future
- It's possible to enjoy things, and I can experience this again.
- I can have control over my experiences by doing the things I enjoy more often.
- If I can help others now, I can do more in the future.

the opportunity to check the accuracy of these guesses, updating the Recovery Map in the process.

You can uncover the beliefs that are most significant to a person by asking questions during activities that activate the adaptive mode, such as:

- "What's the best part of playing this game?"
- "What's it like when you're teaching me this recipe?"
- "How does it feel to be doing this right now?"

You can also notice what they say during those activities:

- "This is fun."
- "I know everything there is to know about birds."
- "You guys really would have been out of luck if I wasn't here to show you how to build that!"

Figure 3.6 shows the process of updating Jackie's Recovery Map. The new information appears in italics.

Through low-pressure, consistent, and predictable opportunities to connect, individuals can experience not only the behavioral change and energy that comes with the adaptive mode but positive beliefs ultimately become more and more accessible.

Recognizing the role that beliefs have when someone is in the adaptive mode can also inform your planning of strategies and interventions—for instance, the positive beliefs activated are often in direct contrast to those activated when challenges are present. If you know what negative beliefs people hold about themselves (e.g., "I am worthless"), consider presenting opportunities that activate the adaptive mode (e.g., helping run a clothing drive for people experiencing homelessness) and activate the opposite belief (e.g., "I can help others and am valuable").

ACCESSING AND ENERGIZING THE ADAPTIVE MODE	
Interests/Ways to Engage: • Arts and crafts • Jewelry making *Latest successes:* • *Giving advice on jewelry materials* • *Possibly wants to help others who are lonely (nursing home project)* • *Moves with others* • *Music*	**Beliefs Activated While in Adaptive Mode:** • Guess: I am capable or skilled • Guess: It's worth being around and spending time with others when we're doing things I enjoy *Other possibilities:* • *I am helpful* • *Others appreciate my skills* • *It is worthwhile to do projects with others* • *The more I do that I enjoy, the better I feel and the easier it is to help others* • *I can connect and it's worth doing things with other people* • *I get more energy by doing things I enjoy*

FIGURE 3.6. Jackie's updated Recovery Map: Accessing and energizing the adaptive mode section.

POSITIVE ACTION AND EMPOWERMENT	
Current Strategies and Interventions: 1. Identify ways to activate the adaptive mode • Ask for advice about craft projects • Ask for help setting up crafts and other activities • Ask Jackie and her family about things she used to enjoy doing 2. Identify and enrich aspirations • Create recovery image	**Beliefs/Aspirations/Meanings/Challenge Targeted:** 1a. Beliefs about capability • I am capable and can be connected • The more I do that I enjoy, the better I feel • I can enjoy more than I thought and can still do the things I used to enjoy 1b. Reduce isolation 2. Beliefs about the future • Hope and purpose for the future

FIGURE 3.7. Jackie's updated Recovery Map: Positive action and empowerment section.

The new, more elaborated positive action and empowerment section of Jackie's Recovery Map is shown in Figure 3.7.

First, Jackie's team knew they needed to learn more about her interests and tap her energy before pursing aspirations or addressing challenges, so they selected interventions that met her in her room, with low-demand questions. These provided an early opportunity to contribute successfully. They sought her input, which increased both connection and possibly capability. When Jackie came up with a way to help others, the staff turned that into an intervention to shift possible beliefs of being useless to those about her having value and being helpful. Given the success of this approach, the team can use the understanding of beliefs to inform future interventions—for example, are there other ways Jackie can be helpful in the residence, in the community, or with her family?

Drawing Conclusions

Accessing the adaptive mode makes positive beliefs more accessible. However, having a good experience by itself does not guarantee that an individual will *notice* that they are connected, capable, or anything else of value. When the experience is over, opportunity can be lost to tap into the potential power of these meanings. This is one of the reasons that the adaptive mode is dormant for many individuals—the potential of their good experiences has gone mostly untapped.

To strengthen the underlying positive beliefs, we make statements and ask questions that draw attention to these valuable meanings during the accessing activity. Important considerations are *when* to use guiding strategies, *which types* of inquiries are best based on the targeted beliefs, and how much energy or other cognitive resources the individual has.

When to Guide: During the Peak or Soon after an Activity

Drawing conclusions when individuals are still in the adaptive mode is important because they are experiencing positive emotions and beliefs in real time, making it particularly easy to notice and draw conclusions. We are catching the positive emotions and beliefs when they are hot! The greater the time elapsed between the peak of the activity and guiding, the more difficult it will be for the person to find the beneficial emotions and beliefs. This will be especially true if they have returned to the "patient" mode.

The best time to notice is when the activity is peaking, which you can tell by the person's level of excitement and energy. As the experience is cresting, you might say, "I love this song. How is it for you? More fun than you thought?" or "This is a great walk. How does it feel for you? Do you have more or less energy than before we began?"

Draw Attention to the Value of the Activity

It's important to highlight the value of activities to aid individuals. The conclusion you want them to draw is based on (1) the intended effect of the activity and (2) seeing whether the individual experienced the effect. To do that, you can ask questions, such as "Did you have more or less fun than you thought you would?" and "Is it better to do things with other people?"

Accessing the adaptive mode is also a chance for the individual to make many useful observations and conclusions that will enable future connection and activity with others:

"I share similarities with others."
"Time with others is worthwhile."
"Time with others is fun."
"Talking with others feels better than time alone."
"Connecting with others can give me purpose and a role."
"I can learn from and help others."
"Talking with others gives me more energy."

Ultimately, you want to help the person discover that engaging in certain activities with others has great personal benefit, and that these types of things are worth doing. These conclusions are the gateway to energizing the adaptive mode.

Open-Ended versus Closed-Ended Questioning

"What does that say about you?" This is a terrific question for drawing conclusions about the positive meanings of an interaction, in terms of self, others, and the future. However, broad questions such as this can easily reactivate the "patient" mode, defeating your purpose in accessing the adaptive mode. Open-ended question can require extra energy. If posed before a person has identified a strength (e.g., I'm capable), they may experience self-doubt or anxiety and not respond to the question. They might also expect that they're going to get the answer wrong.

To keep the person in the adaptive mode while drawing conclusions about the experience, you can use a strategy of starting with less effort-demanding, closed-ended questioning and moving to more open-ended questioning over time. This begins with sharing observations, floating a conclusion, and seeing whether the individual agrees (e.g., "I'm so glad you gave me that great idea! You're a pretty helpful person. What do you think about that?"). As you build trust and strengthen the adaptive mode, you can shift to asking broader questions about the experiences and how the person sees themselves (e.g., "What does it mean about you that you did this?"; "What does it mean about your ability to connect to others?").

Considering Jackie, the team hoped to strengthen beliefs about her being *capable, connected,* and *valuable,* and that the more involved she was in enjoyable pursuits, the more *energy* she had and the *better she felt.* Given these belief targets, the staff helped Jackie notice in a manner that increasingly fit her energy and trust:

- Guiding her attention to staff observations.
  - "I noticed you were smiling while you were helping me pick out beads. Do you enjoy working on this project?"
- Gradually posing more open-ended questions about what it means for Jackie when she's in the adaptive mode.
  - At first:
    - "Wow—you came up with a great idea and everyone is having fun doing it. You're really helpful, aren't you?"
    - "I have so much more energy when we're working on this project. How about you?"
    - "If it feels good while we do this, do you think we should do it more or less often?"
  - Over time:
    - "What does that say about you that you came up with the idea for our service project?"
    - "What does it say about you that it has been successful and brought people closer together?"
    - "What has it been like for you now that we've been making jewelry for the nursing home more often?"

ENERGIZING THE ADAPTIVE MODE

Once you have identified interests and activities that can reliably access the adaptive mode, the next step is to do these things more often. Because the adaptive mode is often dormant and the "patient" mode is correspondingly overactive, we need to build up the person by energizing the adaptive mode in this way. Repeatedly accessing the adaptive mode together feels good and strengthens your relationship. Helping the person access their adaptive mode more often every single day enriches their life and propels them toward thinking more about the future and what life could look like.

Repeated Experiences

Energizing requires accessing the person's adaptive mode over and over in a manner that is predictable for them. This can be done informally. It might involve planning increased activity on units or on residential milieus. Or, it might entail generating action plans individually that involve scheduling more activity into the individual's week. Frequent and consistent opportunities to engage in preferred activities increases time spent in the adaptive mode. As individuals increase the amount of time in the adaptive mode, there are fewer opportunities for challenges to become intrusive. There are also more opportunities to strengthen beliefs about their ability to be energized and connect with others.

Positive Action Scheduling

Some like a structured approach to energizing the adaptive mode. Positive action scheduling, a variation of activity scheduling (Beck, 2020; Beck et al., 1979), involves planning for activities that activate the adaptive mode. It is a process of building up the person's life to increase energy, improve mood, and reduce the amount of time challenges are present. The person has additional opportunities to see that action is worthwhile, and to strengthen positive beliefs about the benefit of action with other people. The steps of positive action scheduling are presented in Figure 3.8.

Experiencing the Benefit of Activity Together

The time you spend with the individual can demonstrate the benefits of taking action together. Among them are enjoyment, increased energy, success, belonging, and more. Even better, you

Purpose: Plan enjoyable, aspiration-driven activities that bring meaning and purpose into every day!

Experience	Experience the benefit of doing an activity together (e.g., listen to music)
Observe	Observe the benefits of an activity by doing it more during the week
Schedule	Schedule an activity during the week
Target	Target the schedule for specific challenges (i.e., certain times of the day, certain types of stressors, etc.)
Refine	Refine the schedule by increasing frequency and type of activities
Strengthen	Strengthen positive beliefs related to action

FIGURE 3.8. Positive action scheduling.

can draw the individual's attention *in the moment* to the benefits they're experiencing. You can also suggest they try the same activity on their own ("Wow that was some walk and we both said we felt more energized. When can you do it again?"). Positive action scheduling helps you plan activities that activate the adaptive mode more frequently. Here's one way it can look:

> PROVIDER: How much energy do you have today?
>
> INDIVIDUAL: Ehhh.
>
> PROVIDER: Not a lot?
>
> (*Individual nods.*)
>
> PROVIDER: I could use some energy, too. Let's walk!
>
> INDIVIDUAL: Okay.
>
> (*During walking*)
>
> PROVIDER: How do you like walking?
>
> INDIVIDUAL: It's good.
>
> PROVIDER: I like it, too. Do you feel like you have a little bit more energy? Do you feel a bit better?
>
> INDIVIDUAL: Yeah, I do.
>
> PROVIDER: Me, too! So, we went for a walk together, and now we feel better. I guess when you do a little bit more that you enjoy, the better you feel and you have a little more energy?
>
> INDIVIDUAL: Yeah, I think so.

Positive action scheduling starts with the individual's own experience with you. They develop new ideas about how life can be better (e.g., that doing things you enjoy with others can make you feel more energized).

Seeing the Benefit of Action in Daily Life

Capitalizing on your successful action together, you can help the person plan to do the activities at other times and see whether the same great feeling occurs. For example:

- "You sure enjoy music! Do you ever listen to music at other times?"
- "You sure have more energy when you talk about sports. Do you ever talk about sports at other times? Who else could you talk with about sports?"
- "Those dance moves sure make you feel better and have a little more energy. When can you try it again?"
- "Can you show your brother that funny video?"

Start with enjoyable or meaningful activities that produce the largest impact on energy.

Scheduling Activity

You can collaboratively create a schedule with individuals using any number of tools, based on the individual's preferences. You want the schedule to make it more likely that they will succeed in activating their adaptive mode more often. It has to work for them. The experience should be uplifting and feel good rather than be a burden or source of feeling like a failure—features that will bring back the "patient" mode and defeat the purpose of positive action scheduling. Instead of an itinerary of mundane tasks, the schedule focuses on appealing activities that bring out the person at-their-best.

Start by focusing on memory. We all can struggle to remember things. How would they like to remember the plan to do more of their preferred activity? Do they want to write it down? Use a planner, make a calendar on the computer, use art supplies? Do they want to use technology, such as a tablet or cell phone? Do they want to create a picture or meme? The schedule itself can be any format—a little collaborative creativity can make all of the difference. Figure 3.9 is just one example of a positive action schedule. A blank positive activity schedule form can be found in Appendix E.

Targeting Specific Challenges with the Schedule

As the benefits of activity accrue, you can consider those parts of the day when it might be important to get into the adaptive mode (e.g., in the morning to jumpstart energy, or ahead of times when stressors or challenges might be more likely to come up). If a person has difficulty gathering the energy to get up and start the day, the two of you can schedule energy-boosting activities to help. You might ask, "If you felt more energized while listening to music, are there times you feel less energy and can use music to help?" You then add listening to music to the schedule at a time it seems most helpful—early in the day. Even if the scheduled activities alleviate some challenges, the focus is on bringing about the adaptive mode. Scheduled activities should not be oriented around "patienthood"—such as taking medication, attending to grooming, or going to therapeutic groups.

Refine the Schedule by Increasing Frequency and Type of Activities

As the person benefits from doing activities more often, focus on increasing the amount and diversity of pursuits—for instance, if an individual has successfully used music to feel good in the morning once during the week, perhaps it would be worth doing it again on another day. If music was effective, is it possible that other activities will also help with energy? Having a variety of appealing active experiences can help extend the amount of time spent in the adaptive mode. Consider activities the individual has stopped doing but would like to start again, as well as something completely new. You can return to ideas for accessing the adaptive mode, such as those listed in Table 3.1 and Appendix D, to identify additional interests.

Accessing and Energizing the Adaptive Mode 51

> PRO TIPS:
> - Be creative! It doesn't have to be a chart or look boring!
> - Use technology, notebooks, or whatever a person can easily access
> - Create it collaboratively WITH the individual

Weekly Activity Schedule

Sunday	Monday	Tuesday	Wednesday	Thursday	Friday	Saturday
			8:30 am – Read inspirational quote in community meeting			
	1:00 pm – Watch videos of animals with staff					
					6:00 pm – Participate in card-making club for Veterans	

Aspiration:

1. <u>Become a social worker</u>
2. <u>Be an advocate for animals and take in rescues</u>

Meaning:

1. <u>Help people; useful member of my community; accomplished; inspire hope; have purpose</u>
2. <u>Helpful; nurturing; show patience, care, and affection; make the world better</u>

FIGURE 3.9. Positive action scheduling example.

Strengthening Beliefs

As individuals engage in more and more personally appealing activities every day, you can regularly check on successes. You can further strengthen positive beliefs about success, capability, energy, and the benefits of planning activities—for example, you can draw the individual's attention to the fact that the more they do during the week that they enjoy, the better they feel and the easier it becomes to do even more preferred activities.

Positive action schedules can also be modified to make it easier to draw conclusions—for example, you can add a column where the person notes how they feel while they're doing certain activities and whether or not they'd like to do them again. The feedback they give can help inform your guiding questions (e.g., "You said you felt proud helping take care of your sister's dog, and that it's worth doing again. What was the best part about that? When might you help her again?") See Figure 3.10 for an example of a modified schedule.

Positive action scheduling is not limited to planning pleasurable activities. It can also be used to plan meaningful action steps toward aspirations. We revisit the use of positive action scheduling and how it evolves as we uncover and develop aspirations in Chapter 5.

	Activity	Feel?	Voices/ stress/pain?	Want to do it again?
Monday		good bad just okay helpful proud annoyed strong sad	Yes No	Yes No
Tuesday		good bad just okay helpful proud annoyed strong sad	Yes No	Yes No
Wednesday	Take sister's dog for a walk; play fetch	good bad just okay helpful proud annoyed strong sad	Yes No	Yes No
Thursday		good bad just okay helpful proud annoyed strong sad	Yes No	Yes No
Friday		good bad just okay helpful proud annoyed strong sad	Yes No	Yes No
Saturday		good bad just okay helpful proud annoyed strong sad	Yes No	Yes No
Sunday		good bad just okay helpful proud annoyed strong sad	Yes No	Yes No

FIGURE 3.10. Weekly activity schedule used to draw conclusions.

ENERGIZING THE ADAPTIVE MODE WITH JACKIE

Energizing Jackie's adaptive mode involved the staff making observations about increased mood, energy, and connection to others in the house. They said things like "It seems like you've really helped us all by showing us how to make jewelry. What do you think? If making jewelry helps and makes you feel good, what do you think about doing it more often?" With Jackie's agreement, the staff asked her when she would like to do it again and how often. Together, they planned to make jewelry twice a week. Over time, they added some other activities, like going to the store with the staff for supplies, joining other residents to watch movies in the common room, and listening to more music. With an energized adaptive mode, Jackie's life was beginning to expand.

IMPACT OF ACCESSING AND ENERGIZING ON THE RECOVERY MAP

As you move through different stages of CT-R, your understanding evolves and you will update the individual's Recovery Map accordingly. With much more information about what helps Jackie access her adaptive mode and with plans to help her energize this mode of living, her team revised her Recovery Map, which now looks like Figure 3.11. New developments are noted in italics.

ADDITIONAL CONSIDERATIONS

The Process Can Take Time

The process of discovering what an individual is doing when they're in the adaptive mode doesn't have to happen all at once. You may try talking about or playing music for a few minutes one day and try again with the same topic briefly the next day, but if it doesn't seem to be a person's interest, you can try something different in the next interaction. Accessing the adaptive mode is about *meeting people where they are* and being genuinely curious about their experiences and interests. Many individuals have been disconnected from others for a long period of time and sometimes have had life experiences that reinforce that they should stay away from others. Others might be disconnected because extensive periods of inactivity and isolation make even the idea of connection exhausting. We have found that *you should keep trying*. It might take many attempts before you find the right strategy.

Accessing the Adaptive Mode Can Be Returned to at Any Time

Accessing the adaptive mode is not just an initial move; it is an ongoing process with the individual. Over the course of treatment, individuals may ebb and flow between the adaptive mode and the "patient" mode. When you see signs that the individual is beginning to lose energy or is increasing the expression of challenges, you can return to using methods of activating the adaptive mode.

Recovery Map	
ACCESSING AND ENERGIZING THE ADAPTIVE MODE	
Interests/Ways to Engage: • Arts and crafts • Jewelry making *Latest successes:* • Giving advice on jewelry materials • Possibly wants to help others who are lonely (nursing home project) • Moves with others to music	**Beliefs Activated While in Adaptive Mode:** • Guess: I am capable or skilled • Guess: It's worth being around and spending time with others when we're doing things I enjoy *Other possibilities:* • I am helpful • Others appreciate my skills • It is worthwhile to do projects with others • The more I do that I enjoy, the better I feel and the easier it is to help others • I can connect and it's worth doing things with other people • I get more energy by doing things I enjoy
ASPIRATIONS	
Goals: • Not known yet—need to develop further • What might her belief about bringing people back from the dead mean? Is there something desired there? • Would she like to be involved in creative activities in the future? *Guess:* • Help other people?	**Meaning of Accomplishing Identified Goal:** • Guess: Connection? • Guess: Power or importance? • Guess: Capability? *Guess:* • Value?
CHALLENGES	
Current Behaviors/Challenges: • Paying attention to voices to the point of reduced awareness of her environment (e.g., walking into the street) • Isolation • Difficulty with verbal communication (disorganization) • Delusions around bringing people back from the dead and generating body parts	**Beliefs Underlying Challenges:** • I have no control • What's the point of doing things with others, I will fail anyway • I can't enjoy the things I used to anymore • People don't like me • People can't understand me • The world is unsafe • I have nothing to offer, I'm incapable • I'm unimportant and have little value
POSITIVE ACTION AND EMPOWERMENT	

Current Strategies and Interventions:
1. Identify ways to activate the adaptive mode
  • Ask for advice about craft projects
  • Ask for help setting up crafts and other activities
  • Ask Jackie and her family about things she used to enjoy doing
2. Identify and enrich aspirations
  • Create recovery image
	Beliefs/Aspirations/Meanings/Challenge Targeted:
	1a. Beliefs about capability
	  • I am capable and can be connected
	  • The more I do that I enjoy, the better I feel
	  • I can enjoy more than I thought and can still do the things I used to enjoy
	1b. Reduce isolation
	2. Beliefs about the future
	  • Hope and purpose for the future

FIGURE 3.11. Jackie's updated Recovery Map.

Methods of Accessing the Adaptive Mode Are Not Rewards

Because the activities and interests that bring about the adaptive mode are so often typical, everyday, enjoyable events, we say that *the best treatment doesn't always look like treatment*. In CT-R, activities such as music, games, going outside, gardening, doing art, going on walks, and so on are part of accessing the adaptive mode and are a foundational element of treatment. They also target specific and personal beliefs. Therefore, it is important that these activities be incorporated into the treatment plan and made available, and not be provided as rewards for demonstrating desired behaviors. Rewards invoke a power dynamic—a break in connection—that the *rewarder* controls and the individual must comply with—an unwitting way to trigger and sustain the "patient" mode.

Repetition Helps Strengthen Beliefs

Repeated successful, energizing, connecting experiences and repeated drawing of conclusions about those experiences strengthens positive beliefs. Many of the negative beliefs about the self, others, and the future have permeated individuals' ways of seeing the world for a very long time. You may hear individuals say things like, "Well, that was fun yesterday, but it was a fluke. I can't get myself energized like that again." This is just one reason it is especially important to have repeated experiences when you can help the individual notice their power and capability. You may find that you pose the same type of guiding question frequently (e.g., "You seem to have a lot more energy when you're making jewelry, don't you think?"; "If making jewelry gives you more energy, what does that mean about whether or not you should do it more often?"; "Do you feel more energized when you're making the jewelry? It looks like it to me, too"). In CT-R, repetition is not redundant—it is part of strengthening that enhances an individual's resilience.

Accessing the Adaptive Mode in Highly Restrictive or Low-Resource Settings

Sometimes engaging in activities that access and energize the adaptive mode is simply not an option due to the setting someone is in. Examples might be forensic or corrections facilities, or facilities that are lacking in resources. In these situations, you may have to be very creative. One method you can use to access the adaptive mode is visualization or imagery to help a person imagine preferred activities. Building the image can involve questions such as "What is the activity you imagine doing?"; "What does it look like?"; "Where are you?"; "What are the sights, smells, and sounds?"; "How does it feel to be doing the activity?"; and "How does it feel right now to be imagining it?" As a person develops a rich image and gets into the adaptive mode, you can ask strengthening questions and those that lead to energizing: "If it can feel this good and energizing to imagine this now, would it be worth thinking of these things again?" and "When can you plan to do that?"

For individuals in these restrictive or low-resource settings who have a very difficult time with conversation, and for whom visualization or imagery might be too much, find ways to bring fun and energy into any interaction. This might include coming in and asking whether they know the TV theme song that's been stuck in your head, which you then begin to hum, or you can present simple choices related to areas of interest or ways to help you (e.g., "So! Burgers or pizza?" or "Who makes the best cheesesteak?"). All of these options pull for the adaptive mode, but no materials or in-depth conversation are required!

Respect Your Own Comfort Level and Boundaries

Because the activities and conversations that can bring about the adaptive mode may not look like traditional therapy interventions, some providers may feel uncomfortable or worry that they are crossing professional boundaries. If you have concerns such as these, be assured that you can still uncover an individual's adaptive mode and stay authentic to your own needs for boundaries and privacy. *Genuine* curiosity is the best asset you can bring to the table—for example, instead of asking advice about something you could do outside of work, you can ask for some suggestions to spruce up your office space. You don't need to sing or dance or exercise with individuals to ask what moves they might teach someone else. You can also use other methods for an activity, such as using technology (e.g., watching videos on a computer), or inviting the individual to teach someone else. In some cases, using visualization and imagery strategies is sufficient. In any of these situations, it is most important that you make consistent efforts to connect.

WORDS OF WISDOM

BOX 3.1. Genuine Relationship or How "You Believe in Me" Becomes "I Believe in Me"

When asked what helped them improve, individuals will often say something like "You believed in me," instead of naming specific therapeutic strategies. Similarly, when individuals are asked the meaning of going through a chain analysis of a scary situation, they might say, "It is good to have a friend."

Genuinely asking individuals for help (about health, cooking, working out, sports) and working on a project together are two superb approaches that support the individual in concluding "Wow, someone really respects me"; "She has faith in my instructions"; and so on. Your enthusiastic expression of satisfaction when the individual completes a project or reaches a milestone shows that you are being friendly and supportive. Knowing that "You have confidence in me and my ability to achieve my aspiration," bolsters the drive to success.

A key element of CT-R is that the therapeutic relationship should be highly authentic and genuine—you achieve this through identifying with the individual in a holistic and humanistic way.

Individuals may attach great significance to your verbal and nonverbal behavior toward them—for example, when an individual has sustained a setback or has accomplished a challenging task, your sympathetic understanding or pleasure regarding their success has important meaning to them. You build genuineness through curiosity, wanting to know their interests, values, history, family, yearnings, stories, and remembering them.

This mutual relationship of genuinely helping each other leads naturally to successes and confidence building. Supported by friendly questioning this helps "You believe in me" become "I believe in me."

The Adaptive Mode as the Gateway to Aspirations

The energy, connection, cognitive flexibility, and distance from distressing experiences that occurs when an individual is in the adaptive mode provides a gateway to uncovering meaningful aspirations and hope for the future. Sometimes, the idea of sharing desires and dreams can make people feel vulnerable, afraid, or defeated. However, when connection and trust are established, it can be easier for people to share meaningful possibilities for the future. The genuine curiosity you use to uncover interests and skills helps you smoothly transition to curiosity about aspirations. The momentum that builds when energizing the adaptive mode and taking action can grow meaningful aspirations.

The next chapter elaborates on how to identify and enrich aspirations and further develop the adaptive mode.

SUMMARY

- The adaptive mode is an achievable, concrete clinical target every individual has the ability to access. You can identify times when individuals are in the adaptive mode by answering the question "What are they like at-their-best?" Every individual has at-their-best moments.
- Accessing the adaptive mode may take time and persistence; the process looks different for each individual.
- The decision trees can help you adjust your approach to succeed in accessing the adaptive mode when you do not initially succeed.
- Accessing the adaptive mode can be a chance for individuals to strengthen positive beliefs about *action*: "I share similarities with others," "Time with others is worthwhile," and "Time with others is fun," and about *themselves*: "I am knowledgeable," "I can connect with others," "I am capable of creating my own energy," and "I am capable of enjoying things."
- We can energize the adaptive mode by providing multiple experiences to engage in meaningful, pleasurable, connection-driven activities and helping the individual draw conclusions along the way.
- Accessing and energizing the adaptive mode are the foundational steps of CT-R. They bring to life the recovery dimension of connection.

CHAPTER 4
Developing the Adaptive Mode
ASPIRATIONS

Jackie and the other residents made quite a bit of jewelry over several weeks. The staff thought it was time to find a place where they could deliver it. They invited Carl, another resident, to help them locate and call nursing homes in the area that might accept the gifts. Carl never made any jewelry with the others, but was motivated to help his housemates find a place "so they can make other people happy," he said.

When they went to make the first delivery, Jackie was one of the first people up, dressed, and ready to go. They listened to music in the van on the way over, and the staff noticed Jackie smiling and singing along at times. While they were at the nursing home, Jackie's speech was clear, she talked with some of the jewelry recipients about how she made the pieces, and asked people whether they liked what she made.

Later that night, back at the residence, the staff asked Jackie whether she'd like to make and deliver jewelry again. To their surprise, Jackie responded by repeatedly saying, "I need to bring everyone back from the dead and heal them." She did, however, continue to make jewelry the next day. A week or so later, the group went to make another jewelry delivery to a different nursing home. Jackie was fully in the adaptive mode once again.

This time, as soon as the residents got in the van to leave the nursing home, a staff member asked, "What was the best part of doing that just now—delivering the jewelry?"

Jackie said, "Helping people and making friends."

Carl said, "They see we care about them."

Jackie added, "They won't be lonely."

The staff member then said, "So should we plan to do this again?"

Everyone enthusiastically responded, "Yes!"

The staff shared the experience of the outing with Jackie's outpatient therapist, so that the therapist might continue drawing conclusions with Jackie about the positive experience and begin exploring other desires she has for the future.

So far, we have uncovered quite a lot about what Jackie is like at-her-best—her adaptive mode—and about the types of experiences that she's been able to add to her life. Now, her team can start to use the energy and momentum of the adaptive mode to discover hopes, desires, and possibilities for the future. This chapter focuses on how to develop the adaptive mode to identify and enrich aspirations. These help individuals build a rich, full life of their choosing. First, we define "aspiration." We then distinguish aspirations from other stated goals. Next, we describe when and how you can elicit these aspirations. Techniques for enriching and discovering the meaning of aspirations are then introduced.

DEFINING ASPIRATIONS

When an individual is increasingly spending time in the adaptive mode, it will be a natural extension of your work to begin identifying life aspirations. We use the term "aspirations" with great intention. Aspirations expand on the concept of goals, emphasizing the importance of long-range, meaningful pursuits. The word "aspirations" does not replace the word "goals"—rather, it is a broader concept.

Some persons with lived experience have told us that being asked about their aspirations rather than goals made them think differently about their answer. In their mind, the word "goals" was reserved for treatment needs, while aspirations evoked more life-oriented ideas. Aspirations are highly valued by the individual—they connect to belief systems and reflect how they want to see themselves as a person and how they hope others will see them (Callard, 2018). Aspirations provide internal sources of motivation and are topics that help clinical staff better collaborate and connect with individuals and are central points around which positive action can be planned. Aspirations can serve as a guiding light that increases the sustainability of the adaptive mode and can be pursued over time. Discovering and building treatment around aspirations helps *develop* the adaptive mode—nurturing a sense of hope, which is a major component of wellness and recovery (Harding, 2019).

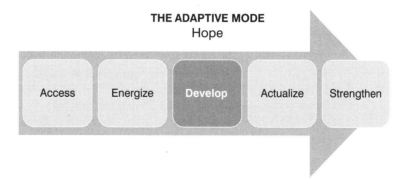

Many individuals with serious mental health conditions have given up on dreaming about the future. The aspiration-generating process rekindles their dreaming, expands their horizons, and uncovers their untapped potential. Sometimes the idea of reimagining a future, and especially sharing that vision, can make people feel vulnerable. Perhaps they have beliefs such as "I can't have dreams anymore because this is as good as it gets," "Others will judge me," or "The future is hopeless."

Accordingly, it is essential that you not move to aspirations until:

1. You have a well-established relationship with sufficient connection and trust.
2. The person is in the adaptive mode.

Both of these conditions are formed through activities that access and activate the adaptive mode (see Chapter 3). The adaptive mode provides a foundation for safety and enthusiasm in sharing ideas about the future.

When you discover a truly meaningful aspiration, the individual's adaptive mode becomes even more activated. Similar to accessing the adaptive mode, you will be able to see that you have hit on the right target by the person's behavior. Signs include increased:

- Energy in affect, speech, and body language when talking about the aspiration.
- Spontaneity and elaboration of speech regarding the aspiration.
- Off-the-cuff planning and problem solving for the aspiration.

> **Aspirations:**
> ✓ Expand on the concept of goals
> ✓ Extend the adaptive mode into the future, providing hope
> ✓ Are meaningful and give insight into a person's values
> ✓ Provide information about one's desired self-concept
> ✓ Provide internal motivation
> ✓ Enhance collaboration with providers
> ✓ Are the anchor points for treatment
> ✓ Provide the context and rationale for increased action and working on challenges

In short, aspirations are exciting and provide important information about a person's values and the greater purpose or mission they seek.

The progression you will follow when working with aspirations is illustrated in Figure 4.1.

You first identify what the person says they want. You then use techniques to enrich the vision for the future. Next you uncover the meaning and beliefs underlying the aspiration, and then you collaborate with the individual on action steps to achieve either the target itself or the meaning underneath it. We created a decision tree to help guide you through the process of developing powerful and effective aspirations (see Figures 4.2, 4.4, and 4.5).

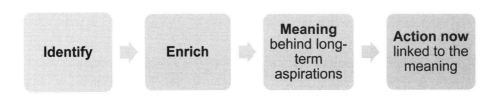

FIGURE 4.1. Developing the adaptive mode: aspirations process.

ELICITING ASPIRATIONS

When to Do It

Eliciting aspirations requires trust, energy, and mental flexibility. You want to access the person's adaptive mode (see Chapter 3) when you go for aspirations. The resulting interpersonal connection makes it easier and safer for the person to share personal strivings. An activated adaptive mode also increases the mental resources needed to project the mind into the future and consider new possibilities and questions.

Sometimes, the person comes out of the adaptive mode when answering future-oriented questions. They may respond without emotion. They might say, "I don't know. Nothing," or providing vague aspirations (e.g., "something better"). Others may have difficulty focusing on the future or feeling safe to share their dreams, because they feel demoralized or defeated by challenges (e.g., "I've lost everything and everyone I love!"; "I can't do anything because I hear voices"; "My therapist isn't actually interested in what I want"). Each of these responses reflect the "patient" mode and mean that you should shift your approach back to energizing and connection-driven interventions.

For example, you might try going for a walk or talking about something the individual enjoys doing to activate the adaptive mode and elicit aspirations. Importantly, these interventions can be returned to at any point throughout the process of developing aspirations to recharge and refocus.

What to Ask

To elicit aspirations, you begin with the question "If everything was how you'd like it to be, what would you be doing or getting?" Some other questions to elicit aspirations include:

- "Once you are discharged from here, what would you like to be doing or getting?"
- "Before all of this [i.e., challenges] started, what did you want to be doing or getting?"
- "What is something your family would want to be doing or getting?"
- "If I could snap my fingers so that nothing was bothering you and nobody was in your way, what would you be getting differently or doing differently?"
- "When you were little, what did you dream that you'd be able to do?"
- "If you weren't here right now, at [e.g., 1:00 P.M. on a Wednesday], what would you like to be doing?" [For the individual in inpatient treatment.]

Figure 4.2 is a decision tree to help guide you to eliciting the best aspirations that have the most possibility for living and sustaining a desired life.

DISTINGUISHING ASPIRATIONS FROM OTHER TARGETS

People often express exciting desires in response to the question "If everything was how you'd like it to be, what would you be doing or getting?" However, sometimes individuals may share

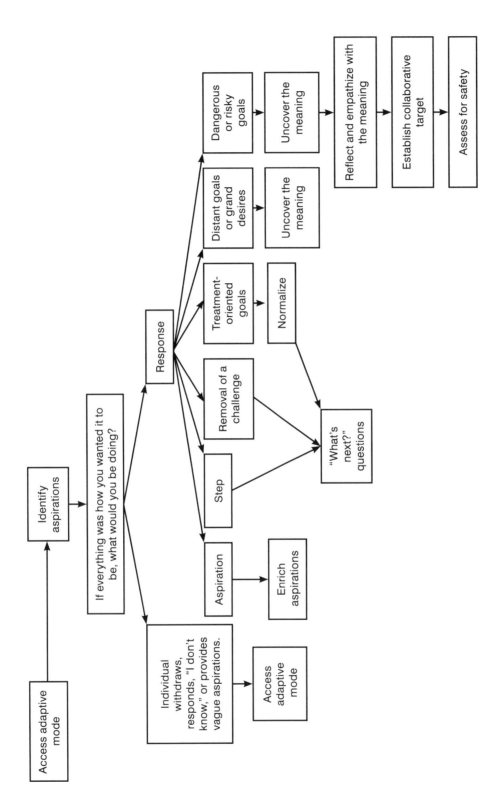

FIGURE 4.2. Identifying the best aspirations.

Developing the Adaptive Mode

ideas for the future that may sound like highly valued goals but are not quite aspirations. These may include:

- *A step.* Something that, once accomplished, does not provide a reason for ongoing pursuit (e.g., get a driver's license, get discharged from the hospital, housing).
- *Treatment-oriented goals.* Goals based solely on treatment-based activities or addressing challenges (e.g., attend therapy group, take medicine, shower daily).
- *Removal of a challenge.* Focusing what is *not* wanted rather than what *is* (e.g., stop hearing voices, stop cutting, sobriety).
- *Grand desires.* Goals that are rooted in what might be considered delusions or that are incredibly difficult for anyone to attain (e.g., wanting to be a professional athlete, return to their 20 mansions, bring people back from the dead).
- *Distant goals.* Aspirations that may take a long time to accomplish and involve many steps (e.g., be an entrepreneur or surgeon, own a home).
- *Potentially dangerous or risky goals.* Goals that may lead to harm of self or others (e.g., kill myself, continue or return to substance use).

You can collaborate with the individual to transform any of these responses into powerful aspirations that hold considerable value for them. Let's consider each.

Steps

Sometimes, an individual's expressed goal is really a step to an aspiration. Steps are not typically exciting enough to sustain motivation in the long run. Steps are goals that are discrete and help move toward an aspiration, but often lack great meaning and are not pursued any further when they are completed.

For example, getting discharged from a hospital or acquiring an apartment are great steps. They involve effort to achieve, and people want them very much, but by themselves, they do not lead to continued positive action. Steps can, however, lead to bigger aspirations, such as becoming a filmmaker who educates others or being a caregiver for an aging parent. Transforming steps into aspirations is important because when challenges arise (e.g., attending to cruel voices or reduced access to energy), a stronger source of motivation is needed to take action. Basically, the bigger and more value driven the aspiration, the better.

If an individual indicates they want a step, you can ask questions that extend beyond its completion, such as "That sounds great. What would be the best part about that? Once you achieve that, what would you be able to do or get?" For example:

> PROVIDER: What would be good about having an apartment? What would you be able to do when you have the apartment?
>
> INDIVIDUAL: I could get a dog and set up a space to do my art.
>
> PROVIDER: That sounds really nice! What would be the best part of that for you?
>
> INDIVIDUAL: I'd feel like I would be able to enjoy things again and maybe even teach my niece.

Asking "What's next?" types of questions puts steps into a broader context and helps uncover multiple points of energy and motivation. The process is similar to the downward arrow technique in traditional cognitive therapy (Beck, 2020; Beck et al., 1979), except that rather than a core belief, the process reveals core valued pursuits.

Treatment-Oriented Goals

When asked about aspirations, some individuals share goals that focus predominantly on the role of being a patient whose desires have a treatment focus (e.g., I want to take medications, attend more groups, go to a treatment program). This may reflect beliefs they have about themselves (e.g., "I'm broken," "This is all I'm able to do"), or a desire to say what they think you want to hear.

Treatment-oriented goals, like steps, are quite narrow. They also focus on patienthood and illness rather than the whole person and a desired life. Ultimately, it can be challenging to follow through on treatment-related goals when these are not linked up with something bigger.

When the person expresses wanting a treatment-oriented goal, acknowledge the value of the response, then ask what doing those activities would allow the individual to do—for example, "Taking your medicine and going to groups sounds good. What might you like to do while you're taking care of those things?" or "If you were to do those things, what would you be able to do or get?"

Here, you continue to elicit until you get a good aspiration. You might find that some people are especially anxious to give the *right* answer, that they cannot be shaken from these more rehearsed responses. If so, you can take the following approach:

PROVIDER: It sounds like going to group and taking your meds is really important to you—and to lots of people. I guess what I'm wondering is, besides ideas related to therapy or other treatment, what do you want to be doing or getting? What are some of your dreams for your life—maybe even things you haven't thought about in a while?

INDIVIDUAL: Really?

PROVIDER: Yeah, really!

INDIVIDUAL: My dad and I used to belong to a model railroading club and I always liked that. I'd like to find one in this area.

PROVIDER: That sounds cool! Can I help with getting to that? What kinds of trains?

In this example, the provider acknowledges and reassures the individual that their answer was good, but then encourages them to identify a richer aspiration, expressing genuine curiosity to learn more.

Removal of a Challenge

Similar to treatment-oriented goals, individuals might desire reduced challenges, such as not hearing voices anymore, staying sober, or not feeling so angry or afraid all the time. These may be significant challenges, or the person may be telling you what they think you want to hear.

There are a few points regarding why removal of a challenge will not function as an effective aspiration:

- It may not be possible to remove the challenge completely.
- Empowering relative to the challenge is a step rather than a life striving.
- Focusing so much on the challenge has the unintended effect of emphasizing the "patient" mode and beliefs of being defective.

Focusing on future potential (e.g., becoming a nurse who gives people hope) is likely to produce more motivation and activation of positive beliefs (e.g., capability, importance, connection).

To guide the response from challenge to aspiration, you can say, "That challenge sounds really important, and we should help with that. If it weren't in your way, what would you be able to do or get?" For example:

INDIVIDUAL: I want quiet from the voices.

PROVIDER: Absolutely, it sounds like they're very upsetting to you. I'm curious. If you were less bothered by hearing voices, what would you be able to do or get?

INDIVIDUAL: I could go to Friday prayers again with my community.

PROVIDER: That sounds so important. Can we work on that, too?

You start by empathizing with the distress of the challenge. But rather than focus on the momentary distress, you elicit what the empowerment would allow for in terms of bigger desires for life.

Some individuals are completely overwhelmed by challenges. They have spent so much time living with distress or identifying themselves as "ill" that their visions of the future are limited. The person might want a job, but at the same time thinks, "I am stupid, defective, or broken." The person may fear rejection for being different or expect that others can hear their voices. You could then ask about aspirations while developing a plan to get rid of the challenge—for example, "What if you felt you were able to focus more and you did not need to worry about the voices stressing you out? What job would you want then? What do you think about us working on that job and finding some tricks so those concerns don't limit you? Does that seem worth trying?"

Grand Desires

Sometimes individuals answer the call for aspirations with responses that are expansive or rooted in improbable beliefs (e.g., bringing people back from the dead), or difficult for anyone to attain (e.g., becoming a famous rapper or rock star). Grand aspirations are often expressions of more basic yearnings in an exaggerated form. The person may be expressing these desires to compensate for feeling controlled by and alienated from other people. Grand desires might also be a way for them to catch up in life or to make up for feeling diminished by others.

These desires can create a tension for you. The difficulty, if not outright impossibility, of achieving them is matched by the importance these desires have for the person. If you try to scale back ambition, then you risk demoralizing the person and harming your relationship. To let them go for it seems to set them up for failure.

> **BOX 4.1. Not Cutting Down Dreams**
>
> The individuals we work with have untapped potential. For a variety of reasons, they have not been able to realize what they are capable of. In CT-R, our aim is to help them tap into this wellspring of inner strength and possibility. We will be most effective in this mission if we meet them where they are. Our role is to collaborate with them to identify the meaning of the aspiration and focus on pursuits they can achieve now that also have that meaning. They might remain steadfast in their pursuit of an aspiration that is difficult to attain, or you might find that the aspiration shifts as the individual finds the underlying meaning through other means.

The way forward is to focus on the underlying meaning (e.g., being respected, listened to, and connected) that *would* be experienced in attaining the grand desire.

To get the meaning, you can ask, "What would be good about that? What would you be able to do or get if you accomplished that?" You can then focus on pursuits that meet this meaning or need in the here and now—for example, when Jackie's therapist asks her what would be good about bringing people back from the dead, Jackie says, "I can help them and other people will be happy." Jackie's therapist can then reflect on the meaning in here-and-now terms: "It sounds like helping others and making them feel happy is really important to you. Do I have that right?"

Being a helpful person or good person are important meanings she can always pursue—they are value driven and aspirational.

Distant Goals

Distant goals, such as owning a business, completing education, or becoming a homeowner are desires that often take considerable time and planning for anyone. The challenge here is the far-off quality, which can make it difficult to maintain enthusiasm, hope, and drive over time.

To help the person get the most from these desires, consider how replete they are with meaning. What would owning a business say about a person? What would be good about being a homeowner? For some, it might be about being accomplished or successful. For others, achieving these desires means they can better help others in their family or community—helping and connection being the valuable meanings.

You want to learn as much as possible about these meanings and collaborate to find ways of experiencing them now and in the future as the person takes steps toward their long-range aspirations.

Nothing succeeds like success to spark the motivation to pursue a more distant dream—for example, volunteering regularly at a food bank, individuals care for others, which enhances their resolve to continue prerequisite studies for nursing school to help people even more. In this way, individuals develop an appetite for success that helps to sustain their pursuit of distant goals.

Potentially Dangerous or Risky Goals

Individuals occasionally express aspirations that have the potential for harm and can be concerning (e.g., kill myself, kill my treatment team, cut myself, continue substance use, live on the street). When an individual suggests one of these desires, you have the opportunity to gain helpful information about the individual's needs.

What would they gain through the high-risk actions? What is the meaning? After finding the benefit, you can propose an alternate method to obtain those benefits that doesn't include the dangerous behavior—for example:

> PROVIDER: Do you mind me asking, what would be good about killing yourself? I want to make sure I'm understanding it from your perspective.
>
> INDIVIDUAL: I wouldn't hurt so much anymore.
>
> PROVIDER: Hurt? Hurt how?
>
> INDIVIDUAL: Focusing on how much I have lost and can't do. And I wouldn't mess up my mom's life anymore.
>
> PROVIDER: So, you wouldn't hurt anymore from not being able to get things done and you wouldn't see yourself messing up your mom's life anymore. Those seem painful. Do I have that right?
>
> INDIVIDUAL: Yes, very much.
>
> PROVIDER: Anything else that would be good about killing yourself?
>
> INDIVIDUAL: I wouldn't have to hear those messages from the TV anymore about my life being a failure.
>
> PROVIDER: I can understand wanting all of those things to end. What if we could accomplish your not being bothered by messages, not seeing yourself as messing up your mom's life, getting stuff done again, and maybe even not hurting so much without having to kill yourself? Would you like that, even if that sounds like an impossible idea?
>
> INDIVIDUAL: Yeah, I guess.
>
> PROVIDER: And, if you were able to not hurt like this anymore, what would you be able to do or get?

Validation of the individual's pain and distress is the first step. You follow this empathy by proposing amelioration by other means—instead of acting on the dangerous behavior. The pivot to aspirations comes when you have the person consider what is possible and what they would want if they were feeling better.

Table 4.1 is a quick guide to transforming stated goals into aspirations. The left side includes the types of responses you might get when asking about aspirations, whereas the right side can prompt you to recall the best strategy for each.

BOX 4.2. Dangerous Aspirations

Finding the meaning of the dangerous desire can be a useful opening to the safety assessment protocols in your setting. Doing so increases understanding of a person's experiences, which by itself can increase connection with the person and possibly reduce the risk of them acting on these desires. Also, being connected and understood can make it more likely the individual will participate in safety planning and assessments collaboratively with you.

TABLE 4.1. Transforming Goal Targets into Aspirations

Response	Strategy
Step	"What next?" questions
Removal of a challenge	"What next?" questions
Grand desires	Uncover the meaning
Distant goals	Uncover the meaning
Treatment-oriented goals	Normalization and "What next?" questions
Dangerous or risky goals	Uncover the meaning, reflect and empathize with meaning, establish collaborative target, and assess safety

ELICITING JACKIE'S ASPIRATIONS

For Jackie, the staff initially worked to develop her desires for the future by floating the idea of making jewelry again. Thinking about this possibility for the future excited Jackie and energized her adaptive mode. Having one concrete activity provided a starting point for Jackie's therapist to identify even more desires for the future. Importantly, her therapist also asked about the best part of delivering the jewelry to the nursing home residents. Jackie's response was powerful: helping and connecting to others.

The therapist said, "It sounds like helping people is really important to you. Is that something you'd like to do more of?" Jackie agreed that she wanted to help people, but that "it's most important that other people aren't lonely and that they feel cared about." This is a key meaning. How might Jackie help people to not be so lonely? Jackie said she'd like to spend more time volunteering at one of the nursing homes. The therapist added this to the Recovery Map, as shown in Figure 4.3.

You'll notice that even with confirmation of a future desire and meaning, the therapist and team kept their ideas and guesses on the Recovery Map. This is because Jackie may have other desires that they do not know. The team will want to try to understand more about her. Because they now know some of Jackie's aspirations, they have crossed off the item "Not known yet."

ASPIRATIONS	
Goals: • *Volunteering at a nursing home* • What might her belief about bringing people back from the dead mean? Is there something desired there? • Would she like to be involved in creative activities in the future—*Yes!* Guess: • *Help other people*	**Meaning of Accomplishing Identified Goal:** • Connection, helping—people won't be so lonely, they'll see someone cares • Guess: Power or importance? • Guess: Capability? • Helping? Guess: • *Value?*

FIGURE 4.3. Jackie's updated aspirations with new guesses and confirmed goals.

ENRICHING ASPIRATIONS

After an individual has shared a desire for the future, you want to enrich it. Enriching is the process of discovering the value the aspiration holds in a person's life and why it is so exciting or energizing for them. You enrich aspirations by:

1. Using imagery.
2. Eliciting feelings associated with possible achievement of the aspiration.

Figure 4.4 contains a decision tree to guide your enriching efforts.

Enriching Aspirations through Imagery

Aspirations can be enriched by creating vivid and elaborate *recovery images* that make it easy for the person to project themselves into the future. Mental images are advantageous

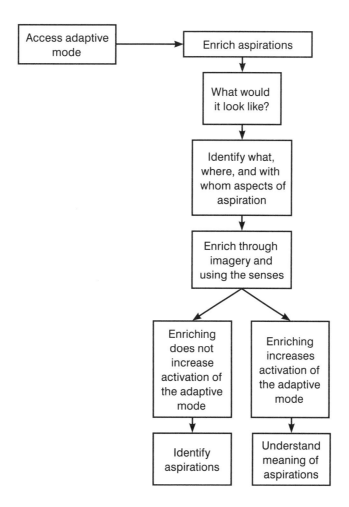

FIGURE 4.4. Enriching aspirations.

because they enhance access to emotion and aid memory (Hackmann, Bennett-Levy, & Holmes, 2011). Many individuals experience images that prompt unpleasant emotions and negative beliefs about themselves. Using imagery for aspirations turns this liability to advantage, making for a strength, as the image sparks positive emotions and a hopeful vision of their future.

In this step, you are aiming to answer the question "What would it be like?" The more vivid and specific the image, the more effective it is to create positive emotion and boost hope. It is also easier to call to mind. Someone could say they want their own place. Contrast this largely informational target with a recovery image: "I see myself in a brownstone. I am on my laptop, drinking a cup of tea and petting my dog. I am talking with friends online. We are about to play a game."

To create a recovery image with an individual, you can use the five senses (seeing, hearing, smelling, tasting, feeling), memories, social connections, plans, and other details to collaboratively envision what life might look like. For example, if the individual wants to have their own place, you can ask:

- "What would be the best about having your own place?"
- "Tell me more about it; what would your house look like?"
- "What food would you cook and what might it smell like?"
- "Who might you invite over?"
- If something stands out (e.g., a particular room in the house, a place to go with a romantic partner, a particular occasion for meeting with family), spend time focusing on it ("Tell me more about this room," "What kind of music will you play?").
- "Paint me a picture of what life might look like."

For an individual who wants a significant other, you might ask:

- "What would they be like?"
- "What would you do together?"
- "Where would you want to go? What would be your favorite thing about having a partner?"

In creating an image, place emphasis on developing the aspects that contain a social role for the individual—for example, getting a car is a fine aspiration, but getting a car so the individual can take their son to school every day is stronger; it has a *role* embedded in it and perhaps has the meaning of being a good father or relative. Imagining this role is exciting and taps into important personal values, making the aspiration seem more possible and linked to the person's best self.

The recovery images you create collaboratively can then be referred to throughout the course of your work together to ignite excitement and hope and to check whether these are still important areas of focus for the person.

Accessing the image can be very helpful. The person can call it to mind when they are feeling the tug of stress. It can help them stay the course when life becomes more challenging. It can also be useful to experience daily. To help individuals recall the image, you can be creative and collaborative. They can write it down, create vision boards with pictures or words, create a mutually agreed-upon word or phrase that reminds the person of the image (e.g., listening to Frank Sinatra or Tupac), among other possibilities

Enriching Aspirations by Identifying Positive Emotion

When you collaboratively build a rich recovery image, you will want to elicit how it would feel to experience the aspiration. You can ask, "What would it feel like to have your aspiration?" The more specific you can be, the better:

- "What will it feel like to have a girlfriend?"
- "What will it feel like to be cooking in the kitchen for your neighbors in your own place?"
- "How do you imagine you would feel to be driving to the concert with friends?"
- "How will you feel when you teach your daughter to hit a baseball?"

You might also notice that the person smiles, has a more relaxed posture, or gets excited as they share their image. You can ask questions to help the person notice this in the moment, too:

- "As we're talking about this, I noticed you smiling. Does just thinking about it make you feel happy? Excited?"

Drawing attention to this present emotion can further support the use of the recovery image in the future. For example:

- "If this feels good and energizing just sharing your image, would it be worth finding a way to remember and think about it on days when getting energy feels tougher?"

Eliciting the positive emotions serves several purposes. These feel good and can add to the momentum and motivation to strive. They are also good memory cues for the benefits of the aspiration. In addition, you can use the emotion as a starting point to consider other activities that would feel the same and might be worth pursuing.

DISCOVERING THE MEANING OF ASPIRATIONS

After you've identified the aspiration, built an image of what it would be like, and linked it to a feeling, ask questions that aim to discover its deeper *meaning*—beliefs about the self, others, and the future that are associated with the aspiration. Figure 4.5 contains a decision tree that guides you to find the meaning of each aspiration.

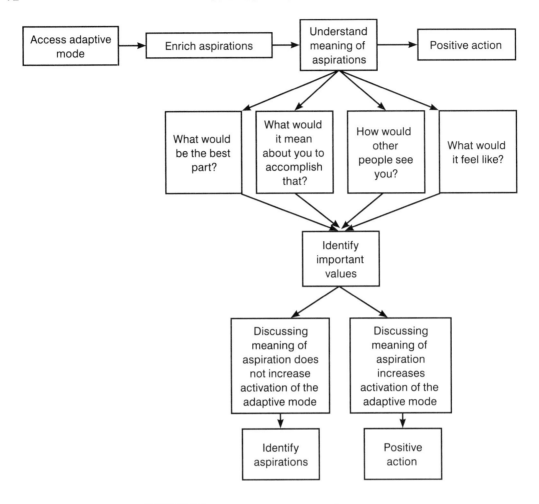

FIGURE 4.5. Finding the meaning of aspirations.

A key question is "What would be the best part?" You might also ask:

- "What's the most important part of doing that?"
- "How would you see yourself if you achieve that? Would you see yourself as capable? Worthy? Helpful?"
- "How might others see you?"
- "What would this say about you as a person?"

Meanings are incredibly important. They can be pursued regardless of the stated aspirations or restrictiveness or limitations of the setting (community, inpatient, forensic). There are infinite ways to be helpful, useful, a leader, and so on. The desire to meet any of those values is bigger than any one action.

This is why you do not need to worry about judging whether or not an aspiration is realistic for a person—because meanings, positive emotion, and the beliefs they bolster are very real and quite attainable every day. Figure 4.6 provides a summary of suggested questions.

Developing the Adaptive Mode

Identifying →	Enriching (imagery) →	Identify the meaning →	Difficult to attain/ delusion
Identify a meaningful vision about a way that an individual wants to live their life	What, where, and with whom; enrich through imagery and using the senses	Find the meaning underlying aspirations to identify values and target beliefs	We can still learn a lot when individuals share expansive or difficult aspirations
"If everything was the way you wanted it to be, what would you be doing?" "Before all of this started, what did you want to be doing?" "If I could snap my fingers so that nothing was bothering you, what would your day look like?" "I have noticed that [insert activity] is something you enjoy to do . . . is that something you would want to do more of in the future?"	"What will your day look like?" "Where do you see yourself doing that?" "Who will you be doing things with?" "How do you think it would feel to do that?" "Paint me a picture, I want to imagine it how you see it."	"What would be the best part?" "What would it mean about you to accomplish that?" "How would other people see you?" "What would it feel like?"	"What would be the best part about [aspiration]?" "It seems like [meaning] is important to you; am I getting that right? What is the most important part about it?" If we can work together to feel more [meaning/ belief], would it be worth trying?"

FIGURE 4.6. Suggested questions for aspirations.

ENRICHING AND MEANING WITH JACKIE

Jackie had identified an initial aspiration that she'd like to volunteer at a nursing home. Her therapist knew that helping and caring for others were two important values Jackie held, but she wanted to learn more about the specific meaning of volunteering.

The conversation evolved using imagery first, then feeling, then meaning.

Imagery

THERAPIST: Volunteering at the nursing home sounds awesome! What would that look like? What might you do?

JACKIE: Maybe I could just talk with them or play cards. They are just so lonely.

THERAPIST: So you'd talk or do different activities with them. Is that right? Sounds like things that would be very helpful to them.

JACKIE: I hope so.

THERAPIST: When you imagine doing that, what does it look like? What would you be doing? What would they do?

JACKIE: I'd bring my favorite games and they would smile. Maybe we'd talk about where they were from.

Feeling

THERAPIST: I notice you are smiling while you're telling me about this. What are you feeling right now?

JACKIE: Happy. I really want to help them.

THERAPIST: How do you imagine feeling if you volunteered?

JACKIE: Happy.

THERAPIST: Are there other times you have felt that feeling?

JACKIE: Helping my family.

Meaning

THERAPIST: What do you think would be the best part of volunteering?

JACKIE: Making people feel happy. I'd be a good friend.

THERAPIST: Sounds like having friends and being connected with people is also really important. What would it say about you if you made the nursing home residents happy?

JACKIE: I can do good. I'm friendly. I'd really be helping.

The therapist is now able to update the Recovery Map with the aspiration and the value it brings to Jackie, as shown in Figure 4.7. Both are important meaningful targets for Jackie.

The process of enriching aspirations is one that can take a while, often over several meetings with an individual. Give yourself enough time to build up the aspirations and learn about their meaning before moving to the next stage: action planning. With the right amount of detail and meaning, the aspiration can help activate the person's adaptive mode, which then leads to more action toward—and realization of—their desired life.

By pursuing aspirations, the individual begins to live the life of their choosing, a life that is like other people's and not defined by an illness or being a "patient." These aspirations actualize the fulfillment of yearnings, such as restoring dignity, becoming part of the community, making a difference, and being in control of one's own life. Abstract principles of wellness and recovery—hope, efficacy, independence, and connection—become realized in their everyday life and thinking (Harding, 2019). Aspirations provide the guide to action that realizes one's best self everyday (Condon, 2018).

ASPIRATIONS	
Goals: • Volunteering at a nursing home • Continuing to make jewelry • What might her belief about bringing people back from the dead mean? Is there something desired there? • Help other people	**Meaning of Accomplishing Identified Goal:** • *Connection, helping—people won't be so lonely, they'll see that someone cares* • *Feel happy* • *Being a good friend* • *"Doing good"*

FIGURE 4.7. Jackie's updated aspirations with confirmed meanings.

ADDITIONAL CONSIDERATIONS

Aspirations as a Way to Build Resiliency and Empowerment

Aspirations are specific to the individual and crystallize their vision of a meaningful life. They form the foundation of resiliency and empowerment, because the best aspirations are pursuits that an individual continues to want in life. Individuals find it worthwhile to regularly engage in actions in pursuit of the meaningful aspiration (e.g., talking with friends, waking up in the morning to practice mindfulness). The more the individual takes steps toward aspirations and experiences success, the more positive beliefs about the self, others, and the future are reinforced. Aspirations provide the *why* to continue doing what helps a person overcome challenges; they can also provide the reason to bounce back if and when challenges reappear.

Aspirations as a Link among Multidisciplinary Team Members

Aspirations can be collaborative targets that connect members of multidisciplinary teams to one another and to the individual. Every member of a team has the opportunity to learn not only what a person wants in life but also what meaning it holds. With this knowledge, team members can work together to determine which part of an aspiration can be targeted by which team member based on their respective roles—for example, a person who wants to help kids might work with their peer specialist to research community organizations that need volunteers or donations. At the same time, the individual might work with their psychiatrist on ways to shift attention away from voices so that they can focus better on helping. Collaboration with a housing specialist may now seem worthwhile because the individual wants to be closer to the community they would like to contribute to. When everyone is oriented around the aspiration, there is greater consistency and individuals may have greater buy-in to working with the team.

Aspirations in Highly Restrictive Settings

Aspirations are incredibly important, regardless of treatment setting. Even individuals who are incarcerated or who are not expected to return to life in the community can benefit from a meaningful reason to engage with others and in life. You can ask the same questions you'd ask in any setting about what a person would like their life to look like. The focus of the conversation should then lie largely on the underlying meaning—for example, you can acknowledge that while it may be difficult to achieve the aspiration as they ideally see it, there may be some ways for them to still feel like a productive, contributing, helpful, good person—or whatever the meaning might be.

Many providers have shared with us creative ways that individuals have achieved these meanings: jobs on their cell blocks, creating art to send home to loved ones, teaching exercises to other restricted individuals, studying and pursuing distance learning opportunities, participation in advocacy committees, and so on. There may be several steps required to access these opportunities in restrictive settings, such as achieving certain levels of privileges. In this case, you can work to visualize and create images as vividly as possible to build energy and desire to eventually engage in personally meaningful action. In this way, aspirations ignite and maintain hope.

Changing Aspirations

Some individuals change their aspirations through the course of treatment. This reflects a process anyone might experience as they evaluate what they want to do in their lives—for example, an individual may have an aspiration of getting a job. Across meetings, they might state different occupations (teacher, therapist, tech support, grocery store clerk, social worker) as their plan. You might find a common meaning underlying the aspiration (e.g., being helpful or useful) and make that a pursuit. You can also focus on the common pathways to accomplishing the aspirations, such as going back to school, increasing connections, or becoming active. By targeting the common factor in these different aspirations, you can combine them into a category (e.g., getting a career) and start the action steps to achievement. During the process, the individual will gain more information about these different areas and have a clearer sense of the paths they wish to pursue.

You might find that some individuals shift aspirational ideas to avoid failure. Some individuals protect against making even the smallest mistake (defeatist beliefs). In an attempt to avoid disappointments, the person might jump from aspiration to aspiration without investing much time or effort in any specific one. This avoidance ultimately has the unwitting effect of strengthening the belief of being a failure, because the individual constantly exerts effort but never succeeds. In these situations, you can enrich the aspiration to find the truly valuable meanings sought, work with the individual to have successful experiences that counter the defeatist beliefs, or use strategies that increase activity and energy, so the individual can reengage in the aspiration development process.

Multiple Aspirations

Individuals often have more than one desire—in fact, this is preferable. Considering that aspirations motivate change, multiple aspirations ensure continuous sources of motivation—for example, the individual may be trying to date, get a job, return to prayer, or get an apartment. If the dating life hits a "soft" patch, the job pursuit and apartment can make up for the lost momentum. This can lead to strengthened resiliency beliefs ("Well, dating might be tough, but at least my boss is happy and the apartment application is complete"). Diversifying aspirations is a good approach and should be encouraged.

When Aspirations Are Really Big

You might be concerned about giving individuals false hope about the future. However, our experience is quite the opposite: big dreams or desires that would take a while to achieve harbor great potential for catalyzing recovery. These aspirations help individuals tap into their desires, and the energy behind them can bring out talents and potential we might not have otherwise known about. Aspirations are long-term, ongoing pursuits. Developing an aspiration is not a contract with the individual to deliver the desire within the week. What is critical to maintaining motivation is the meaning of the activity—to be connected, capable, valuable, loved, and so on. Every activity, like starting to work out or date, moves toward deeper desires that have important meaning to the person (e.g., having a family). Meeting the desired meaning of aspirations on a regular basis in conjunction with breaking the aspirations into positive action steps allows individuals to maintain motivation and savor small and meaningful successes. This maintains and grows hope: every successful engagement in an activity is one step closer to the aspiration and these successes act as motivation for further action.

Chapter 5 focuses on action that achieves the meaning of aspirations to realize one's best self every day.

WORDS OF WISDOM

BOX 4.3. "CALL TO ARMS" TO CREATE DYNAMIC ASPIRATIONS

Far from being epiphenomena or just superficial froth, words such as "values" and "mission" are major motivators for action and can be tied to an individual's aspirations. As an example, in the typical "call to arms," a nation becomes mobilized to fulfill broad but personalized objectives, such as freedom, fraternity, and equality. When there is a common "enemy," the activation of collective spirit and values may override other values, such as personal safety. Patriotic songs such as *"La Marseillaise"* (French) or competitive games can also add "juice," as it were, to the general motivation. Thus, abstract words, while ill defined, can capture the team or group spirit.

In our work, the motivating force of "call to arms" can be found in aspirations. We want to elicit the positive meanings underlying the aspiration ("I am a good person," "I am competent," "I have confidence in myself," "I am friendly and other people regard me with respect"). These meanings tend to fall into categories: connection, control, competence, and compassion. The power of aspirations arises from activation of these meanings, which mobilize motivation, cognition, affect, attention, memory, and problem solving.

Not only do aspirations serve as an organizing principle for charting one's behavior but they can evoke and strengthen the adaptive mode, enhance hope, enrich connection, and develop one's best self. Here are the steps to dynamic aspiration building:

1. *Discover* the aspiration collaboratively.
2. *Detail* the meaning of the fulfilled aspiration. What is the best part? Connection, belonging, taking charge of one's life, making a difference, helping others, achieving?
3. *Imagine* the fulfillment of the aspiration in great detail. Ask questions so that you can see it the way they see it.
4. *Experience* the fulfillment as though it is happening right now.
5. *Focus* on the feelings associated with fulfillment: content, happy, excited, proud.
6. *Draw attention* to the personal attributes needed for the aspiration: likable, effective, strong, sociable.
7. *Act now!* Think of an activity right now that could have a similar meaning and emotion.

SUMMARY

- Aspirations are the driving force in recovery-oriented cognitive therapy. They are value driven and consist of what a person would like their life to look like; they provide a reason for working on challenges that may come up.
- The meaning of aspirations—the "best part"—provides an understanding of the positive beliefs individuals hope to hold about themselves, others, and their future.
- The meaning of an aspiration can be achieved no matter how difficult it may be to attain the stated aspiration itself, no matter how restrictive a setting.
- Developing aspirations should happen when the individual is in the adaptive mode. Aspirations should not be broken down into action steps until they are sufficiently enriched using imagery and meaning.

CHAPTER 5
Actualizing the Adaptive Mode
POSITIVE ACTION

Jackie and her team uncovered her aspiration of volunteering at the nursing home and the valuable meanings it would provide for her. They worked together to find opportunities for her to realize this desire. Jackie and her therapist created a vision board with pictures they found of games, people smiling together, jewelry, and music notes. The staff at her residence invited Jackie to help them organize weekly game nights in the house—meeting her desire to be helpful and build connection among people through an activity she really enjoyed. They continued the jewelry making as well, with Jackie in the role of material distributer.

One day when they delivered jewelry to one of the nursing homes, Jackie asked whether they needed any volunteers to keep people company during the week. She was invited to come by every Wednesday.

After you develop one or more aspirations and have identified their meaning, the focus turns to action. Positive action refers to activities that help people take steps toward their aspirations or that meet the underlying meanings. The steps of positive action include frequent review of the aspiration, breaking down the aspiration into steps, planning aspiration-focused action, and tracking progress and successes. This process *actualizes* the adaptive mode and brings about a sense of purpose, which is an important determinant of wellness and recovery (Harding, 2019).

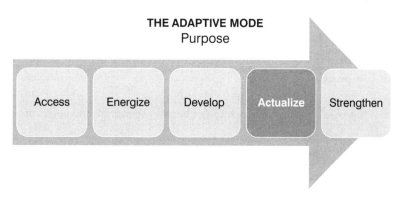

INCREASING POSITIVE ACTION TOWARD ASPIRATIONS

Reviewing Aspirations in Each Interaction

Aspirations can sometimes seem so far away that individuals don't believe they can ever reach them. Defeatist beliefs (Grant & Beck, 2009), such as "Why try? I'm just going to fail anyway" and "It is just too much effort" can sap motivation and energy and make action planning more challenging. So, the first step before taking positive action is to review the aspirations and meanings in every interaction with a person. This creates energy, generates hope, and develops momentum to pursue dreams.

> **Positive action:**
> - ✓ Turns aspirations and meanings into steps
> - ✓ Includes ways of meeting aspirations day-to-day
> - ✓ Provides meaningful markers of progress
> - ✓ Provides evidence of success that helps strengthen positive beliefs
> - ✓ Brings about purpose, which is important for wellness and recovery

You can say, "We're still working together to get you to that apartment with the art space, right? Remind me again what the best part of that will be!" or "I know we talked about possibly going back to school, working, and dating. Are those still most important to you? I remember you said feeling accomplished and in control of your life was a big part of that. Is that right?"

You can list the meanings of aspirations each time you are with someone and use this to activate the adaptive mode throughout action planning.

Breaking Aspirations into Steps

Once the individual's yearning is invigorated, you can link exciting long-term aspirations to current and specific positive actions. This can make even the earliest steps exciting: "You mean if I get up every day in the morning, I can get closer to becoming a world traveler? I can do that!" By breaking the aspiration into enough steps, the individual realizes the target is attainable. Seeing the pathway bolsters effort and resolve along the way.

You can be flexible when recording steps and progress toward a person's aspirations. Use a whiteboard, sheet of paper, or some visual aid that can allow both of you to draw out the recovery achievement path. One example of how to break an aspiration into steps makes use of the chart in Appendix F. You can print or draw the chart. The aspiration goes at the top of the steps on the right; the motivating meanings go on the left. This visual representation of the action plan can be a way to track progress, checking off a step as it's completed, even if repeatedly.

To identify the steps, start with a question such as "What do we have to do to get there? What would you need to do before becoming a nurse?" Talk over each step and where it goes in the pathway that leads to the long-term aspiration.

You can repeat the process as often as needed to develop a plan for action. The dialogue below illustrates this process:

> PROVIDER: What would you need to do to get back to school to become a successful entrepreneur?
>
> INDIVIDUAL: I have to get out of the hospital.
>
> PROVIDER: Okay. What else do you need to do to get back to school?

INDIVIDUAL: Well, I have to get a loan.

PROVIDER: Would you need to get the loan before or after you get out of the hospital?

INDIVIDUAL: After.

PROVIDER: Okay. What else would you need to do to get back to school?

INDIVIDUAL: I need to decide on my major.

PROVIDER: Where would that go? [*shows the individual the chart of the steps*] Do you need to decide that even before you get back to school?

INDIVIDUAL: No, I guess not.

PROVIDER: We could put that later. [*individual nods*] What else would you need to do?

INDIVIDUAL: I need to strengthen my brain, because I can't stay on things for long.

PROVIDER: Okay. When could you do that? Do you have to wait before you get out of the hospital?

INDIVIDUAL: It can wait until after.

PROVIDER: Ah, I'm curious. If you started working out your brain here, how strong will it be by the time you're ready to go back to school?

INDIVIDUAL: True. I guess that step goes before, huh?

PROVIDER: Yeah, I guess it does. So it sounds like we're starting to come up with an order.

You then help the individual organize the steps into a sequence. You can keep eliciting steps with the individual until the road map has enough steps to link up the present with attaining the aspiration. It's important to think broadly—no step is too small to include. Routine steps toward achieving the meaning can also be included. Below are a few examples:

Going to School to Be a Nurse Who Advocates for Others
1. Exercise in the morning for energy.
2. Study for the general equivalency diploma (GED).
3. Look up schools.
4. Figure out how to pay for it.
5. Look up classes.
   Daily: Find someone to help—ask others: "What can I help you do today?"

Have a Romantic Relationship
1. Join the community meeting to meet people on the unit.
2. Talk to people.
3. Think of where I'd want to go to meet people with my same interests.
4. Get discharged.
5. Go to places in the community where there are people.
   Daily: Imagine what I'd cook for my family one day as a good partner and caretaker.

Finally, you can collaborate with the individual to develop daily plans that will help when pursuing the aspiration:

- Setting and responding to an alarm to get up early helps in getting used to a work schedule.
- Planning out meals can reduce stress when in school or working.
- Practicing exercises to increase energy at the start of the day.
- Practicing mindfulness or prayer to unwind and relax at night.

Figure 5.1 shows an example of what this looked like for an individual who wanted to be involved in a meaningful relationship. For this person, getting out of bed in the morning was the most challenging step for a while, but it was helpful to see that every time he was able to take that step, it got him that much closer to the meaningful relationship he desired.

Note that it is not necessary to fill in all of the steps on the chart—rather, just enough to make the link seem plausible and to track progress. Also, as the person begins to succeed, more specific steps will become apparent.

This step-building activity can also be used in group therapy sessions—Chapter 14 illustrates how.

Positive Action Scheduling for Aspirations

Positive action scheduling (Beck, 2020; Beck et al., 1979), introduced in Chapter 3, can support the pursuit of aspirations. Together with the individual, plan activities that move them closer to achieving aspirations. These activities can vary from steps, such as reading more, going to a free lecture, or visiting family, to broader pursuits, such as volunteering, getting a job, or caring for an older adult. They can also include different ways of fulfilling important meanings, such as helping someone each day.

Positive action scheduling for aspirations takes the schedule beyond activities that energize, and adds motivating activities aligned with greater life fulfillment.

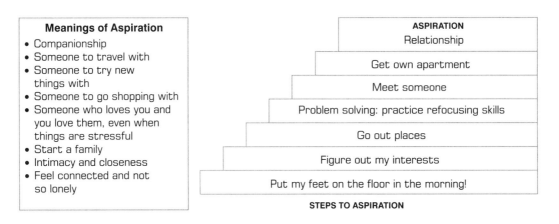

FIGURE 5.1. An example of breaking aspirations into steps.

If you are using Appendix E (or an equivalent), you can now enter the person's aspirations and associated meanings into the chart. Then, you can view together how the planned activity of each day links to the person's desired life. This is a concrete way to help them experience purpose daily, drawing their attention to what this says about their capability, connection with others, and ability to make a difference (see Chapter 6).

Gradually Build the Positive Action

The aim of positive action is *not* to ensure that every moment of someone's day is full or that they are active all the time. As exciting as aspirations are, and as ambitious as anyone might want to be in achieving them, positive action planning is most effective if it is slowly built up over time, ensuring success. The risk of overscheduling is that not accomplishing planned tasks can be disappointing and frustrating, triggering defeatist beliefs. However, as individuals successfully accomplish steps, they will likely identify times that could use a boost in action.

EVALUATING PROGRESS AND DRAWING CONCLUSIONS FROM POSITIVE ACTION

As individuals successfully complete positive actions, draw conclusions that help them notice progress, strengthening positive beliefs about self, others, and the future. To evaluate progress, you can use the schedule itself or create visual tools, such as the steps chart in Figure 5.1. Indicate what has been accomplished by filling in a progress bar, making check marks, or whatever method the individual prefers.

Each successful step can be acknowledged or celebrated. Individuals can hang a copy of the steps chart and their progress so they can see it every day. The aim is to see how they're moving toward the life they want, and that today's actions connect them to their desired life. For example:

> PROVIDER: You have been really busy this week. Look at all of those activities you have done! How does it feel to be out there that much?
>
> INDIVIDUAL: Really good!
>
> PROVIDER: You aren't tired with being that busy?
>
> INDIVIDUAL: No, I feel great!
>
> PROVIDER: Awesome! By going to the library, helping your brother with the yard work, and getting to church, do you have more or less energy than when you weren't doing these things?
>
> INDIVIDUAL: I have a lot more.
>
> PROVIDER: I wonder whether this gets you closer to or further from your aspiration of being a really great uncle.
>
> INDIVIDUAL: Much closer. I feel closer to my family right now and I know my niece and nephew like having me around more.

As individuals take positive action, draw their attention to positive beliefs. These may include:

- *Aspirations can be achieved with planning.* Aspirations are not unattainable or unrealistic; they just require consistent application of effort. When challenges are encountered, an opportunity arises to problem-solve and plan to triumph.
- *Meaningful action produces energy.* The individual does not need to conserve energy—rather, the more a person does—things they enjoy—the more energy they are likely to have. You can help the person notice that on the days they did more, especially when the activity was aspiration oriented, they had more energy than on the days they did less or a less meaningful activity.
- *Meaningful action and mood are connected.* The more exciting and meaningful the activities, the more of an impact they will have on energy and mood.
- *Every step I take gets me closer to my aspirations: I am capable, competent, and in control.* When individuals successfully plan and take action, what does it say about them and their ability to control their own lives? Drawing attention to this strengthens self-efficacy.

POSITIVE ACTION FOR JACKIE

Jackie, her therapist, and the staff at her residence worked together as a team to bring her dreams to reality. They also developed ways for her to fulfill the meanings associated with her aspirations. This was not just in attaining the desired goal of volunteering but also about maximizing opportunities to see herself as helpful, caring, connected, and happy. Her updated Recovery Map reflects this progress, as shown in Figure 5.2. Any guesses that turned out to not apply have been removed.

ADDITIONAL CONSIDERATIONS

Identifying Challenges along the Way

After meanings and action steps are developed, you can begin to consider what challenges might interfere with achieving aspirations. You can ask about the overall aspiration: "What is getting in the way of doing what you want?" or you can ask about the immediate action step: "What could make it tough to go to the library tomorrow?" Individuals may indicate low energy, beliefs about being incapable, becoming aggressive in certain situations, fears of hearing voices, and so on. Address challenges only to the extent that they impede action toward a person's aspirations. Interventions, such as stress management and refocusing techniques, may now seem worth trying because they are in the service of achieving a meaningful desire, and as such, they can be built into the action steps. Specific interventions for challenges are discussed in Part II, Chapters 7–11.

Recovery Map	
ACCESSING AND ENERGIZING THE ADAPTIVE MODE	
Interests/Ways to Engage: • Arts and crafts • Jewelry making • Music	**Beliefs Activated while in Adaptive Mode:** • Guess: I am capable or skilled • Guess: It's worth being around and spending time with others when we're doing things I enjoy
ASPIRATIONS	
Goals: • Volunteering at a nursing home • Continuing to make jewelry • What might her belief about bringing people back from the dead mean? Is there something desired there? • Help other people	**Meaning of Accomplishing Identified Goal:** • *Connection, helping—people won't be so lonely, they'll see that someone cares* • *Feel happy* • *Being a good friend* • *"Doing good"*
CHALLENGES	
Current Behaviors/Challenges: • Paying attention to voices to the point of reduced awareness of her environment (e.g., walking into the street) • Isolation • Difficulty with verbal communication (disorganization) • Delusions around bringing people back from the dead and generating body parts	**Beliefs Underlying Challenges:** • I have no control • What's the point of doing things with others, I will fail anyway • I can't enjoy the things I used to anymore • People don't like me • People can't understand me • The world is unsafe • I have nothing to offer, I'm incapable • I'm unimportant and have little value
POSITIVE ACTION AND EMPOWERMENT	

Current Strategies and Interventions:
1. Identify ways to activate the adaptive mode
  • Ask for advice about craft projects (successful intervention, keep using)
  • Ask for help setting up crafts or other activities
  • Ask Jackie and her family about things she used to enjoy
2. Continue methods identified that activate her adaptive mode and seek other interests (jewelry, music, ask for help, movie night)
3. Identify and enrich aspirations
  • Create recovery image
4. Opportunities for Jackie to be in a helpful role and a role that helps bring others together
  • Weekly game night lead
  • Jewelry making
  • Volunteering 1x/week
5. Strengthen positive beliefs
  • Draw conclusions after participation and success
	Belief/Aspiration/Meaning/Challenge Targeted:
	1a. Beliefs about capability
	  • I am capable and can be connected
	  • The more I do that I enjoy, the better I feel
	  • I can enjoy more than I thought and can still do the things I used to enjoy
	1b. Reduce isolation
	1c. Value and helpfulness
	2 and 3. Beliefs about the future
	  • Hope and purpose for the future
	4. Roles
	  • All of the above
	  • Hope and purpose for the future
	5. Positive beliefs
	  • Strengthen and develop beliefs about being helpful, connected, caring, liked by others, capable, valuable, safe, and successful

FIGURE 5.2. Jackie's updated full Recovery Map.

> **WORDS OF WISDOM**
>
> ### BOX 5.1. Keeping the Ball Rolling
>
> Establishing aspirations and a mission leads naturally to action. It is here that individuals' multiple defenses, inhibitions, and safety-making behaviors emerge (e.g., paranoid thinking, avoidance, hypervigilance). We can invigorate the person to sustain motivation in the face of various challenges. Total engagement in achieving aspirations is the way to do so. Meaningful action spurs the adaptive mode that activates positive characteristics and beliefs (e.g., self-confidence, trust, hope). This steadfast focus and mental investment in the positive traits, strengths, talents, and beliefs shifts the focus away from negative aspects (e.g., apathy, inhibition, suspiciousness, sense of failure, rejection) and tends to deactivate them.
>
> Examples of specific strategies to counter challenges are:
>
> - Insecurity → doing together
> - Paranoia/hypervigilance → doing together and group belonging
> - Rejection → group participation
> - Inhibition and avoidance → successful experiences with others
>
> Successful experiences and meaningful activities increase confidence in the self and enhance self-competence and control. Interpersonal relationships prime positive attitudes and beliefs. Team spirit and group spirit stimulate the desire for group belonging and a valuable social role.
>
> Activities translate into personally valued meanings of self-worth and being respected. The person progresses as participation in group or individual activities increases the positive components of their personality and diminishes the negative ones. Individuals respond terrifically to commonplace activities that line up with the meaning of their aspirations (e.g., decorating the unit, working in a garden, helping out in an animal shelter). The individual's specific interests, talents, and capabilities are often reawakened after being latent for extended periods of time. Each success consolidates the individual's positive attitudes and assets and weakens access to the negative.
>
> From time to time the individual may find a particular activity too challenging. You can be a consummate collaborator by drawing their attention to the positive emotion and aspirational meaning of the task. Call on the adaptive mode to access motivation and willpower. Individuals can best meet a challenge in the context of achieving their ultimate objectives and aspirations. As Mary Poppins says, "A spoonful of sugar helps the medicine go down!"

SUMMARY

- Aspirations and the value they hold for a person provide powerful internal sources of motivation. Aspirations help providers connect with the individual and can be the driving force for taking action.
- Aspirations and their meanings can be broken down into practical steps and acted on every day. This action can empower individuals to see their capabilities and feel more in control of their lives.
- Breaking aspirations and meanings into steps should only be done once the aspiration is sufficiently developed (see Chapter 4).
- As individuals have repeated success completing steps toward aspirations and their meaning, it is essential to draw their attention to what it means about them to have done so.
- Challenges are addressed only when they interfere with a person taking action toward their aspiration and its underlying meaning.

CHAPTER 6
Strengthening the Adaptive Mode

Jackie has been making and delivering jewelry to the nursing homes for over 2 months now and also volunteering at one facility for the past 2 weeks. She spends more time with her housemates, and visits with her family are lasting longer and longer. She still sometimes expresses a desire to bring people back to life but has had far fewer experiences of leaving the house in distress.

As a team, her therapist and the staff at the residence want to be sure Jackie notices her capabilities and successes, and sees herself as strong, competent, helpful, and worthy. They've tried to strengthen these beliefs and others throughout her treatment, even when times are more stressful.

One day, Jackie's therapist asks her, "You've been involved with the jewelry project for a while now. What does that say about you?" Jackie replies, "I'm making their day and making friends. I'm good." The therapist then asks, "On days that don't feel so good, or when there's not much going on, would it be worth thinking about how you're good—a good person who helps others?" Jackie smiles and says, "Sure."

Succeeding interpersonally, making a difference with other people, getting the life that you want—these are all opportunities to strengthen positive beliefs about oneself. Recovery-oriented cognitive therapy is an experiential process whereby individuals come to believe they are capable, lovable, can enjoy things, and can connect; other people appreciate them, want to know them, and are caring; and they can make a difference in the future. A key part of the CT-R approach is drawing attention to these positive beliefs to strengthen them.

Of course, as an individual begins to live the life they desire, they'll run into stressors and things that won't always go the way they want them to. When life is more difficult, challenges emerge, such as negative symptoms, hallucinations, delusions, aggression, and self-injury.

Resiliency is about discovering and developing a sense of empowerment with regard to these stressors and experiences. It is a human expression of strength. Resiliency is knowing that you can withstand these things and not have them get in the way. Developing resiliency beliefs is another essential part of CT-R.

Jackie experiences connection, enjoyment, and capability, but she may not immediately recognize these changes. Shifts in beliefs, such as from "I'm worthless" to "I'm helpful," or "It's

Strengthening the Adaptive Mode

not worth spending time with others" to "It can be fun to connect with people," can lead to more frequent vitalizing action. This, in turn, supports resilience even in the face of setbacks.

In this chapter, we focus on how to elicit beliefs activated during positive experiences and those that contribute to challenges. We also address how to strengthen positive beliefs and develop resiliency beliefs through guiding. These procedures are used in each stage of CT-R to help individuals draw meaningful conclusions about themselves, others, and the future. Strengthening the adaptive mode brings about resilience, an important aspect of wellness and recovery (Harding, 2019).

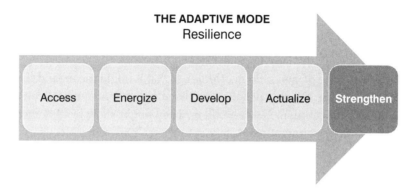

ELICITING BELIEFS

Drawing conclusions from experiences is a systematic process. The goal is to:

- Recognize strengths.
- Develop or enhance helpful beliefs (e.g., ones that help move someone toward their aspirations).
- Build resilience beliefs that are more accurate than the beliefs that fuel challenges.

First, we need to identify positive beliefs that can be strengthened. Beliefs that drive challenges are also important targets for change. You can capture these beliefs in the "Accessing and Energizing the Adaptive Mode" and "Challenges" sections of the Recovery Map (see Chapter 2).

When individuals are in the adaptive mode, positive beliefs become more accessible and can be strengthened. You can ask the person, "What is the best part of doing this activity? What does it say about you as you do it?"

> **BOX 6.1. Be Flexible**
>
> It can be challenging for individuals to describe the beliefs they have about themselves, others, or the future. Many interventions in this chapter can be performed with minimal need to talk, though some require more in-depth conversation. Be flexible in choosing an approach—meet each person where they are to maximize opportunity for true belief change.

You'll aim to weaken negative beliefs related to challenges, replacing them with more accurate resiliency beliefs. You might want to ask, "When this challenge comes up, what are some of the thoughts you have about yourself or other people?"

Keep in mind that answering such open questions requires a lot of energy and abstract thinking, which can be difficult for some people. If verbal questions like these don't help you gain new information, there are other approaches you can take. You might start with making guesses about beliefs and then move to sharpening their accuracy.

Methods that help identify these central beliefs include making observations, floating conclusions, and doing a chain analysis.

Noticing in the Moment

Start by observing what the person is doing, thinking what it might mean, and then helping the person notice that meaning. When a person is in the adaptive mode, what are they doing and saying? They may be interacting more with others. They might show bright emotions: smiling, laughing, talking more. They might say, "This is fun!" or "Do we have to stop already?" You might guess that the person feels happy, is experiencing enjoyment, or is feeling socially connected.

To elicit the positive beliefs of the adaptive mode, you can ask:

- "When you're doing that, what's the best part about it?"
- "What does it feel like?"
- "I noticed you were smiling and told John you were having fun. What does it mean that you're able to have fun with him?"

If the person has difficulty answering open-ended questions, you can get even more specific:

- "What's the best part about it? Is it the energy you get or sharing your knowledge with others?"

The same process can be applied when an individual is really struggling with a particular challenge—for example, they might be distressed and say, "Everyone leaves me; none of you people actually care about me!" or when invited to participate in an activity, they might say, "What's the point of joining you? I'm just going to mess it up anyway."

Noticing phrases such as these is valuable and informs your understanding of the person and gives a glimpse of what is likely getting in the way of pursuing aspirations.

To confirm that these are important beliefs, summarize back what you heard, and empathize with what that must be like—for instance, "I hear you saying no one cares. Have I got that right? I imagine that might make you feel lonely and disconnected. Is that your experience?"

Floating a Possible Belief

Next, try to determine whether your guess about their belief is correct. You can ask the individual directly. This approach has several advantages:

- It is collaborative and puts the individual in control of sharing and confirming their experiences.
- It helps individuals who struggle to put their thoughts into words.
- It reduces the amount of energy it takes to answer.
- It can help the individual see that they aren't strange for having certain thoughts, as others can understand and verbalize them.

Considering possible positive beliefs, you might say, "Wow—you've taught me so much. You must be a pretty good teacher. What do you think?"

Prompts you can use to float possible positive beliefs include:

- "Have you ever noticed that . . . [the more you do what you enjoy, the better it feels]?"
- "Sometimes I feel . . . [closer to people when we are doing something fun together]—have you ever thought that?"
- "Some people really see themselves as . . . [capable when they complete a step]. Is that your experience?"

In trying to understand a challenge, you might ask, "I wonder whether you think to yourself that the voices are telling the truth, so you have to listen to them?" "So is it that the voices are telling the truth, or that they are never going to stop talking and you have no control of what they say? Or is it something else?"

Prompts you can use to float possible beliefs about challenges include:

- "Have you ever felt like . . . [people just don't understand; the energy will never come; failing partway is the same as being a complete failure]?"
- "I know it's sometimes hard for me to get moving if I think to myself . . . [people don't really want to see me; it's too much effort]. How about you?"
- "Some people I know think . . . [there's no point if success isn't guaranteed; other people don't care and just judge them], and it keeps them from doing things they really enjoy. What do you think?"

Chain Analysis

There are times it can be helpful to identify a belief activated by a specific event. *Chain analysis* (Beck, Davis, & Freeman, 2014) is one procedure you can use to discover these beliefs. It can be used for both positive and negative events.

For positive events, this can be an opportunity to slow down the event and determine all of the good thoughts the person had during the process. You can draw the person's attention to make these beliefs stronger and more accessible.

As to negative events, this is your opportunity to determine what beliefs get activated that might inhibit action toward preferred activities or aspirations.

Before considering a chain analysis, you need to have built a good relationship with the person. At the time you attempt it, the person should have energy and cognitive resources for the conversation. You should use strategies for accessing the adaptive mode before using any extensively verbal or explorative approaches. Imagery is key to getting the right results. Get the person to imagine the scene and then see how they felt and what that means.

Example for a positive experience:

PROVIDER: When you help people you feel better, right?

INDIVIDUAL: I do.

PROVIDER: When did you last help people?

INDIVIDUAL: At the soup kitchen, Thursday.

PROVIDER: Help me see what you saw.

INDIVIDUAL: I poured soup for a lady.

PROVIDER: And what was on her face?

INDIVIDUAL: A smile.

PROVIDER: What did you feel?

INDIVIDUAL: Happy.

PROVIDER: What did it mean about you as a person?

INDIVIDUAL: I am a good person.

PROVIDER: How much do you believe that?

INDIVIDUAL: A whole lot.

Example for a negative event:

PROVIDER: So when you hear the voices, you get really upset. When was the last time it happened?

INDIVIDUAL: I was in my room last night and I heard it.

PROVIDER: So, you are in your room. What were you doing when you heard the voice?

INDIVIDUAL: I was on my bed and had been reading but stopped and started staring at the wall.

PROVIDER: So you are in bed, reading your book, and you stopped and stared at the wall. And that's when you heard the voice. What was it saying? How did you feel?

INDIVIDUAL: Yeah. It kept saying I was going to die. I got really scared.

PROVIDER: So, you are sitting in your bed and reading and start to zone out. As you are zoning out, you hear the voice say you're going to die and this, understandably, scares you. When you hear this, what do you tell yourself about what it said?

INDIVIDUAL: I better get my act together because they are coming. This is for real. Then I stay up all night waiting.

PROVIDER: So when you hear it, you think to yourself, "It is telling you the truth"?

INDIVIDUAL: Yeah! It's always telling the truth.

PROVIDER: That sounds really scary. When you tell yourself that it is telling you the truth, you keep yourself awake. Must be tiring to do that every night. I am so sorry for that.

In these examples, the provider walks through the situation with the individual to fill in the details as the person revisits the memory in the moment. Care can be given to make sure that the beliefs and feelings are accurate, and you can check with the individual. You can celebrate successes and empathize with stress. The beliefs elicited will help you collaboratively strengthen the person's best self.

For example, to strengthen Jackie's adaptive and positive beliefs around helping, the staff at the residence sought her out to help them lead game night. This same experience helps counter her beliefs that she's worthless, which they suspect contributes to her expansive beliefs of bringing people back from the dead.

GUIDING FOR POSITIVE AND RESILIENCE BELIEFS

As CT-R is highly experiential, you have ample opportunity to help individuals notice when things are going well, when they are going better than expected, and what it means that the actions *they* took made it so. These beliefs will be held more strongly and are more likely to be retained by the individual when the person discovers them for themselves (Beck, 1963; Beck et al., 1979). You can use questioning or reflecting on experiences with the individual to achieve this.

Table 6.1 contains examples of questions you can use to help people notice that they have more energy, capability, control, and connection than they may have otherwise thought. Next, we describe how you use these, and other questions, as you conduct CT-R.

TABLE 6.1. Strengthening the Adaptive Mode: Sample Guided Discovery Questions

Energy	Capability	Connection	Control
"Wow, I have more energy now than when we started. How about you?"	"Since you were able to do that, do you think it's possible you might be able to do it again? Or to do [different activity]?"	"Looks like by working together we were able to do a lot—it's pretty worthwhile to do things with others. What do you think?"	"What does it say about you that by doing this, you weren't bothered by voices?"
"Man, it seems like the more we were dancing, the more awake we felt, don't you think?"	"You were really able to accomplish a lot. You're pretty hardworking, aren't you?"	"That was fun, seems like you and [peer] are pretty connected. It's good to have a friend, don't you think?"	"Is it possible you've got more control than you thought?"
"Did you enjoy it? Would it be worth trying again?"	"Seems like working on this with your friends was a success. Should we all do it again?"	"If you are able to connect with [me/peer], is it possible to make friends at [other community place; e.g., church]?"	"It's so cool you were able to do that! Do you think it gets you closer to [insert aspiration here]?"
"Did this go better than you expected?"			

Accessing and Energizing the Adaptive Mode

Initial opportunities for drawing conclusions come from observing benefits during engagement in the activities that activate and energize the adaptive mode—for example, an individual who goes for a walk with a peer specialist might draw the conclusion she had more energy after the walk than she had at the start. Similarly, conclusions can be drawn during a group activity—for instance, in a residence with a garden:

> PROVIDER: Look at you! How many tomatoes did you pick today? How many did you eat with Sally?
>
> INDIVIDUAL: I lost count.
>
> PROVIDER: Sounds like it was fun.
>
> INDIVIDUAL: It was!
>
> PROVIDER: I know when we were about to start you said you thought no one would want to do this with you, but Sally did, didn't she?
>
> INDIVIDUAL: Yeah.
>
> PROVIDER: Did it go better than you expected?
>
> INDIVIDUAL: Actually, yeah.
>
> PROVIDER: That's great! So it sounds like gardening with someone else is really enjoyable and doing things alone would have been less fun?
>
> INDIVIDUAL: Yeah, it would have been.
>
> PROVIDER: So, if gardening with others is fun, I wonder if doing other things would be fun, too. Would it be worth trying?
>
> INDIVIDUAL: Sure.
>
> PROVIDER: Who could you do something with and when could you do it?

This conclusion represents a shift in perspective: it's fun and good to spend time with others, and others may be more interested in spending time with me than I previously thought. And this is something that can be noticed at other times.

Here are key guiding questions you can use during adaptive mode activities:

- "When were the times you felt better/worse?" Draws attention to the fact that the adaptive mode activity was better than not engaging in activity.
- "In what ways did you have more/less control (e.g., over voices, urges)?" Draws attention to the fact that a person feels in control when they do things they enjoy or are skilled at.
- "Did this go better or worse than expected?" Draws conclusions to shift expectations and help a person notice that they can, in fact, anticipate positive experiences.
- "You seem to have more energy than earlier; did you notice that?" Draws conclusions that by doing enjoyable or skillful activities individuals can create their own energy.

Questions that can be asked when energizing the adaptive mode include:

- "Would it be helpful to do more or less of this?" Draws conclusions that continued action is worthwhile because it feels good or leads to something valuable.
- "What does it mean about you that you accomplished all of this?" Draws conclusions about capability, strength, and competence.

Aspirations

Individuals can be guided to more empowering beliefs as they move toward their aspirations (e.g., ability to be successful, chance for success in the future, can make a difference). Learning from small successes prompts the person to go for pursuing larger aspirations. This is strengthened even further as individuals have repeated success and get progressively closer to realizing their dreams—for example:

- "Your son visited for the weekend? That sounds fun and tiring at the same time. Do you think he had fun?"
- "So if the two of you had that much fun, does that make you a good dad, or not?"
- "What does that mean about you? If you can be successful as a dad, can you be successful in other ways?"

The amount of progress observed toward the aspiration can be used to further strengthen beliefs:

PROVIDER: Do you remember our first meeting? You didn't think you would ever get out of the hospital.

INDIVIDUAL: Yeah.

PROVIDER: And what did you just do?

INDIVIDUAL: Enroll in college.

PROVIDER: What does that mean about you that you are enrolling in college?

INDIVIDUAL: I can do things.

PROVIDER: Was it easy?

INDIVIDUAL: No. It took a lot of work, and I took one thing at a time.

PROVIDER: So what does that mean about whether you can accomplish things in the future?

INDIVIDUAL: I can succeed. I just need some help from friends and to go slow and steady.

PROVIDER: That sounds about right to me. Can we start and see?

Positive Action and Resilience

Meaningful activity provides some of the best opportunities for turning the person outward toward pursuits they find enjoyable and purposeful. As the person engages in these activities, they may experience a corresponding reduction in distress. This shows that they don't have to wait for problems to dissipate before getting what they want in their life.

You can ask:

- "When you were [engaging in this activity], did you feel more or less stressed?"

You can compare this to other times that have been more difficult in the past:

- "How about when you were in bed all day—was that more or less stressful?"

You can then guide individuals to the conclusion that activities put them in control to reduce stress:

- "So it sounds like when you were doing the things you really enjoy, you felt good but also you weren't nearly as stressed—you heard fewer voices and didn't have the urge to hurt yourself. Do you agree?"
- "What does that say about you that you were able to do this and be less stressed?"
- "Do you have more or less control over stress than you might have thought?"

Your strategy can evolve from noticing empowerment to predicting it—for example, "If the voices stop bothering you when *we* talked about your grandmother's recipe, could you try talking to your *brother* about another recipe? If the voices stopped with us, then what do you think would happen with your brother?"

You can then evaluate the effectiveness together:

PROVIDER: So how much did you hear the voices while talking with your brother about family recipes?

INDIVIDUAL: Not at all.

PROVIDER: What was it like before he visited?

INDIVIDUAL: Oh, the voices kept telling me how he spits in my food.

PROVIDER: That sounds terrible. So what happened?

INDIVIDUAL: When we started talking, they stopped!

PROVIDER: That's awesome! Would you like that more often?

INDIVIDUAL: Yeah!

PROVIDER: What can you try more?

INDIVIDUAL: Talking to people?

PROVIDER: If you talked to your brother and they stopped, then who is in control of when they come and go?

INDIVIDUAL: I am. For sure.

This is the foundation for developing resilience beliefs. If individuals can have more control over some of the challenges they experience, they can persevere when things get tough. This is the definition of discovering inner empowerment and building it up.

We can ask questions that emphasize this even further:

- "What does it say about you that even though you still heard some voices, you were able to get all of your schoolwork done?"
- "I know she made you so angry that you wanted to hit her, but I wonder—would that get you closer to or further from getting out of the hospital and being an awesome aunt?"
- "What does that say about you that you didn't hit her? Who is the stronger person?"
- "What does that say about your ability to take control when you really care about something?"

REMEMBERING POSITIVE AND RESILIENCE BELIEFS

As individuals start considering new possibilities about themselves, it's good to plan for how and when they will bring the ideas to mind—for example, "Now that we have seen you can succeed if you keep trying, how might we remember this when you need it?" Some methods include teaching others, positive action scheduling, and creating empowerment cards.

Teaching Others to Strengthen Positive Beliefs

Teaching others has the benefit of strengthening positive beliefs about interpersonal capability (Koh, Lee, & Lim, 2018). And it is one of the best ways to connect with others—for example, if an individual learns something new (e.g., a dance move, a recipe, a knitting stitch, deep breathing, yoga, mindfulness), teaching it to others, such as a parent, friend, or housemate, would involve recalling and understanding:

- The rationale (e.g., fun, reduced stress).
- Times that doing it has been helpful (e.g., first thing in the morning, before a job interview).
- The best time for trying it (e.g., before the stressful event).
- The steps to doing it successfully.

The person's own actions moves them into the adaptive mode. They can notice having control, freedom, and strength. Also, as the person helps family members, friends, housemates, or acquaintances, they can recognize their own capability, feel appreciated, and know they are making the world a better place. Many conclusions can be drawn—for example, an individual teaches mindfulness to her father. As her dad describes a meeting where he grabbed a cup of coffee and focused on the heat, smell, and bitter taste, the individual realizes she is able to help her father to reduce stress. The provider can help draw those conclusions by saying, "So, you taught your dad about how to take a time-out from a running brain? And it helped? Wow, you must be a good teacher and helpful."

Positive Action Scheduling

Another way to solidify the modified belief is to add practice of it to the individual's positive action schedule (see Chapters 3 and 5). The individual can do this in two ways:

1. Identify activities in their daily schedule that activate the positive belief (e.g., "Time with my children, working, or attending Friday prayers lets me know I'm a good, loving person"). You can then check on the *strength* of these beliefs. Ask the person how much they believe it now—"I am a good and loving person" on a scale of 0–100% (or give a range of "a little" to "a lot") and compare that to previously.

2. Set a time to review the events of the day and determine whether they support the empowering belief—for example, an individual previously believed voices that said her boyfriend was going to kill her. Though she was successful (in school, apartment, dating, volunteering at a soup kitchen), she continued to have moments of worry and frustration about the voices. At one point she posed the question "Could I ever be like other people?" After reviewing the facts with her provider, she concluded that she could. They set up a time at the end of the day to review the facts of the day, asking whether this was like other people's days. Doing this repeatedly provided opportunities for her to recall and strengthen the conclusion that she was living life like anyone else. The more she did this, the more she believed it, and the more empowered she felt to pursue her dreams.

Empowerment Cards

An empowerment card is terrific for aiding memory of positive and resilience beliefs. This "card" can take many forms: index card, text messages, memes, videos, signs, jewelry, colorful posters—whatever way catches the individual's attention. The more engaging the empowering memory aid, the easier it will be to use. The purpose of the reminder is to create a tangible version of the conclusions drawn during or after positive experiences. Here are four ways you might use empowerment cards:

1. *Motivational.* These cards contain content that has strongly appealing ideas and emotions. These can include the aspirations, with steps to attainment. It can be an expression like "You got this!" It can be an image that helps the person feel at their best. You can create the information using pictures, videos, music, words, or any other materials.
2. *Action plans.* These cards set a specific activity or set of activities, helping the person remember what they wish to do. They can be elaborate, including steps to follow, reminders about the associated beliefs, and plans for pleasurable activity during the day—for example, a card might read:

> *The Plan Is to Get Back to Being a Great Dad*
> 1. Read the game plan during the day.
> 2. Listen to the music playlist first thing.
> 3. Remember: Once you get your heart moving, the body and mind follow.
> 4. Get a coffee after you finish the first half of the plan.

3. *Challenges.* The purpose of these cards is to remind the individual of what to do to activate their empowerment—for example, the individual might have a card that reads:

> *"The Voices Toolkit":*
> *The Plan Is to Refocus Away from the Voice to What Matters*
> 1. Talk to your neighbor about cooking.
> 2. Get your headphones on and rock out.
> 3. Describe the fruit you are about to eat.
> 4. It doesn't matter what they say. You don't need to listen.

4. *Accessibility.* As the individual strengthens and develops beliefs, you can collaboratively develop cards that record these conclusions and review them daily (e.g., "The more I do what I enjoy, the better I feel" vs. "I need to wait for the energy"; "My kids are worth getting going for" vs. "As long as people are stalking me, I can't do anything"). These are used like study cards that prime the person's positive and accurate outlook.

Empowerment cards can be adapted for individuals who have difficulty reading and writing, since plans and conclusions can be depicted in picture form. When creating plans for future action, develop them collaboratively with the person. This way, the person's preference is crafted into each card so they will want to use it. See Figure 6.1 for examples of empowerment cards.

ADDITIONAL CONSIDERATIONS

Turn Compliments into Questions

Use questions, such as the ones in this chapter, rather than simply complimenting individuals on successes or jobs well done—for example, many people dismiss compliments, saying, "Well, I guess it was okay this time, but that was just a fluke." The individual might also attribute the success to others. Posing compliments as questions (e.g., "Wow, you must be pretty clever to figure that out, don't you think?" or "What does that say about you that you solved that problem?")

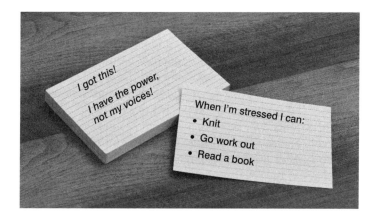

FIGURE 6.1. Sample empowerment cards.

provides the opportunity for the person to draw their own conclusions, which makes it stronger and helps them notice something they may have otherwise missed.

A tip to remember: Anytime you want to give someone a compliment, add a question at the end. Adding short questions to a compliment, such as "You are a really helpful person, don't you think?" or "You can do more than you realized, did you notice that?" can help you practice these guiding strategies.

When It Comes to Guided Discovery Questions, Meet People Where They Are

Big, open-ended questions may help some individuals draw meaningful conclusions from experience—however, sometimes you will need to adjust your approach to meet someone where

---

WORDS OF WISDOM

BOX 6.2. Responding to Stressors and Building Resilience

Individuals have been subjected to an unusual number of negative traumatic events. They also regularly encounter many minor stressors reflecting society's attitude toward them as being "maladjusted," "broken," and "not worthy." As a result of this stress onslaught, they develop an ugly picture of themselves as worthless, useless, ineffective, and helpless. Over time, these images become exaggerated and they tend to withdraw from purpose-bringing activities and community participation. The person may think "I am worthless" in response to frustrations on the job, "I am useless" to slurs from other people, "I am unlikable" to others' social rejection, "I am unsafe and vulnerable" from others' intimidation, and "I am helpless" when feeling controlled.

Focusing on the meanings that the individual attaches to major and minor stressors is the royal road to resilience. You may find the meaning by directly asking or by noticing that the person's voices say, "You are stupid . . . weak . . . useless . . . worthless." The individual's reaction to the negative meanings can take the form of regression and total passivity, avoidance and inactivity, increased suspiciousness, hostile reactions including getting into fights, or self-harm.

To empower the individual against such reactions, it is useful to conduct a chain analysis of the sequence. The chain can reframe the meaning of the event and change the individual's reaction to one that supports personal empowerment, resilience, and pursuit of aspirations. Once the sequence of self-derogatory meanings and problem-causing actions are detailed, then it may be feasible to conduct a role play in which the individual rehearses the original reaction and then subsequently, a different, more adaptive one.

Have handy common phrases, such as "When you're in a hole, stop digging"; "Don't make a mountain out of a molehill"; "You have to make mistakes in order to find the right path"; and "Sometimes the strongest person doesn't react."

As CT-R involves connection, success, and purpose, individuals' resilience increases over time. They develop a sense of safety, worthwhileness, efficacy, connection, and power, all of which work to further buttress resilience. When subjected to the minor traumas of everyday living, hurt to their self-esteem may be neutralized by a number of positive beliefs about themselves, allowing for a more rapid rebound from the slight. They are also less likely to misinterpret other people's attitudes and ambiguous situations. Instead they activate beliefs that help them to not overreact.

they are. This can include narrowing questions, providing choices, or other methods of giving the individual the best chance at strengthening or shifting beliefs. You can make the following adjustments:

- *Make the questions simpler or more concrete.* "When you have more energy does it feel better? Would you like more of that?"
- *Ask questions to get a better definition of an idea.* "So how would I know if a person couldn't get energy? What would it look like if they were energized?"
- *Clarify an idea.* "So to summarize, these are the ways I would know whether a person had no energy?"
- *Adjust the original question to guide in the desired direction.* "If you were able to generate your own energy when you wanted, would it make it easier to go out and be less worried about what people might think?"
- *Ask more direct or closed-ended questions.* "When you tell yourself that, does it make it easier or harder to go out? Is it possible that you have plenty of energy but just haven't used any of it?"
- *Summarize information already presented, with the purpose of refocusing.* "So to summarize [review information], what would happen if we tried the opposite? Would it make it easier to go out?"

Repetition, Repetition, Repetition

People typically do not strengthen or shift beliefs based on a single positive experience; most people do not typically endorse a different way of thinking after one guiding question. Often you will need to repeat questions many times and help people notice the same strengths and resiliency beliefs again and again over time. Beliefs that keep people stuck, such as defeatist beliefs, beliefs about inadequacy, self-stigma, and so on, have often been built up and strengthened over a considerable amount of time. It will be through repeated experiences and repeated guiding that individuals may discover and develop their own inner empowerment.

SUMMARY

- People do not often modify beliefs from positive experiences spontaneously.
- It's important to identify beliefs when the person is in the adaptive mode or when impeded toward valued action.
- Successful experiences provide in-the-moment opportunities to guide individuals to empowering beliefs about themselves, others, and the future.
- Success can be positive personal experiences or the handling of stress. Conclusions regarding both support individualized empowerment.
- Strengthening positive and resiliency beliefs requires repetition.
- Planning future positive action provides a multitude of experiences to strengthen beliefs and bolster empowerment.

PART II
EMPOWERMENT FOR COMMON CHALLENGES

This section takes you through the CT-R approach to challenges. Our process is represented here:

PROCESS FOR ADDRESSING EMERGING CHALLENGES

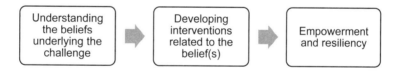

Challenges are addressed when they impede progress toward aspirations.

First, you develop a cognitive understanding of the beliefs that fuel the challenges. Then you develop interventions related to these underlying beliefs. You then strengthen resiliency beliefs, which empowers individuals relative to the challenges they face. In CT-R, you address challenges as they impact progress toward aspirations. In these chapters, we aim to balance the experience of many individuals, the formulation, and the approach to action and empowerment. We will do this for:

CHAPTER 7. Empowering When Negative Symptoms Are the Challenge 105
Reduced access to motivation, energy, and connection

CHAPTER 8. Empowering When Delusions Are the Challenge 116
Strongly held beliefs that may be difficult for others to understand

CHAPTER 9. Empowering When Hallucinations Are the Challenge 133
Perceptions that can consume attention and prevent action

CHAPTER 10. Empowering When Communication Is the Challenge 143
Speech that is limited in quantity or hard to follow

CHAPTER 11. Empowering When Trauma, Self-Injury, ... 155
Aggressive Behavior, or Substance Use Is the Challenge
Individuals' responses to trauma and their search for safety

CHAPTER 7
Empowering When Negative Symptoms Are the Challenge

> Maria spends most days in her room lying in bed with the lights out. She comes out for meals and medications. When in the hallway, Maria paces back-and-forth, frequently running her finger along the wall. She does not speak much, especially not spontaneously. She declines showers, and others are concerned that her hair has become a single clump. When people try to strike up a conversation with her, she tends to say, "No," and walks away. When invited to the treatment team meeting, she typically announces, "I'm fine," and either doesn't attend or immediately leaves the room.

Maria displays a set of challenges labeled "negative symptoms," which can be quite tricky for the individuals who experience them and for mental health professionals. The designation *negative* implies that these are symptoms that reflect the reduction or diminishment of what is assumed to have been previously present—a reduction in energy, affect, and so on. This is in contrast to *positive*, which implies the addition of an experience, such as voices (Crow, 1980). The accepted psychiatric terms for negative symptoms can be a little misleading because they imply a complete lack of motivation ("amotivation" or "avolition"), a lack of social desire ("asociality"), a lack of pleasure ("anhedonia"), a lack of speaking ("alogia"), or a lack of emotion ("flat affect") (American Psychiatric Association, 2013; Blanchard & Cohen, 2006; Galderisi, Mucci, Buchanan, & Arango, 2018). We know this strict lacking language isn't accurate because people can show all of these things in the right context. A more helpful way to think of negative symptoms is in terms of access rather than absence: having difficulty *accessing* motivation, difficulty *accessing* energy, difficulty socializing, or difficulty anticipating and participating in pleasure or joy.

This chapter helps you develop a successful strategy for empowerment for this vexing set of challenges (Patel et al., 2015). We begin with what it might feel like to experience negative symptoms. This leads into a discussion of associated underlying beliefs. We then suggest specific actions that access, develop, realize, and strengthen the person's best self.

WHAT NEGATIVE SYMPTOMS MIGHT FEEL LIKE

The challenges that fall under the umbrella of "negative symptoms" embody disconnection. You may no longer feel like being around other people like you used to. You might have difficulty finding energy to put up with others. You don't ever seem to feel comfortable socially. Nothing seems right. Your life may have been full of letdowns, leaving you to expect the worst. People might have called you lazy. They don't seem to understand how hard things can be for you, how different you feel from them. Again and again, people appear to have made promises and not followed through. They don't seem to care. And you have been so hurt by people repeatedly. How can you trust anybody? So, you stay to yourself. This feels safe. You say "No" to each opportunity. This can last for months, years, decades.

And yet, your desire for social connection is still there. While it is good to be safe, you still want to have a friend, to find a partner, and above all, to belong. But it is like there is a wall between you and others. The situation seems hopeless, you feel helpless, and the isolation seems endless.

In addition to this profound disconnection, negative symptoms can negate purpose. Every task seems impossibly challenging. It may be hard to muster energy for the most mundane actions. You may ask yourself, "How can I ever do the bigger things in life?" You feel so incompetent. So unlike others. Even the smallest thing not working out feels like a huge failure.

So you don't try, or if you get started, you give up quickly. You might be waiting to feel right again, get the energy, feel motivated. The molehills of your life have become mountains, and the only thing you can see. So you wait and do the minimum required of you. Life appears to be going on but you are not a part of it.

Ever since you were a kid you wanted to make the world a better place. This is still true. You want so much to be a part of something bigger than yourself. To make a difference. To help others. But you feel utterly incapable, not at all like others—sure to fail at absolutely everything. Though it wasn't always this way, you now feel defeated, helpless, broken.

Common beliefs underlying negative symptoms include:

✓ Difficulty accessing motivation or energy
  - Why bother?
  - Failing partway is the same as failing all the way
  - I have to wait to do things until I have the energy
  - The future is hopeless

✓ Difficulty socializing
  - Nobody likes me
  - No one will like me

✓ Difficulty anticipating pleasure or joy
  - I can't enjoy this
  - I won't enjoy this

✓ Limited speech or difficulty communicating
  - People won't understand me
  - People don't care what I have to say
  - People will judge me

As if sapping connection and purpose weren't bad enough, negative symptoms can also take the fun out of everything. Who thought pleasure would be hard to find or out of reach? Other people appear to be effortlessly having the time of their lives, but enjoyment seems so distant, so unlikely for you. So much work for so little—or no—payoff. So, you don't try for fun.

From the inside, everything seems so globally off. Life is dominated by your sense of inability, which is like gravitation, keeping you at rest. It seems impossible to get the energy, the access to motivation, to turn things around. How could you possibly do anything? Connection, purpose, and pleasure seem out of reach, perhaps forever.

HOW TO THINK ABOUT NEGATIVE SYMPTOMS

The person experiencing negative symptoms is caught in the gravitational pull of beliefs that promote inaction as a way to remain safe (Grant & Beck, 2009a, 2010). These beliefs limit access to motivation and energy; they make it hard to see social success or anticipate participating in pleasure or joy. The resulting isolation—for example, staying in bed most if not all of the day—promotes an inertia that can seem impossible to break.

However, the person still has desires and the ability to dream. And there are times, too, when the flattening is temporarily lifted, when things feel right, and the person is in the adaptive mode. It might be during karaoke, a sporting event, a birthday party, or a picnic. During these moments, things don't feel so hopeless, there is a sense of capability and possibility, however fleeting.

Out of this dichotomy—of safe isolation, on the one hand, and unrealized desire, on the other—we have our way forward. The individual's defeatism and difficulty mustering motivation are coming from powerful beliefs, which emerge from distrust, from a sense of inability, inevitable failure, and shame. However, we know the person is not incompetent, nor as incapable as their beliefs would suggest. They have talents and untapped potential, but there is little opportunity for that "best self" to be realized.

WHAT TO DO—EMPOWERMENT

Accessing the Adaptive Mode—Finding the Hook

With this understanding in mind, you have to locate this best self and help the person cultivate it. You need to access and energize the adaptive mode (see Chapter 3). You do this through asking about shared interests, or by having them help you, and consistently and predictably making opportunities available to experience energy, connection, motivation, and success.

Recovery-oriented cognitive therapy uses human connection to counter profound and debilitating disconnection. Yet, as important as positive social and success experiences are, they are not enough, in themselves, to potentiate and sustain the person's desired life. To counter the pull of the negative beliefs you need to draw individuals' attention to the fact that they are, in fact, energized, connected, and successful—a combination of accessing the adaptive mode and strengthening it. You do this during the experience itself, rather than just reflecting on it afterward. You want an individual to begin to notice positive emotion and experience it *in vivo*, when the experience of success or enjoyment is most immediate and accessible. With enough repetition of doing activities together and noticing the impact, the person will develop more access to energy and motivation. They will also begin to trust you, as you have done things with them, and helped them see how much better life can be.

Initially, you may not have a lot to go on in terms of what gets the person into the adaptive mode. It is important to be persistent and move by trial and error. The negative beliefs that underlie the person's disconnection are strong, but with a sufficiently appealing activity, you can access their adaptive mode. You will know when you have it right because of the change in their interaction with you.

When filling out Maria's Recovery Map (see Figure 7.1), the team does not know much yet for accessing the adaptive mode or aspirations. What they do know falls under challenges: negative symptoms and beliefs. The action plan in the fourth row of the map centers on trying to access and energize the adaptive mode.

A team member begins bringing in magazines and playing music. Maria initially rejects all of these efforts—turns the music off, doesn't want to look at the magazines, leaves them unopened meeting after meeting. During each time together, when Maria has had enough, she kicks the team member out or gets up and walks away.

The team member continues to come predictably, trying different types of music, different magazines, different topics. On one occasion, Maria responds to a dog on one of the magazine covers. The team member asks whether she likes dogs. The change is dramatic—Maria becomes very animated talking about her childhood dog. Dogs become the first hook and access point to her adaptive mode. Before leaving, the team member asks, "It seems like talking about dogs gets us both pretty energized, would you like to do this more?" Maria gives a quick nod before turning away.

This is an example of how brief, frequent, and predictable attempts at connection can be effective. Other strategies and interventions, such as offering choices—"Should we look at this magazine or that one?"—and staff activity scheduling (see Chapter 13) are good alternatives. The team member makes a quick observation to highlight the impact and checks on worthwhileness. Appendix G is a one-page summary of these steps.

Energizing the Adaptive Mode—More Hooks, More Often

Once you have the activity that accesses the adaptive mode—the hook—and have established it's worth doing again, you need to do at least two things. First, make this accessing activity a regular occurrence with the person. This helps to energize the person's adaptive mode and provides repeated occasions to strengthen positive beliefs about capability, energy, and success,

CHALLENGES	
Current Behaviors/Challenges: • Staying in bed; not coming out of room • Short answers; ending treatment early; saying "no" • Not showering	**Beliefs Underlying Challenges:** Guess: • Why bother? I am not capable. Waiting for others. Others don't care • I am not safe
POSITIVE ACTION AND EMPOWERMENT	
Current Strategies and Interventions: 1. Identify ways to activate the adaptive mode • Play music • Look at magazines 2. Make meetings predictable to energize adaptive mode 3. Connect outings to aspirations and to community • Go to coffee shop	**Beliefs/Aspirations/Meanings/Challenge Targeted:** 1. Activate adaptive mode • I am capable and can be connected • Reduce isolation 2. Beliefs about control and others • I have control • People care 3. Beliefs about the future • I can pursue goals—the future is hopeful • I can be part of the community

FIGURE 7.1. Maria's initial Recovery Map.

Negative Symptoms

as well as beliefs related to connection and trust. Second, make efforts to expand and find other interests and activities that you can do with the person to fire up the adaptive mode. This consistent broadening of activity builds the person's life space out, increasing the experience of positive emotion, enjoyment, and meaning. This is the basis of empowerment as the person moves decisively away from a limited state when negative symptoms have been their default mode.

> As the encounters continue, it becomes clear that Maria knows a lot about dogs and really cares for them. She begins to teach the team member. What are the different breeds (the ideal breed is a boxer)? How to care for them (grooming and feeding)? What to do when they are sick (go to the veterinarian)? Sessions grow longer, the energy of interaction increases; Maria is brighter, she elaborates more, she is connecting.
>
> During one of these meetings, the team member asks about coffee and learns that Maria's favorite is mocha. She subsequently brings mocha java to each encounter, which continue to occur predictably, and are kept short. Maria still ends sessions abruptly, but each meeting is a little longer than the one before.
>
> At this point, the team is able to fill out the top row of the Recovery Map, including possible beliefs to target in the midst of the appealing activity, as shown in Figure 7.2. The action plan changes to energizing the adaptive mode, drawing conclusions, and discovering and enriching aspirations (see Chapter 4).

Going for It—Dreams and Aspirations

As the person spends more time in the adaptive mode, you can begin to consider the question "What are their aspirations?" The time is right when the person has more available energy and mental resources to think about a future. The person should also trust you enough to share their dreams, which may have been dismissed by others in the past.

You need to pick an opening question. You may start by asking whether the person wants to do more of the activities that bring out their best self: "We have a lot of fun talking about your family recipes, are there other things like this you'd like to be doing?" Basketball, for example, could pull up an aspiration regarding coaching or important meanings of wanting to help young people. Cooking could lead to an aspiration of wanting to become a chef or to volunteer in a soup kitchen. It is also an option to simply pose a general question about what the person wants to do or get.

> The team member asks Maria, "If you weren't here, what would you be doing or getting?" She answers that she would be somewhere surrounded by mountains and trees while fly fishing.
>
> When asked what would be the best part, Maria says, "It would be fun to be some place beautiful in nature and exciting to catch a fat fish." When asked how she would see herself if she did that, she says, "Relaxed and skilled." When asked what might be getting in the way of doing it, she replies,

ACCESSING AND ENERGIZING THE ADAPTIVE MODE	
Interests/Ways to Engage: • Dogs • Mocha coffee	Beliefs Activated while in Adaptive Mode: • Guess: I have something to offer • Guess: Other people are interested in me

FIGURE 7.2. Adding ways of engaging to Maria's Recovery Map.

ASPIRATIONS	
Goals:	**Meaning of Accomplishing Identified Goal:**
• Go fly fishing in a scenic location • Learn Tae Kwon Do • Teach Tae Kwon Do	• Capability • Capability • Helping person; good person

FIGURE 7.3. Adding new aspirations to Maria's Recovery Map.

"I am stuck here and I used to want to do it and I don't know if I can." The team adds the aspirations, meanings, positive beliefs, and defeatist beliefs to Maria's Recovery Map (see Figure 7.3).

Sessions focus on dogs, fly fishing, and scenic places to vacation. Again, the team member learns from Maria, who is the expert. A new interest emerges at this point: martial arts. They begin to do activities together involving kicks and stretches and moves. Martial arts turn out to be an aspiration: Maria wants to learn Tae Kwon Do herself and teach it to others. When asked what the best part of learning Tae Kwon Do is, she says, "To be a master of something, to be an expert." The best part about teaching Tae Kwon Do is "helping others, making the world a better place." The team adds these to the Recovery Map, as shown in Figure 7.3.

Actively Actualizing the Adaptive Mode—Getting Purpose into Every Day

Aspirations provide a cornucopia of goodness for people who experience negative symptoms. The specific ideas the person develops are a source of hope for the future. They provide the opportunity to strengthen optimistic beliefs about getting and achieving the life one wants. Aspirations deeply involve individuals' sense of purpose and what brings their life meaning. This big picture empowers the person to keep going, sustaining motivation and action in the face of daily hassles and frustrations.

Aspirations can function like an organizing principle for the person's life. The meaning of the aspiration gives it propulsive power. You want to collaborate with the person to get that meaning into each day. Purpose is lived. It is a matter of planning action, doing it, drawing conclusions. Life grows outward.

Tae Kwon Do becomes a focus of daily action for Maria and the team. She watches videos and practices moves, ultimately setting regular times each day to do Tae Kwon Do. Others notice her doing the moves and ask to join. Initially, Maria says no. After repeated requests, she has a change of heart, allowing members of her team and other individuals to learn Tae Kwon Do from her. A team member draws Maria's attention to what it means about her that she is mastering martial arts ("I can do things if I put my mind to it") and teaching it to others ("I am helping people").

During this period, Maria begins going outside with others. She is seen kicking a soccer ball around, smiling broadly, laughing, clearly enjoying the experience, quite a contrast to the mode of her life previously, in which she did little, said little, stayed to herself, paced the hallways, and mostly stayed in bed.

Strengthening the Adaptive Mode—Building Resilience

Because of the strong pull of the negative beliefs, you need to help the person draw conclusions repeatedly regarding all of the benefits of being active, doing things with others, and the meaning of success (see Chapter 6). Empowerment is ultimately reflected in two kinds of beliefs:

1. Positive beliefs about the self and one's role in the world—"I can create my own energy," "I am a good person," "I am a helping person," "I can make a difference."
2. Resiliency beliefs about one's ability to handle daily hassles and stress—"Even if I don't feel like doing it, if I keep going, I feel better and can succeed"; "I might not succeed at first, but if I keep at it, I will."

Positive beliefs are usually already a part of the person's adaptive mode and become active and accessible when they are in that mode. However, resiliency beliefs tend to be new and can be developed in your work with the person. Both sets of beliefs strengthen the adaptive mode. Positive beliefs enhance the accessibility and durability of the adaptive mode, while resiliency helps the person shift back to the adaptive mode when the negative beliefs of the "patient" mode become active.

> Maria's team repeatedly and gently point out her emerging ability to learn difficult martial arts forms: "What does that say about you that you are learning so much Tae Kwon Do?" They help her draw conclusions about what this means for her future: "If you can do that here, what other things can you do?" They also collaboratively notice the impact of her successful teaching upon others: "Wow, you are learning so much and having fun. What does it say about you as a teacher?"
>
> The possibility of discharge emerges, but Maria is not interested. The team speculates that the idea of leaving might be overwhelming for her, stoking up beliefs about not being capable, not being likable, and not having control. The team then works with her to consolidate all of her progress:
>
> TEAM MEMBER: What are the things that make you feel the best?
> MARIA: Nice dogs, mocha coffee, Tae Kwon Do.
> TEAM MEMBER: How can you remember these things, even when you are not here?
> MARIA: Pictures, drawing, make a list.
>
> The team begins to include new staff from the community into the action planning with Maria. While initially declining to let them join, Maria warms when these people bring mocha coffee and want to talk with her about her interests: dogs, Tae Kwon Do, fly fishing, beautiful mountainous places to travel. They begin joining her class. Then a member of her new team floats the idea of going out to participate in Tae Kwon Do in the community. They make field trips to get coffee, go to pet stores, and join Tae Kwon Do classes. Eventually, Maria begins to say she wants to leave, and begins talking about her family. The new team updates her Recovery Map (see Figure 7.4). Ultimately, Maria decides to make the transition.

ADDITIONAL CONSIDERATIONS

Negative symptoms have been historically difficult for both individuals and providers. These experiences can cut people off from the most valuable features of life, and also contribute to disability and early mortality (De Hert et al., 2011; Saha, Chant, & McGrath, 2007). We have a powerful understanding and strategy for empowering people challenged with negative symptoms. Nonetheless, the experiences can be tough. The following points are a guide to maintaining optimism and effectiveness when collaborating with someone who experiences negative symptoms.

Recovery Map	
ACCESSING AND ENERGIZING THE ADAPTIVE MODE	
Interests/Ways to Engage: • Dogs • Mocha coffee	**Beliefs Activated while in Adaptive Mode:** • I have something to offer • Other people are interested in me
ASPIRATIONS	
Goals: • Go fly fishing in a scenic location • Learn Tae Kwon Do • Teach Tae Kwon Do	**Meaning of Accomplishing Identified Goal:** • Capability • Capability • Helping person; good person
CHALLENGES	
Current Behaviors/Challenges: • Staying in bed; not coming out of room • Short answers; ending treatment early; saying "no" • Not showering	**Beliefs Underlying Challenges:** • Why bother? I am not capable. Waiting for others. Others don't care • I am not safe
POSITIVE ACTION AND EMPOWERMENT	

Current Strategies and Interventions:
1. Identify ways to activate the adaptive mode
   • Play music
   • Look at magazines
2. Make meetings predictable to energize adaptive mode
3. Connect outings to aspirations and to community
   • Go to coffee shop
	Beliefs/Aspirations/Meanings/Challenge Targeted:
	1. Activate adaptive mode
	   • I am capable and can be connected
	   • Reduce isolation
	2. Beliefs about control and others
	   • I have control
	   • People care
	3. Beliefs about the future
	   • I can pursue goals—the future is hopeful
	   • I can be part of the community

FIGURE 7.4. Maria's completed Recovery Map.

Remain Cheerful and Persistent

The negative beliefs and biases that underlie the experience of negative symptoms can be difficult to break through. The person is defended against disappointment and failure. The individual may have been out of the flow of doing activities with others for a considerable amount of time. This means that it can be hit-and-miss when trying new things with them, and you might encounter a lot of refusals to try. Keep a cheerful optimism. Know that much of the reluctance is a matter of the person wishing to remain safe. The person may also be out of interpersonal practice. Know that what you are seeing is part of why the person has become stuck. As long as you don't become discouraged, you will prevail. It just takes one spark of success in accessing the adaptive mode to open up a way to a new desired life. They want this life, but do not know how to reach it. The key is inside of them. With a positive, warm, genuine approach, persistence and a little creativity, you will find it together. The result will be transformative.

The Less Your Work Feels Like Treatment, the Better

The negative beliefs linked to isolation and inactivity are quite accessible. The person is well practiced in this mode of living. They may have a long history of being given diagnoses and receiving services of various kinds. They might find the whole treatment thing quite disempowering. Encounters with health professionals can bring out all of the beliefs about personal incapability, the futility of trying, and the impossibility of true connection. For this reason, you will be best served by having your meetings not feel "therapeutic" in the traditional sense.

The person is likely not help seeking, but they may be thirsting to be help giving. Having fun with others is something they might relish. It is this deep yearning that you want to tap into—the experiences that have the most empowerment potential are the person helping you or others and having fun in a group. What could be better evidence that the individual is a good person than helping someone else? How better to see that they are capable and that doing things with others is better than doing things alone? It is in the repetition of these activities that the person's whole life and life view changes.

Many activities that work best could be gathered under therapies called recreational, occupational, life coaching, and self-improvement. But there is a key difference. We understand the beliefs that lead to disconnection, to difficulty accessing motivation and energy. Rather than waiting for energy, we do things that are enjoyable or meaningful, which will produce more access to energy and motivation. Rather than wait, we use tangible human connection to counter the pervasive discontents of disconnection.

No Intervention Is Too Small

What works can be fairly ordinary, especially at the start. A cup of coffee at each meeting might not seem like much, but as we saw for Maria, this is a powerful intervention. The mocha provides a predictable, shared, enjoyable experience. It is the foundation of an emerging connection. It shows that someone cares. It is something to look forward to. Having coffee is a natural time to talk, which allows exploration of Maria's interests, leading to longer encounters, her expertise with dogs and then martial arts emerging.

Feel comfortable starting small. It could be with food or drink, it could be a song, it could be a hobby. A joke could work, maybe current events or politics, a place in the city or world, or simply going for a walk. The list is endless.

Though we might start small, we do not stay small. Empowerment requires that we go big, especially when negative symptoms are the challenge. Aspirations are about the person's purpose, their mission. This is as big as it gets.

Don't Be Deterred If Progress Is Slow

Because we are working with very practiced, ingrained ways of being and thinking, it is to be expected that progress might be slow. It takes time to find the right hook to get started. Then as you begin building up activity, access to energy, and motivation, this also takes time. Caution can be hard to overcome, with the person slowly opening up more and more to taking risks and living more. Friends take time to find and develop, as do relationships. The most meaningful aspirations are long term. It might take some time to find and develop the right ones and more time to locate the right opportunities to propel forward.

Recognize these potential limits on how much change you see. Maintain your vigilance to notice even the slightest advance. What might seem small to others is actually huge from the inside. Being able to regularly share one's expertise about dogs is a giant leap from lying in bed all day.

Don't Be Surprised If Some People Just Take Off

Everyone is different. This surely holds for those who experience negative symptoms. While you need to be ready for slow progress, there are some people who respond quickly to the program of connection, aspiration, and action. They move quickly from inactivity to a rich and colorful life. Research suggests that people who are younger and have spent less time living with negative symptoms are more likely to show rapid change (Grant et al., 2017)—however, people with a lifetime in disconnection can also progress quickly (Grant et al., 2017; Savill, Banks, Khanom, & Priebe, 2015). They just need a little spark to reignite their interrupted life, and then there is no stopping them. The potential is within each person. We continue to be surprised by each person who realizes their best self and brings it into the world, whether this be rapid or slow.

WORDS OF WISDOM

BOX 7.1. Meanings, Motivation, and Affect

We have observed individuals completing a set of requested activities and still lack energy and animation. We have observed these same individuals become spirited by going for a walk, showing how to cook a dish, or demonstrating a dance step.

This difference in affect and access to motivation centers on the meaning of the activities. When the individual perceives the task as mechanical, something they are expected to do that could be judged, energy is hard to muster. When the task has a personal meaning, energy, positive affect, and motivation are much easier to come by. It is not "The more you do, the better you feel"—rather, it is "The more you do that you enjoy or is meaningful to you, the better you feel."

Pay attention to the expectations the individual has about potential activities. Do they believe "I won't have the energy for the activity," or "I won't enjoy it," or "People will reject me"? Because these beliefs are global and extreme, you have a near guarantee that the actual experience will counter this negative anticipation. Experiences of enjoyment or acceptance can translate into positive beliefs about the self, the outside world, and the future.

Research supports the idea that, through a repeated series of successful experiences, you can help the individual see themselves as more capable and acceptable, others as more supportive and accepting, and the future as promising and desirable (Grant et al., 2018). When the task seems formidable and challenging, you can be supportive and encouraging, which can greatly influence the meanings the person draws.

If the Person Retreats, Return to Accessing and Energizing the Adaptive Mode

Recovery is not linear; life is not linear. There are ups and downs. We have harder and easier periods. Because negative symptoms promote a sense of safety from hurt and hassle, we can reasonably expect these experiences to become more prominent when the person is having a rougher time. The person might feel that it is all too much. They might start to see that their progress is just too little, or they might feel they are setting themselves up for failure. For these and other reasons, they can begin to withdraw from others, from interests, and from pursuit of their aspirations.

Because our methods can reach people when they are the most disconnected, you can remain hopeful and meet the person where they are. Return to a focus on the activities that first accessed and then energized the adaptive mode. If upon discharge Maria began to remain in bed again, her new team could arrange to bring mochas and ask questions of her because they need help with their dogs, or they could watch fly-fishing videos online.

SUMMARY

- Negative symptoms can be understood as difficulty with access rather than a lack of energy or ability.
- Individuals who experience negative symptoms often have strong, negative beliefs about themselves, their capability, and the way others view them. These beliefs can prevent individuals from living the life they want by limiting their access to motivation and energy.
- The best ways to counteract negative symptoms are to access the adaptive mode through attempting to connect over shared interests or inviting the individual to help us learn. Once the adaptive mode is accessed and energized, aspirations are identified and become the powerful motivator to sustain and grow activity and interactions with others.
- Consistency and repetition are key in working with an individual to tackle negative symptoms due to the stronghold of negative beliefs.
- While individuals are in their adaptive mode and making meaningful steps toward accomplishing their aspirations, you can help them to draw conclusions about themselves and others, which directly counter the beliefs that feed negative symptoms.
- Empowerment is realized through an expanding life space of connecting and purposeful activity accompanied by positive and resiliency beliefs.

CHAPTER 8
Empowering When Delusions Are the Challenge

Jonathan is a middle-aged man, living by himself in a major city. He is inactive most of his days, going out little. Yet, he is pleasant and welcoming to those who visit, mostly members of his case management team. Often the team finds sitcoms from the 1960s playing on his television. Jonathan lets all visitors know he is God, a kind one who gives away his food and possessions to help others meet their needs, even if this leaves him without these things. When they ask whether he needs anything, Jonathan says, "No, don't worry, I am God. I don't need to eat because I am God." His team reports that all conversations return to his being God, which makes doing any clinical work or case management challenging. Jonathan does take medications delivered by his team. When the team asks what else he might want for his life, he says, "I'm fine—because God serves others."

Delusions are hotly contested beliefs. To loved ones, service providers, and most (if not all) others, the beliefs seem hopelessly (and sometimes frustratingly) false. To those who hold them, however, the beliefs aren't beliefs at all but truths, important truths, neglected truths, world-defining truths. Nobody likes to be called delusional. So this divide easily leads to conflict, entrenchment, or impasse. The person who holds the beliefs is disconnected from others precisely by these beliefs that are so personally important, becoming isolated and ostracized as one who is not of sound mind. How do you collaborate on a person's desired life given all of this?

In this chapter, we describe an approach to these beliefs and experiences that skirts conflict and ultimately gives everyone—individual, loved one, service provider—a good chance at getting what they want. We first consider what it feels like on the inside. We will see that these beliefs give us a powerful understanding of what the person values and wants in their life. Empowerment will come through getting that meaning into everyday life and drawing conclusions to build resilience as we go.

There is a long history in the psychiatric literature of typing the beliefs labeled as delusions. We focus on two rough categories: beliefs that compensate for an underlying sense of inadequacy (often termed "grandiose") and beliefs that reflect an underlying sense of vulnerability, threat, and concern for the safety of self or others (often termed "paranoid"; Kiran &

Chaudhury, 2009). Our understanding and strategy will differ depending on which type of belief we are working with. In each case, we consider the need being expressed—for control, a sense of value, connection, purpose, safety—and alternative ways to meet this need.

GRANDIOSE BELIEFS AND THE EXPANSIVE MODE

What It Might Feel Llike

You are in the hospital when you first realize it. Things don't seem right. They say you were kicked off the football team, kicked out of school, disowned by your family. They say you have an illness and must take pills. But this can't be right.

Everybody loves you. You have always known you were special. But wow. How special! And how strong. You are Bruce Lee, damnit! Mightiest man in the world. Best fighter. Savior to the weak.

Your doctor says that Bruce Lee is dead. But this only makes you want to show her how tough you are. You smile as you flex your muscles in the hallway and do kung fu moves. Everybody loves you. You are the best ever. It feels so good to be you.

> Common beliefs underlying grandiose delusions include:
>
> *About the Self*
> ✓ I am incapable.
> ✓ I am inadequate or inferior.
> ✓ I am defective.
> ✓ I am worthless.
> ✓ I am stupid.
>
> *About Others*
> ✓ People don't like me or don't care.
> ✓ People disrespect and reject me.
>
> *About the Future*
> ✓ The future is hopeless.
> ✓ I will never contribute anything of value.

How to Think about Grandiose Beliefs

Given the importance of the beliefs in the person's life and the ever-present potential for unhelpful conflict, you need to tread lightly. Keep in mind that you should focus only on these beliefs when they are getting in the way of the life the individual wants—for example, when they interfere with forming relationships, spending time with others, and pursuing life ambitions. Sometimes these beliefs might get people mixed up with systems (e.g., criminal justice) that can cause further isolation and withdrawal from society.

With grandiose beliefs, the person's life is pervaded by a sense of lacking (Beck et al., 2019; Knowles, McCarthy-Jones, & Rowse, 2011). Things are not as they should be—the person has not accomplished what they feel they should and others do not seem to appreciate and value them. Beneath grandiose ideas may be beliefs such as "I am worthless," "I am insignificant," or "I am broken"; "Others do not respect me," "Others do not care about me," or "I am unlovable"; and "I'll never amount to anything," "I am never going to do anything meaningful," or "I will always be a useless piece of crap."

These negative beliefs about self, others, and the future give rise to unpleasant and uncomfortable emotions. The grandiose belief compensates for this personal and social sense of utter deficiency. Awful feelings and ideas are replaced with great feelings and ideas and the person enters a more expansive mode. As the saying goes, "It is good to be the king." The scope and size of the belief may help you understand just how bad the person feels when the underlying beliefs get fired up—owning the state, being God or being a supreme world leader. How bad must you feel if you need to be God to feel good?

Understanding a person's grandiose beliefs can also give you a good sense for what the person values and wants in their life. You can start by asking yourself, "What would be good about holding the belief? What is the best part about being God or royalty?" In the case of being divine, you would be supremely important, others turn to you for help, they listen to you, you know everything, and you have created the world. As a royal you are at the top of the social ladder, people listen to what you have to say, they respect you, look up to you, and you can make things happen. A sense of social importance and accomplishment comes through in both cases. It's not necessarily so that all of these values are important to the person, though it's likely one or more will be. And it is easy to guess that underneath, the person is feeling pretty insignificant, incapable, and alone.

You can conduct this type of thought exercise for any grandiose or improbable idea: being a famous person or loved by one, owner of a sports team or a business, inventor of an important discovery, or writer of an influential book or song. This way of thinking helps you get started. You will have useful guesses as to the type of experience that you want to have with the person—what their values are, what positive beliefs could be activated, and which negative beliefs are contributing to the delusion being expressed.

As you progress with the person and develop your relationship, you may be able to pose the question "What is the best part about _____?" directly and sharpen your understanding of the meaning.

Jonathan's team starts to understand his expansive mode by asking themselves, "What might be the best part about being God?" Members of the team have several ideas:

- That everybody likes God.
- They listen to God.
- They respect God.
- God does good things for everyone.

Being God could be an effort-free way to connect with others that is guaranteed to succeed every time, since God is supremely appealing and never fails. Giving away food and being nice would also fit in with the idea that Jonathan wants to be a good and helpful person who is appreciated by others. It seems reasonable to suppose that underneath it all Jonathan feels incompetent and worthless, his life imbued with an unbearable loneliness.

Indeed, for Jonathan, loneliness is next to godliness. The more alone he feels, the stronger he needs to be God. The more inferior he feels, the more he needs to tell people that he is God and give

CHALLENGES	
Current Behaviors/Challenges:	**Beliefs Underlying Challenges:**
• Referring to self as God • Isolation • Inactivity • Giving away belongings • Not eating	• I am alone • Others leave me • If you are really nice, people won't leave you • I can't do things until I have the energy for them • I am in danger, so I should stay inside

FIGURE 8.1. Jonathan's initial Recovery Map.

them gifts. The team conjectures that they unwittingly fire up Jonathan's expansive mode when they visit. He would see them as coming to see God, he would give them gifts, and would declare that he does not need any help. What the team needs is a way to access his adaptive mode that doesn't also activate his vulnerabilities around inferiority and incapability. Jonathan's challenges and associated beliefs are captured in Figure 8.1.

What to Do—Empowerment

Accessing the Adaptive Mode

Once you understand the meaning of these strongly held beliefs, you can begin accessing the adaptive mode, as this will give you a better sense of what the person cares about. Each time you do activities together, positive beliefs about the self and others are activated. You can draw attention to these. Activities that involve roles that show the person's interpersonal value is the place to start, as these are less likely to activate the expansive mode. Leading a walking club or explaining how to cook a recipe or choosing music for the group—all of these activities show that the person is able to contribute. Beliefs that may arise that you can strengthen include "I am capable," "I can make meaningful contributions to others," and "Others are interested in what I have to say."

> A member of the team meets with Jonathan to try a new tack. Hoping to access the adaptive mode, she asks him about his interests. Jonathan replies in a manner that is hard to follow. He seems to be saying that God is interested in all of his creations. Since speaking is challenging at the moment and might be causing Jonathan to feel vulnerable, the team member tries playing music. This is successful. It turns out that Jonathan loves listening to music with another person. They sing together and then dance, too. Jonathan's energy rises all the while, and he repeatedly smiles broadly. He becomes more talkative, sharing knowledge of the song, the singer, and when the recording was released. Noticeably, during all this shared shouting and grooving, Jonathan does not talk about being God even one time. The team can build on this encounter, as it shows that a mutually enjoyable social activity does not activate the vulnerabilities that fire up his expansive mode, and instead effectively brings about the adaptive mode.

Energizing the Adaptive Mode

You will want to establish predictable activities. These can start with you, but it is best if they include others so that the person has repeated opportunities to see themselves as capable and participating in a meaningful way. The predictability also helps the person feel in control and counters negative expectations that other people do not care. You can support individuals in drawing these useful conclusions about themselves and others in the moment when the experience is peaking. Draw attention to how good it feels and the clear contribution the person is making. If the activity helped you, you can share this with them: "You've really taught us this well. You're pretty helpful, wouldn't you say?" Then you can ask what it means about them that they helped you and other people: "Would you like to do this more? Are there other kinds of contributing that you would want to do?"

All of this repetition energizes the adaptive mode and helps the person experience genuine importance. As they feel important, connected, in control, competent, and energized, they are less likely to go into the expansive mode, because there's no need to compensate for the real thing. Ultimately, you will develop enough connection and trust that you can project aspirations and move your work together to the next level.

> After the initial success with Jonathan, the team shifts focus to repeatedly and predictably connecting with him to energize his adaptive mode. During the next encounter, he and the team member listen to music, dance, and take a walk. On the walk, they run into some of Jonathan's neighbors. The team member comments, "It's great to meet your neighbors, do you like seeing them? Do you ever talk to them at other times? Would it be fun to talk with them during the week?" Jonathan laughs and agrees.
>
> Over the course of the next few weeks, the team member gradually increases activity with Jonathan. Each meeting starts with listening to music and dancing together, then graduates to walks around the park near his apartment complex. Soon, they add strolls to get coffee together, and ultimately getting coffee and meeting up with people in the neighborhood. All the while drawing conclusions about the value of doing activities to gain energy, feel better, and connect with others. (See Figure 8.2.)
>
> As Jonathan's energy goes up, he talks about being God less often. The team is pretty confident that connection and relationships are important to him.

Aspirations and Meaning

When grandiose beliefs and the expansive mode compose the challenge, aspirations are the key to helping the person get more of the life they desire. This is because the value of what the person wants is found in the best part of being God, royalty, a famous singer, very wealthy, and so on. Successful aspirations tap into this same meaning.

To this point you have been building up activity to enable the person to experience being important, to contribute successfully, and to trust you and others. Now, you can trade on the trust and newfound energy to help the person dream. This is a dream of the person's best self. The aspirations provide targets for daily action that bring this most cherished meaning into daily life. Most likely this will be something having to do with making a difference in the world.

> While walking, the team member asks about Jonathan's neighbors. He talks about liking them and agrees that doing activities with them is better than by himself. The team member brings up the possibility of helping the neighbors—helping to take out their trash, perhaps, or walking their dogs. Jonathan is very enthusiastic. He can imagine how good this would feel. The best part is making a difference, doing good. He agrees to bring this up on trash day.
>
> At the next visit, Jonathan is quite excited. He shares how he helped two of his neighbors take their trash out. The team member has him describe in vivid detail how it felt and what everyone said. Jonathan draws the conclusion that he is a helping person, a good person. He explains that one of

ACCESSING AND ENERGIZING THE ADAPTIVE MODE	
Interests/Ways to Engage: • Music (listening, singing, and dancing) • Walks • Talking about friends and helping friends • Getting coffee	**Beliefs Activated while in Adaptive Mode:** • I am connected to others • I am an equal with others • The more I do that I enjoy, the better I feel

FIGURE 8.2. Adding interests and beliefs to Jonathan's Recovery Map.

ASPIRATIONS	
Goals: • Have friends • Get married • Have a job	**Meaning of Accomplishing Identified Goal:** • I can connect with others • I will be connected in the future • I am capable • I am a good, helping person

FIGURE 8.3. Adding aspirations to Jonathan's Recovery Map.

the neighbors has invited him to watch over her dog while she does laundry. This is more opportunity to actualize the adaptive mode.

On their walk the next time, Jonathan explains the great experience and good feeling of helping his neighbor carry the laundry basket and watching her dog.

TEAM MEMBER: What does that say about you that you are helping your neighbors so much?

JONATHAN: I am a helping person, not a hurting person.

TEAM MEMBER: Are there other times you have felt that?

JONATHAN: With friends.

TEAM MEMBER: Wow, sounds like you want to help your neighbors and reconnect. Have I got that right?

JONATHAN: Yeah.

TEAM MEMBER: Are there other things you want, too?

JONATHAN: I would like to see my old friend, go back to the old places, get a girlfriend, get married.

These become aspirations and the focus of the team's work with Jonathan, as shown in Figure 8.3.

Actualizing the Adaptive Mode—Experiencing Best Self in the World

The value of the grandiose belief resides in its meaning. Developing aspirations that realize this same value provides ample opportunity for the most significant and purpose-achieving action. Success breeds success, and the adaptive mode grows to fill more of the person's life space, at the expense of the expansive mode. Because you are being guided by the meaning, and by progress, no action is too small—for example, if the person wants to be a social worker, the meaning may be helping people. This can be achieved anywhere. In the community, they can help their neighbors, in a programmatic residence or hospital setting, they can have a role in-house to help other individuals or staff, and this can achieve the meaning and also be a step toward the larger aspiration.

Brainstorm with the person. There may be constraints given the current situation, but this need not stop you. Allow yourself to be creative. Enable the person to be creative. There are countless ways to meet the meaning of the person's aspiration, once you know it.

The first step toward reconnecting with old friends is to go to the part of town where they live. The team member takes the bus with Jonathan. The return to this familiar location has a big effect upon

Jonathan. His speech is clear and animated. He directs the team member around and tells detailed, interesting stories about the part of town and his life there. Jonathan takes noticeable delight in talking about his old friends. This activity appears to activate positive beliefs about his own capability, the receptiveness of people, and the potential of his future. The team adds these ideas to his Recovery Map (see Figure 8.4).

When it is time to go, Jonathan continues the momentum, suggesting ideas for the next trip, including places to eat and friends to visit. Very thoughtfully, as they leave, he proposes a better bus for the team member to get home more expeditiously.

Over time, Jonathan widens his social network, adding current connections and acquaintances from the past. He sets up meetings with old friends and goes to see them, rekindling the relationships one by one. Helping people and reconnecting with his old friends increases his energy and expands his life space. The team finds him more often in the adaptive mode when they visit. All the while, he talks less and less about being God, ceases giving away his food and possessions, and looks and feels like his best self.

Strengthening the Adaptive Mode—Building Resilience

As you collaborate on the activities that achieve the underlying meaning of individuals' aspirations, it is a great time to empower them to draw conclusions about their strengths. Making a difference, being appreciated, being a good person—these are at the core of the person's best self. Making progress toward the aspiration is another core strength and speaks to capability and being able to persevere when the going gets tougher.

We can help build resilience since we know the situations that are likely to set off the expansive mode—situations that suggest rejection or disrespect or where the person feels insecure. Resilience can be in the form of empowerment beliefs, such as "I am a good person," "Not everyone has to like you," and "I can make a difference." It can also take the form of beliefs that de-catastrophize setbacks: "If I keep at it, I will get it right" and "Even though this did not work, I will still succeed."

> As Jonathan becomes more active, his team repeatedly draws his attention to the personal meaning of these experiences. He concludes that he feels better when he does things he enjoys with others. He concludes that he can make a difference and others appreciate him. When asked whether he wants to give things away, he explains that he is helping people in his building. Figure 8.5 shows Jonathan's full Recovery Map.

POSITIVE ACTION AND EMPOWERMENT	
Current Strategies and Interventions:	**Beliefs/Aspirations/Meanings/Challenges Targeted:**
1. Listen to music and walk together, have Jonathan introduce team member to neighbor	1. Beliefs about being connected to others
2. Planning for social activities to do in the next session and how he can spend time with people between sessions	2. Reducing impact of separation between sessions; establish pattern that social connection will happen in the future; ability to connect with others
3. Rating energy level before and after listening to music and other activities together	3. Beliefs about having to wait for energy to come before doing things

FIGURE 8.4. Adding strategies and positive actions to Jonathan's Recovery Map.

Delusions

Recovery Map	
ACCESSING AND ENERGIZING THE ADAPTIVE MODE	
Interests/Ways to Engage: • Music (listening, singing, and dancing) • Walks • Talking about friends and helping friends • Getting coffee	**Beliefs Activated while in Adaptive Mode:** • I am connected to others • I am an equal with others • The more I do that I enjoy, the better I feel
ASPIRATIONS	
Goals: • Have friends • Get married • Have a job	**Meaning of Accomplishing Identified Goal:** • I can connect with others • I will be connected in the future • I am capable • I am a good, helping person
CHALLENGES	
Current Behaviors/Challenges: • Referring to self as God • Isolation • Inactivity • Giving away belongings • Not eating	**Beliefs Underlying Challenges:** • I am alone • Others leave me • If you are really nice, people won't leave you • I can't do things until I have the energy for them • I am in danger, so I should stay inside
POSITIVE ACTION AND EMPOWERMENT	
Current Strategies and Interventions: 1. Listen to music and walk together, have Jonathan introduce team member to neighbor 2. Planning for social activities to do during the next visit and how he can spend time with people between visits 3. Rating energy level before and after listening to music and other activities together	**Beliefs/Aspirations/Meanings/Challenges Targeted:** 1. Beliefs about being connected to others 2. Reducing impact of separation between visits; establish pattern that social connection will happen in the future; ability to connect with others 3. Beliefs about having to wait for energy to come before doing things

FIGURE 8.5. Jonathan's completed Recovery Map.

PARANOID BELIEFS AND THE SAFETY MODE

Wayne is a middle-aged man who lives in the city. He keeps to himself and doesn't let anybody into his apartment. When members of his case management team come to knock on his door, he shouts loudly at them. He tells them to stop poisoning him. He accuses the team of raping the other people they visit and plotting to kill them. Wayne feels very protective toward people he perceives as weaker, whom he feels are in incredible peril, given this wicked team. He especially distrusts the team psychiatrist, the mastermind behind the poisoning, raping, and murder. Wayne's team cannot get past the door. They are understandably worried for their own safety.

> **Common beliefs underlying paranoid delusions**
>
> *About the Self*
> ✓ I am helpless.
> ✓ I am weak/vulnerable.
> ✓ I am unsafe.
> ✓ I have no control.
> ✓ I am incapable.
>
> *About Others*
> ✓ People are not trustworthy.
> ✓ People will take advantage of me.
>
> *About the World/Future*
> ✓ The world is dangerous.
> ✓ The future is scary.
> ✓ The future is empty.

What It Might Feel Like

You are uncommon. You look out for the greater good. There are so many bad people. It doesn't seem fair at all. But they don't like you. Really don't like you. You can hear them muttering. You can see it in their faces.

You hide in your room, peer out of the corner of the window. The license plate numbers are sent by them. DOT—it means Dead On Time. Dead. They want to kill you. Soon. They send you images of a gang beating you up. It is awful. You can't get it out of your head. It hurts. You can feel their grip around your neck, choking you.

The food tastes strange. Could it be poisoned? You can't eat it. It has been days since you ate. You want to get even, strike back, but this is life and death.

How to Think about Paranoid Beliefs

With paranoia, anxiety is pervasive. The person feels profoundly unsafe. The world is threatening, people have bad intentions, harm seems imminent (Bentall, Corcoran, Howard, Blackwood, & Kinderman, 2001; Freeman, 2007; Freeman & Garety, 2014). And this sense of dire vulnerability is worsened by a deep-seated doubt about being able to stop the bad thing from happening, whether the target of ill will is the self, others, or both. The person goes into safety mode and scours the environment for signs of threat and conspiracy. They may withdraw, refuse to go outside, refuse to eat. In trying to stay safe, they find danger everywhere. They can trust no one. As one man who lived through this said, "Paranoia is like being buried alive."

We see clearly that the person values safety. However, the attempts at securing it can make life very difficult, as the person becomes acutely isolated and agonizingly distressed. At the heart of the safety mode are the themes of vulnerability and incapability, combined with a powerful need for control and value (Beck et al., 2019). The person may believe "I am vulnerable," I am weak," or "I am helpless"; "Others are rejecting," "Others are not trustworthy," or "Others will harm me"; and "The world is dangerous," "I will never be safe," or "My future is bleak."

As you build up your understanding of how things work for the person in the safety mode, you will want to consider: "What lets this person know that the bad thing is happening? Do they feel a tightening in the throat? Is it a queasy feeling in the stomach? Does the heart race?" This will be helpful in terms of developing your understanding, but also your empathy for what it feels like, which will enhance trust. You can also plan to help the person with this distress, which has the double value of easing anxiety and also activating positive beliefs about other people being caring.

> Wayne's team begins to think about how they might collaborate with him. He appears to feel very unsafe and out of control. Not letting them into the apartment might give him temporary relief—he may feel a little safer and more in control of his situation. That he feels poisoned is likely how his belief about others works—they dislike him so much that they want to kill him. How he knows his food is

poisoned is probably because it tastes funny, which might result from his hyperfocus on staying safe and preventing being poisoned. The team's initial understanding of Wayne's challenges are collected in Figure 8.6.

As a clue to what he is like outside of the safety mode, the team notices that Wayne is at his best when he is helping his older adult neighbor. When in the hospital, Wayne helps people who have a hard time moving down the hallway. The team also hears from a former staff member that he used to love to shoot hoops. These observations about his vulnerability, his liking of helping and basketball, inform their strategy for the next encounter.

What to Do—Empowerment

Accessing the Adaptive Mode

For the person who is wary of others and has concerns about vulnerability, your first task is to establish a sense of trust that helps them feel connected, comfortable, and safe. Accessing the adaptive mode is made just for this purpose. As with each challenge, it might not be clear what to try at the outset. If you have a sense of the person's interests, this gives you a head start. It may be listening to music, singing, dancing, or watching funny videos or sports highlights. If the attempt at mutually rewarding activity does not hit right, you can try again. Nothing is lost in the attempt.

Talking about an area of the person's expertise and asking for advice can be an especially effective strategy, as it provides the need for connection while also providing an opportunity for them to have control. When the person is in the adaptive mode, they feel more a part of things, less anxious, and safer.

There are many benefits of the adaptive mode for individuals who experience paranoid beliefs. It temporarily moves them out of the safety mode. They feel better and less anxious. The activity is mutually rewarding, and the positive experience of connection stimulates more positive beliefs about others that counter suspicions of the safety mode, such as "I have things in common with others," or "I can teach my team."

> The team members keep in mind that offering Wayne help might be unwittingly keeping him in the safety mode during their visits, resulting in no entry and yelling. Since helping *others* appears to be a value of his, they decide they should instead try asking Wayne for help. Previous visits show Wayne is acutely alert to defend himself against them; to succeed they will need to lead with a request. The next team member goes to Wayne's door and knocks.

TEAM MEMBER: Hey Wayne, I am not very good at this sports bracket thing. Could you help me out with it?

WAYNE: [*starts to yell*] . . . Oh, you loser . . . [*opens the door*] . . . Show it to me . . . Get in here.

CHALLENGES	
Current Behaviors/Challenges:	**Beliefs Underlying Challenges:**
• Believes team members are plotting against him • Will not let team members in his home	• Other people cannot be trusted • I am in danger

FIGURE 8.6. Wayne's initial Recovery Map.

Wayne turns out to be quite knowledgeable about sports and knows his way around a sports bracket. He is warm and generous throughout the meeting, helping put the bracket together in an expert manner. The team member thanks him and apologizes for being so deficient at brackets. Wayne smiles widely and says, "It's no matter. You got me. Come back any time."

After the successful meeting and accessing his adaptive mode, the team updates Wayne's Recovery Map (see Figure 8.7). The team begins to plan future encounters, focusing on his helping them.

Energizing the Adaptive Mode

Once you have the hook, your focus is to make the activity regular and find more instances that bring out the person's best self. Interpersonal roles that involve leadership do wonders for this process. If the person likes to cook, can they teach others to do it or share recipes? If they like sports, can they talk with others and arrange a sports bracket? If they like to exercise, can they lead a group or class? If they are spiritual, can they share spiritual quotes with people to kick off a meeting or group?

This energizing work highlights the person's interpersonal importance and enables them to overcome suspicion and distrust—helping desire replaces safety concern. You can draw attention to this during the activities, which allows the person to notice how helpful they have been and what this means more broadly about their life. They have been cut off from other people because of their fear. You are helping them bridge that gulf and become the person they always wanted to be.

In some cases, it is best if you directly address relationships where the person perceives themselves to be down in the pecking order. Often the focus is a health care professional or members of the treatment team. Having repeated, positive equalizing experiences together go a long way to diffuse the mistrust that has built up. There are many ways this can look. Having the doctor learn something from the individual, such as how to play cards or learn a different language, works particularly well for transforming the relationship from dangerous to mutually trusting.

The next team member follows the same formula as the first, asking for help with the sports brackets. Wayne responds, "What is wrong with all of you? . . . Okay . . . Come on in." A similar result occurs: warm encounter, expert helping, invited back. Yet a third team member visits and asks for advice about putting together a staff gathering.

TEAM MEMBER: I have to organize the team reception. I don't know what I am doing. Not good at this kind of thing.

WAYNE: [*opening the door*] What's it for? Birthday? Holiday? Baby shower?

ACCESSING AND ENERGIZING THE ADAPTIVE MODE	
Interests/Ways to Engage: • Sports bracket • Playing basketball • Helping others	**Beliefs Activated while in Adaptive Mode:** • I am capable • I am in control

FIGURE 8.7. Adding interests and beliefs to Wayne's Recovery Map.

TEAM MEMBER: [*goes in*] Baby shower.

WAYNE: You gotta make sure that you don't serve any food that a pregnant woman can't eat. Did you know that there are many foods they can't have?

TEAM MEMBER: Wow, I didn't know that. Thank you.

WAYNE: Good thing you have me. What games does she want to have?

The different team members visit during each week, two doing sports, one planning the baby shower. Wayne is warmer each time when he greets them. On one occasion, sports talk branches over to basketball. Wayne talks about playing. He and the team member agree to go and shoot hoops right then. Wayne is pretty good; they have a lot of fun and share a little banter.

After a few trips to the court, the team member mentions that the psychiatrist wants to play basketball better. Would Wayne be interested in meeting him at the court next time and helping? While there is a flash of suspicion, Wayne agrees.

Once you tap into the adaptive mode and as you continue to energize it, you gradually draw attention to its impact: "You've helped me so much, did you notice that?" or "It seems like when we're doing this you don't feel so stressed, is that right? Should we do this again?" or "What does that mean about you that you taught the doctor how to play the game?" These questions get at the heart of strengthening the positive beliefs.

Sometimes, the individual exhibits considerable agitation as a result of fears of being harmed or in danger. In this situation, they may reject engaging in activities that bring about the adaptive mode. To reduce the intensity of the agitation, you will want to demonstrate that you can understand why they would be so upset. Imagine how you would feel if you believed you were going to be harmed and see whether that is how the individual experiences it. You can say, "I imagine I'd feel frightened. Is that how you feel?" Being understood can increase connection, reduce the heightened negative emotion, and make it more likely that you can refocus the energy onto activities of the adaptive mode. A more robust description of a method for summarizing and empathizing when individuals are agitated (summarize, test, empathize, empower, and refocus; STEER) can be found in Chapter 11.

Aspirations and Meaning

Aspirations provide the sustaining quality of the adaptive mode. The safety mode is dominated by vigilance and negative beliefs about one's capabilities and others' intentions. Since the focus is on safety (especially if focused on others), you should consider the possibility that the person wants to make the world a better place. The person's values have been co-opted, so to speak, by the heightened sense of uncertainty and impending peril.

You will be looking for aspirations that make the world and other people better. This could include having a partner and starting a family. It might involve becoming an advocate for disadvantaged people. It might be becoming a chef. It could be caring for animals. The possible ways to achieve the meaning of making the world a better place are diverse and surprising. The key is to help the person dream enough that a rich idea emerges that excites them and becomes a mission that they can orient their life around.

The momentum of the team with Wayne is palpable. They all draw conclusions with him about control and making a difference. He is now welcoming the team at the door and going out to play

ASPIRATIONS	
Goals: • Coaching basketball • Advocating for the homeless and for children	Meaning of Accomplishing Identified Goal: • I am capable • I am a good/helpful person • I can have control

FIGURE 8.8. Adding aspirations to Wayne's Recovery Map.

> basketball and get food. The connection is strong. The team begins asking for other ways he might want to help. In a lively exchange, he describes how important kids are and how they do not get a lot of guidance. Wayne wants to advocate for kids. He had been homeless more than once, and so wants to spearhead a donation drive. In addition, he also dreams of being able to coach kids in basketball. The team feels closer to him and he to them. When they ask him to paint a picture of what it would be like to be a basketball coach, he imagines smiling kids in a photo next to a large trophy. (See Figure 8.8.)

Actualizing the Adaptive Mode—Best Self Replaces Safety Focus

With the aim of the aspiration in mind, individuals can experience their best self on a daily basis. The meaning is the thing, and is most likely related to being a good person who makes things better in the world or someone capable who is more in control of their life. The person has two courses for positive action at this point: taking steps toward the aspiration and also achieving its meaning every day.

Living one's purpose can be captivating, especially for someone who might have been so distrustful and disconnected. You can collaborate to plan the action that moves the person forward, help them experience their mission every day, and draw conclusions about all of this life-affirming activity.

> Wayne begins to get busy at this point. The team begins to have to change appointment times with him because he has so much going on. He pursues several volunteering opportunities. In terms of kids and the homeless, Wayne participates at soup kitchens and shelters. For basketball, he begins to go to the local recreation center to help out.
>
> As Wayne moves into starting a drive to collect clothes, his schedule becomes fuller still. At all of his volunteer sites he begins to raise awareness of his clothing drive. He finds others in the community who are interested. They begin meeting in coffee shops. The group makes signs and gets permission to place donation boxes at the local library and bank. Wayne and his team begin discussing the possibility of stepping off of the team because he is too busy. They all joke that he is firing them. The positive action section of his Recovery Map looks like Figure 8.9.

POSITIVE ACTION AND EMPOWERMENT	
Current Strategies and Interventions: 1. Volunteer at local rec center 2. Participate at soup kitchens 3. Start clothing drive	Beliefs/Aspirations/Meanings/Challenge Targeted: 1. Beliefs about being connected to others 2. Beliefs about ability to help others

FIGURE 8.9. Adding strategies and positive actions to Wayne's Recovery Map.

Strengthening the Adaptive Mode—Building Resilience

As the person pursues aspirations, challenges will emerge. It is useful to keep in mind the underlying vulnerabilities that will provoke the safety mode. Three big examples are perceived or actual disrespect, rejection, or being controlled. You can help the person anticipate and be ready for such unwanted developments—for example, you can ask, "Are there things that might be tricky along the way as you pursue this?" Challenges, such as anxiety, being told they can't join an organization, or having to be around people they haven't always gotten along with, might come up.

Role plays can help the person see that they can handle disrespect or rejection. You can ask, "What might someone do in this situation? What are all the options? Should we play them out and see what we think?" Moving through each scenario, you infuse empowerment: "Would this get you closer to or further from being that awesome mentor you want to be?" You can then support the individual in drawing the conclusion that the strongest person is the one who is in control of their own actions. This also helps them not make a catastrophe out of whatever setback comes along, as they have more effective ways of responding.

Life is a learning process and they can learn the most when things do not work out. This will help them not retreat into the safety mode when life gets tough. Resilience beliefs help them sustain the good that is at the core of living their purposeful life.

> Team members join Wayne for some of his outings, helping him draw conclusions about his success at making the world a better place.
>
> > TEAM MEMBER: Given all of the helping you are doing at the soup kitchen, the rec center, and the clothing drive, what does it say about you?
> > WAYNE: I am a good person
> > TEAM MEMBER: How much do you believe that?
> > WAYNE: Very much.
> > TEAM MEMBER: And how do the people feel about it?
> > WAYNE: They appreciate me. It makes their lives easier.
>
> Wayne's full Recovery Map is shown in Figure 8.10.

ADDITIONAL CONSIDERATIONS

You Don't Have to Go Big

The scope of the expansive mode can be rather daunting. The person believes they are something special, something larger than most people's lives ever are, such as a deity, royalty, or an exceptionally accomplished person. While this expansive mode compensates for how bad the person feels, the solution does not need to share the grand scale. In fact, what you do can be quite small (such as walking, caring for animals), as long as it meets the underlying need.

Do Not Fear If You Get Included in the Belief

It happens from time to time that you might be included in the belief system. This is especially true of the safety mode, where you might be seen as a persecutor. This does not have to disrupt

Recovery Map	
ACCESSING AND ENERGIZING THE ADAPTIVE MODE	
Interests/Ways to Engage: • Sports bracket • Playing basketball • Helping others	**Beliefs Activated while in Adaptive Mode:** • I am capable • I am in control
ASPIRATIONS	
Goals: • Coaching basketball • Advocating for the homeless and for children	**Meaning of Accomplishing Identified Goal:** • I am capable • I am a good/helpful person • I can have control
CHALLENGES	
Current Behaviors/Challenges: • Believes team members are plotting against him • Will not let team members in his home	**Beliefs Underlying Challenges:** • Other people cannot be trusted • I am in danger
POSITIVE ACTION AND EMPOWERMENT	
Current Strategies and Interventions: 1. Volunteer at local rec center 2. Participate at soup kitchens 3. Start clothing drive	**Beliefs/Aspirations/Meanings/Challenge Targeted:** 1. Beliefs about being connected to others 2. Beliefs about ability to help others

FIGURE 8.10. Wayne's completed Recovery Map.

your relationship—rather, it is a sign that you want to return to accessing and energizing the adaptive mode. This shared activity will activate positive beliefs and trust. Similarly, if the person in the expansive mode sees you as their subject or needing their money or benevolence, you can also return to the activities of the adaptive mode.

Another strategy is to reflect that you understand the value in what the individual is saying. You can say something like "It sounds like helping me out is really important to you—what would be the best part about that?" and then refocus activities and interventions on meeting the need of the "best part": helping, caring, capability, or whatever else it may be.

Do Not Fear If You Are Worried about Collusion

The process of understanding grandiose or paranoid beliefs could seem like you are agreeing with the person about the truth of their belief. In recovery-oriented cognitive therapy you pursue a third way, beyond agreeing or disagreeing with a person's belief. For grandiose or expansive delusions, your questioning uncovers their underlying values ("What is the best part about that?")—that are most important to them. And mutual actions bring these important meanings into real life. For paranoid delusions, your question ("What lets you know this is happening?") demonstrates that you can understand the feelings driving the belief (e.g., fear).

This is not collusion. In both cases, you *do not* delve into the details of the belief or challenge the facts (e.g., "Where's the money? Let's call the bank"). This will only serve to increase disconnection and power struggle, and can, in turn, fire up the beliefs that underlie the delusion.

Do Not Fear If Beliefs Have Both Grandiose and Paranoid Features

There are versions of grandiose beliefs that also have a paranoid flavor. The person is Jesus and being persecuted. The person might be a great inventor, while others are stealing their ideas and making all the money. In these cases, both negative modes are likely active. You will be able to access the person's adaptive mode through shared, meaningful activity. Equalizing, trust, and importance can all be developed as you energize the adaptive mode and develop aspirations. In short, multiple beliefs may be addressed through a singular intervention.

WORDS OF WISDOM

BOX 8.1. Beliefs and Transformed Images: Meeting the Need

Emotional beliefs, such as being controlled, devalued, and scrutinized, are pictorially transformed into specific persecutory or grandiose beliefs. Others are seen as devaluing, controlling, rejecting, and dangerous. The person experiences images of being influenced by rays from an influencing machine, being observed by multiple cameras, having their food poisoned, or being threatened by a gang of robbers.

The genesis of these hard-to-understand experiences is the negative self-concept and the negative concept of others: self as devalued, controlled, vulnerable, and helpless; others as devaluing, controlling, rejecting, and dangerous. This negative view of the self and others, combined with the content of the delusional beliefs, activates urges to be valued, in control, safe, and so on. By fulfilling these needs directly, you can propel the individual into the adaptive mode and alleviate the need for the belief.

The grandiose delusions compensate for the sense of feeling diminished, not regarded as important, and being rejected. The delusion of being God, for example, substitutes worshiped for being devalued, omnipotence for lack of control, and all-loving for undesirable. Whether the beliefs are of the persecutory or the grandiose variety, the specific therapeutic strategies help to restore individuals to what is most important to them: belonging, contributing, being safe, and helping others.

SUMMARY

- The strategy for both grandiose (expansive) beliefs and paranoid (safety) beliefs involves understanding the underlying beliefs, and then identifying activities that will fulfill the need expressed in the underlying beliefs.
- Reflecting your understanding of the meanings or needs most important to the person (e.g., being valued, having control) increases connection and reduces power struggles around the validity of delusional beliefs.
- When individuals are engaged in the adaptive mode, and more adaptive beliefs are activated, help them draw conclusions about themselves, their relationships with others, and possibilities for the future.
- Collaborate repeatedly on valued activities with the individual that have the meaning of their aspirations. Draw conclusions that are the opposite of the meanings underlying the expansive and safety mode.

CHAPTER 9
Empowering When Hallucinations Are the Challenge

Tammy is in her 50s. She spends the major part of every day in bed, covers pulled over her head, demoralized by what she hears. "What grandparent lies in bed all day? You're so stupid they must have given you your diploma out of pity. The devil is real and you can't pray him away if you tried. It's your fault Karen killed herself—she was your best friend!" Tammy feels paralyzed by these relentless voices inside her head. She stares off frequently, can't quite hold a conversation for more than a few minutes before she shifts her attention back to what she's hearing. Her brother petitions to take control over her finances. Her daughter won't bring Tammy's grandchildren to visit. The voice says, "Why would they bother visiting—you don't do anything!" Tammy is even demoralized about treatment—fearing she'll probably mess up and that nothing can make this horrible experience stop.

Hallucinations are perceptions that can be quite confusing. Examples of hallucinations include hearing the voice of a deceased parent, of a deity, of the devil. Other examples include feelings of being choked or touched, of giving off an awful odor, and seeing apparitions (American Psychiatric Association, 2013). The experience is private. Others cannot hear, see, or feel what the person experiencing them does. This fact can lead to a profound sense of separateness and loneliness. The experience can, at the same time, be compelling and highly captivating. The person is caught in this divide between an ongoing experience that separates them from others but also seems so vitally important.

In this chapter, we consider what it is like to experience hallucinations, how to understand them as a challenge, and what to do to promote empowerment. As with other challenges, hallucinations are mainly a problem when they get in the way of the life the person desires. Refocusing on that life is the most powerful approach to hallucinations.

WHAT IT MIGHT FEEL LIKE

It got your attention. How does it know that about you? That is shameful. And the things it says about people as you pass them—embarrassing! Do they hear it, too? Hard to tell. You can't help but laugh uncomfortably in public. People look at you in a weird way. So maybe you elect to stay in more often.

Somehow this makes them—there is more than one!—louder and you hear them more often. You don't see them. But they are as real as your heartbeat. You can't control them. They say what they want. When they want.

You feel inferior, belittled, powerless, and trapped. They know everything about you, your biggest fears, and tell you constantly. They say other people hate you, that you are an unlovable piece of crap, worthless and utterly useless, that you should just die, the world would be a better place without you. This makes you angry. You aren't a piece of crap . . . or are you?

It is hard to do much of anything. You start to read and they talk. You want to call an old friend and they yell. You feel bullied and powerless. You stop trying. What's the point?

HOW TO THINK ABOUT HALLUCINATIONS

The research literature and the stories of those with lived experience converge on a useful way to approach hallucinations. The majority of regular voice hearers (as many as 8–10% of the general population) have not been given a diagnosis, and they describe rich relationships and work lives (Beavan, Read, & Cartwright, 2011; Romme & Escher, 1989). What is more, nearly everyone has experienced hallucinations, such as hearing their names called in an empty room or hearing someone talking who isn't there (Posey & Losch, 1984). Notably, these hallucinations are more likely to occur when you are by yourself, more stressed, or falling asleep (Delespaul, deVries, & van Os, 2002).

Common beliefs about voices include:

✓ I have no control over the voices.
✓ The voices are powerful.
✓ The voices are credible.
✓ The voices are external.

These observations tell us that hallucinations are common and not necessarily a problem; many people experience voices and can still live the life they wish to be living. What appears to make voices a problem are the beliefs the person holds about them: believing the voices are coming and going as they please, and feeling ultimately diminished or inferior to them; believing the voices are a reliable source of information, so you need to listen to them to get important knowledge; or believing you have to do what the voice says because it will otherwise harm you (Beck et al., 2009; Chadwick, Birchwood, & Trower, 1996).

Beliefs underlying voice content include:

About the Self
✓ I am incapable.
✓ I am weak/vulnerable.
✓ I am defective.
✓ I am worthless.
✓ I am powerless.

About Others
✓ People are threatening.
✓ People judge you.
✓ People know all of my wrongs.
✓ People don't understand me.

About the Future/World
✓ The world is dangerous.
✓ These will *never* stop.

These beliefs can lead to distressing feelings. The person may shut down in demoralization or fight back by shouting at the voice. The person might listen for hours on end because they feel they have to. They might feel so helpless and low that the only choice seems to be compliance with commands (Romme, Honig, Noorthoorn, & Escher, 1992).

Hallucinations

The beliefs about voices can help us understand how the person feels and what they do in response to their hallucinations. Another important aspect about voices is what they say. For so many people hallucinations are a challenge because the voices are tremendously negative. They put the person down, tell them they are no good, unlovable, wicked, and so on. The content of these types of voices come from the person's own negative beliefs about self, others, and the future (Beck et al., 2019). The experience of having negative beliefs articulated by credible, powerful, and controlling sources may well be a living hell.

If we know the negative content that the voice is saying to the person, this will help when we think about the positive beliefs activated when the person engages with others and not with the voice.

> Tammy spends her days completely consumed by the barrage of awful things her voices say. Her brother finds a therapist and they go to the sessions together at first. Tammy's therapist sees how difficult conversation is for her, but she is forthcoming about what the voices say. The therapist adds this to Tammy's Recovery Map, as shown in Figure 9.1.
>
> Tammy pays so much attention to her voices that she really cannot engage with others around her. The therapist's first move is to foster a sense of connection with Tammy through mutually enjoyable activities. This will access the adaptive mode, give Tammy more control over her experiences, and provide energy to talk a bit about her hopes for the future. The positive action section of Tammy's Recovery Map is shown in Figure 9.2.

WHAT TO DO—EMPOWERMENT THROUGH REFOCUSING

Hallucinations become a challenge as people get caught up in them and stop living their desired life. The strategy you want to foster is for the person to shift focus away from the alluring–annoying voice and ultimately onto activities that connect to aspirations and values. We call this process *refocusing*. It is an active form of empowerment. Individuals go from feeling inferior, weak, and trapped to valuable, strong, and free. They change their beliefs about the voice. It no longer appears to have control or be worth listening to.

CHALLENGES	
Current Behaviors/Challenges: • Attending to voices • Isolation and difficulty refocusing away from the voices	**Beliefs Underlying Challenges:** • I'm a bad grandmother • I'm messed up, bad • This can't be better • I have no control • This will never stop, there's nothing I can do • I'm stupid • Bad things are my fault • Everything I hear is true • What's the point of doing anything? I'm not good anyway • I have to listen to the voices because they tell the truth • My family has already taken everything from me (control), so what's the point?

FIGURE 9.1. Tammy's initial Recovery Map.

POSITIVE ACTION AND EMPOWERMENT	

Current Strategies and Interventions:
1. Increase control over voices
  • Identify interests to help refocus attention in the immediate (Music? Talking about grandkids?)
2. Identify and enrich aspirations to find meaningful target of refocusing—increase hope and purpose
  • Teaching grandkids?
  • Work?
	Beliefs/Aspirations/Meanings/Challenges Targeted:
	1. Beliefs about control
	  • I can have more control over this than I thought
	  • Even if it feels like it'll never stop, there are things I can do to take control and have power over it
	2. Hope and purpose
	  • I am capable of achieving my dreams
	  • When things are stressful, I can refocus my attention onto the things I care about and want for my life

FIGURE 9.2. Adding strategies and positive actions to Tammy's Recovery Map.

Accessing the Adaptive Mode

Accessing the adaptive mode creates a natural shift away from the internal. Finding the person's interest and doing that activity together becomes an initial experience of refocusing. It is a general version of the old saying that you cannot talk and listen at the same time. You cannot engage in an enjoyable, connecting activity and simultaneously focus all your attention onto voices. The adaptive mode comes with positive emotions and beliefs. The activity feels good and is the opposite of the experience of listening to the voices. The pull of the adaptive mode is more powerful than the voices.

The person may have prominent hallucinations that they effortlessly focus on. You will need the right activity, which will likely require trial and error: singing along to music is particularly good and worth trying, watching funny videos, watching sports shorts, playing a fast-paced card game, or tossing a ball back-and-forth. As always, allow yourself to be creative and never give up.

Accessing the adaptive mode and establishing a connection provides a valuable opportunity to draw conclusions. First, you can help the person notice that the voice is less bothersome during the activity. Next, you can zero in on the choice to participate, which begins to establish that the person has control rather than the voice:

THERAPIST: When we're singing along to the music do you notice anything about the voices?

TAMMY: I didn't even notice them at all!

THERAPIST: That's really neat. You chose music for us to sing and they didn't bug you at all. What does that say about your ability to take control of them?

Energizing the Adaptive Mode

There are a variety of reasons why the pull of the voices might be strong. It could well be that the person is so isolated that the voices are the only thing going on in their life. Or they might be worried that if they don't listen, something bad could happen or important information could be missed. Or the voices effortlessly get their attention after years of practice. Whatever the reason, as you energize the adaptive mode with repeated activity, you also want to draw attention to the success of the chosen activity in diminishing the experience of the voice and promoting a sense of control. The Look-Point-Name game illustrates how this might work.

The Look-Point-Name Game

Playing this game involves directing attention outward toward objects in the environment around oneself, pointing to them, and naming what they are. Because you play together in alternating turns, the game can activate the adaptive mode. The person is having fun, enjoying the positive emotion, feeling connected and trusting, and demonstrating control over the voices.

First, you get a rough assessment of how stressed the person is because of the voices: "How stressed are you? A little, a lot, or somewhere in between?" You then introduce the game by saying, "I know a silly kind of game that some people use to bring that stress down a bit. Want to give it a try with me?" You then start the game by pointing to and naming an object, such as a clock. The person will point to a wall. You point to a window. The person points to a door. You point to a picture. The person points to the tile. You point to a book. And so on. Over the course of this back-and-forth, the person gains more affect and energy, and is more focused on the environment around them. If at the start a person is visibly stressed and does not respond to your attempt at assessing it, you can move directly into the game.

At the peak, when the looking, pointing, and naming is going more quickly, you stop and ask, "Are the voices more or less bothersome?" or "Are you more or less stressed?" This gives you a rough reassessment and the opportunity for the individual to notice the difference. You then give the individual credit for taking control over the voices by asking, "Who made them lessen?" or "So while we're doing this the voices are less intense. Sounds like you have some control over them. What do you think?" This helps strengthen those beliefs. Sometimes, individuals will minimize their role by saying that you were the cause because you suggested the activity. In this case, you can simply reply, "Who chose to do it with me, though?"

If the game proves effective in reducing the intensity of the voices and increasing control, you can draw conclusions about whether it is worth doing again: "Since this helped us feel less stressed now, I'm wondering whether we should do it again?" To encourage the individual to use the technique between interactions with you, you can also ask, "Are there other times you'd like to try this or other people you might want to do this with?" Together, you can also come up with the best ways to recall the technique—for example, does the person want to create a poster with pictures to remember the steps? Would a good action plan be to teach their sibling or a roommate the game?

There are many variations on this game—you can be creative. It needs to be interactive and involve things in the environment. Look-Point-Verse can be done with the Bible or Koran. Look-Point-Beautiful can be done on a nature walk. The best adaptations incorporate the person's interests. A graphical representation of Look-Point-Name can be found in Figure 9.3.

More generally, any activity that increases connection and energy—be it sharing videogame tips, playing cards, dancing—can follow this same recipe for accessing the adaptive mode, noticing the voice is not so bothersome, and drawing attention to the choice the person made to participate, thereby giving them control.

Purpose: Refocus attention away from stress (voices, racing thoughts, etc.) and increase sense of control.

Introduction: "It looks like you're maybe feeling stressed out, is that right? I know this silly game that has sometimes helped me and other people I know feel less stressed. Should we give it a try?"

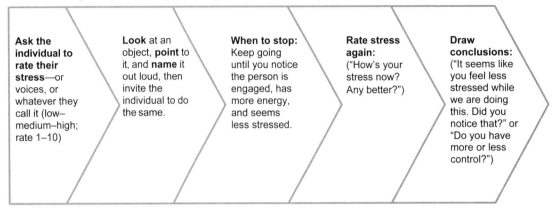

Personalizing the game: There are many variations on this game; you can be creative! Look-point-verse or look-point-read can be done with the Bible or Koran. Look-point-beautiful can be done on a nature walk. Use a person's interests as inspiration!

FIGURE 9.3. The Look-Point-Name game.

Energizing the adaptive mode is building up the person's life independent of hallucinations. It means individuals are filling their days with more and more action, more time engaged with others and not with the voice. Every activity is an act of refocusing away from the hallucinations and toward more valued pursuits. When trust and energy are at the right level, it is time to develop the adaptive mode by eliciting the aspirations.

> Tammy and her therapist start taking walks to the convenience store across the street. They notice that participating in the community has the pleasant result of also reducing the voices. At the store, Tammy buys items so that she can make nice things for her grandkids. They decide these outings would be even more enjoyable by adding music. The two of them repeat the community excursions for a few weeks. During one of these walks to the store, the therapist floats the idea of Tammy trying the outings between sessions at a store near where she lives. Tammy responds enthusiastically to the suggestion and begins making weekend trips into the community, first to the store, then to a local coffee shop, and then to church.
>
> THERAPIST: You've really been doing more and more each week. What do you think about that?
>
> TAMMY: It's been good. I always feel better on the days when I get out of the house.
>
> THERAPIST: That's fabulous! I remember when we first started meeting that the voices often criticized how little you were doing in your life. But you really get out there and do a lot of things. What do you make of that?
>
> TAMMY: That's not me anymore.
>
> THERAPIST: I wonder whether it's possible that when voices say cruel or negative things, maybe they're not that accurate or they're entirely untrue?
>
> TAMMY: Definitely! If you and I wouldn't say it's true, it can't be true.

> THERAPIST: I agree with that. So if we're agreeing that the voices say things that aren't really true, is it worth listening to them when they come up?
>
> TAMMY: Seems like it would be a waste of time.

Energizing the adaptive mode with increased activity not only helps diminish the voices but can also help discredit them. This can lead to the resiliency belief that the voices are not as credible as once thought and are therefore not worthy of time and attention.

Aspirations and Meaning

As aspirations embody the person's values, they become the most powerful source of refocusing. Ideally, the meaning of the aspiration will outshine the draw of the voice. This should make it easier for the person to shift their attention to an activity that achieves the meaning.

Using a recovery image (see Chapter 4) can also help by turning the person's strength with imagery to advantage. Individuals might see themselves sitting in a farmhouse, petting their dog, talking to some friends. They might see themselves walking along the shore holding the hand of a partner. They might see themselves advocating for people with mental health challenges. All of these future-projecting images can act like vision boards to inspire hope, optimism, and also compete with hallucinations. The recovery image is more exciting to think about, and the person cannot listen to the voice and focus on the recovery image at the same time. It is another source of control.

In Tammy's case, it wasn't too surprising to learn that she desired strongly to be a loving and active grandmother. She believed that this was a hopeless endeavor, but it was still the one thing she wanted more than anything. Being a good grandmother would mean she was connected to her family, useful, and capable.

Actualizing the Adaptive Mode

Once you have richly developed aspirations, part of the work of positive action shifts from building up to building out. Over time, as the person gets the meaning of the aspiration into their life and makes progress toward it, they develop a momentum that makes the voice less burdensome and daily life more rewarding. As one person put it, "I now have a family and work as a nurse. The voice is still there, but I don't have the time or desire to listen to it."

> Together with her therapist, Tammy writes out what would help her be a good grandmother: teaching the kids how to cook (starting with practicing making old family recipes herself), sending them cards (starting with going out to the store to pick out supplies to make cards), and creating a scrapbook of family photos (starting with getting up and organizing the boxes of papers and photographs in her room). When Tammy hears the voices, she will put on music to start, and then refocus her attention onto steps toward being a grandmom again.

Strengthening the Adaptive Mode

When the person is less distressed by the voices after doing a meaningful activity together, you can draw their attention to the meanings they can take away from that experience. Questions you might ask include "Were there times when you felt better or worse? Did you have more or less control? Did this go better or worse than expected? Does this get you closer to or further from what you want? Would it be helpful to do more or less of this?" Ultimately, we want the person to see themselves as having control and being a capable and contributing person. The voice is diminished and less important. This is empowerment.

> THERAPIST: What does it say about you that the voices have been nothing more than background noise lately?
>
> TAMMY: They can't have power over me. I can take control back myself!
>
> THERAPIST: And what does that mean about your ability to be an awesome grandmother?
>
> TAMMY: I'm a good one. I don't have time to listen to the voices, I need to be able to do things with the kids.

Tammy's full Recovery Map is found in Figure 9.4.

ADDITIONAL CONSIDERATIONS

Do Not Worry If the Person Calls Hallucinations Something Different

Empowerment does not require that the person identifies the experience as a voice or hallucination. People can call the experience all kinds of names: headaches, people, radio signals, and so on. The goal is to help empower them regardless of how they refer to the experience. Use their language. This is part of meeting people where they are. To move away from labeling the experience all together, you can simply refer to the person's stress. This can serve to normalize the experience, as we all have stress at times.

Refocusing Is Not Distraction

A common misconception about techniques for quieting voices is that all you need to do is repeatedly distract the person away from them (Romme et al., 1992). Distraction does not accurately capture the process that works best and often proves insufficient in maintaining control long term—for example, listening to music to drown out the voices may be temporarily effective, but without refocusing onto something more meaningful the music can become background noise, overpowered by the voices. Refocusing requires an activity that the person enjoys, that is meaningful, or that provides fulfillment of a bigger purpose. It can be the source of shifting energy and attention. If the person is having a hard time refocusing, it is possible that the target activity does not have enough appeal for them. Try other ideas. You will hit on the right thing in time.

When Hallucinations Are Not Voices

Some people are challenged with hallucinations that are not voices, such as visions, feelings, or smells. The same general strategy works: refocusing. Help individuals do what they want to do. Photography or another artistic pursuit can work well for visions. Help the person be less caught up and more in control. Relaxation or mindfulness (Chadwick, 2014), especially when done with another, can help for tactile hallucinations, especially ones related to being touched by others.

Hallucinations

Recovery Map	
ACCESSING AND ENERGIZING THE ADAPTIVE MODE	
Interests/Ways to Engage: • Music • Cooking • Scrapbooking • Family memories	**Beliefs Activated while in Adaptive Mode:** • Energized • Connected to other people/her family • Capable • Control over voices
ASPIRATIONS	
Goals: • Being an active and involved grandmother • Getting control of finances back • Spend more time out of the house with people her age/make a friend	**Meaning of Accomplishing Identified Goal:** • I am not worthless—I have value • I can be connected with my family • I can have a life like everyone else • I can teach and help others
CHALLENGES	
Current Behaviors/Challenges: • Attending to voices • Isolation and difficulty refocusing away from the voices	**Beliefs Underlying Challenges:** • I'm a bad grandmother • I'm messed up, bad • This can't be better • I have no control • This will never stop, there's nothing I can do • I'm stupid • Bad things are my fault • Everything I hear is true • What's the point of doing anything? I'm not good anyway • I have to listen to the voices because they tell the truth • My family has already taken everything from me (control), so what's the point?
POSITIVE ACTION AND EMPOWERMENT	

Current Strategies and Interventions:
1. Increase control over voices
   • Identify interests to help refocus attention in the immediate (Music? Talking about grandkids?)
2. Identify and enrich aspirations to find meaningful target of refocusing—increase hope and purpose
   • Teaching grandkids?
   • Work?
	Beliefs/Aspirations/Meanings/Challenges Targeted:
	1. Beliefs about control
	   • I can have more control over this than I thought
	   • Even if it feels like it'll never stop, there are things I can do to take control and have power over it
	2. Hope and purpose
	   • I am capable of achieving my dreams
	   • When things are stressful, I can refocus my attention onto the things I care about and want for my life

FIGURE 9.4. Tammy's completed Recovery Map.

> **WORDS OF WISDOM**
>
> **BOX 9.1. Hallucinations, Stigma, and Control**
>
> Hearing voices can carry considerable stigma (Vilhauer, 2017). It is perhaps too easy to see hallucinations as abnormal experiences that indicate a mental disorder, a source of shame, or a sign that something is wrong with you.
>
> Typically, when you hear something or see something, you can verify it with another person who is there. Hallucinations are more private than this—they are more like thoughts, but with a difference—voices, visions, and the like are experienced perceptually. Others may not understand what this is like and how compelling the experience can be. They may not recognize similar experiences of their own.
>
> There has been a revolution in the understanding of hallucinations over the past 30 years. The experience of voices in those without a diagnosis is now well documented (Romme & Escher, 1989). Everyone hears voices from time to time and some experience hallucinations on a daily basis. Ethnographic studies show that hallucinations have a significant and positive role in different cultures and at different time periods (Sacks, 2012). There are people who make their living with the experience of voices: psychics (Powers, Kelley, & Corlett, 2017). Those without a disorder—be they teachers, artists, actors, administrators, plumbers, or psychics—all describe being able to stop the experience when they want to (Honig et al., 1998). Control is a key difference for when hallucinations get in the way and when they do not.
>
> Hallucinations are common, relatable human experiences that do not have to be a problem or get in the way of one's desired life. Developing control of the experience and being able to refocus onto activities that are most meaningful form the essence of empowerment.

SUMMARY

- The belief that a voice has the ability to control, has credibility, and has power can interfere with people's ability to live their lives to the fullest.
- The content of voices helps to inform us of the individual's beliefs about themselves and others.
- Refocusing helps to break the cycle of listening to a voice.
- The key to refocusing is drawing conclusions to strengthen positive beliefs about personal control and capability, as well as the voice lacking credibility and not being worth listening to.
- Aspirations provide the target for valued positive action that achieves the meaning of the person's best self every day, which is the opposite of what the voices say. This sustains empowerment long term.

CHAPTER 10
Empowering When Communication Is the Challenge

Christine lives in a programmatic residence. The staff observe that she talks for long periods of time, but they have a hard time following her train of thought—her speech goes seemingly to every topic all at once. At times, Christine walks around quickly in circles, hitting her head with her fist, while talking under her breath. When a staff member asks what she wants for her future, Christine's eyes widen. "The future is very big and complex," she says. "Thinking about the future involves thinking about things. And there was a really good chance about those things that . . . let me give you an example . . . a toddler can have ideas about figuring out ways that they can be better and need opportunities to plan those things out . . ."

Communication is the primary way we connect with others, get our needs met, and help others with their needs. Having difficulty communicating with other people can be profoundly isolating. It cuts you off from potentially meaningful interchanges. Worse, when the simplest of attempts at communication go wrong, it can make you feel like there is something deeply wrong with you.

The communication challenges of individuals given a diagnosis of a serious mental health condition are among the oldest observations in psychiatry (Bleuler, 1950; Cohen & Camhi, 1967; Kraepelin, 1971; Le, Najolia, Minor, & Cohen, 2017; Tandon, Nasrallah, & Keshaven, 2009). These challenges roughly fall into two types: reduced speech, such as one-word answers (often listed as a negative symptom); and speech that flows at a normal rate but is very difficult to understand or follow (often listed as a positive symptom). In this chapter, we include both so-called positive and negative disruptions to communication (Andreasen, 1984). We find that clinically it is helpful to consider them together as challenges to communication and connection.

As we saw for negative symptoms (see Chapter 7), the terminology for these challenges is not particularly helpful. *Alogia* means a lack of language, which is not accurate. Even if the person shows a reduction in speech output, this is certainly not the case all of the time. *Formal thought disorder* (Andreasen & Grove, 1986) suggests that the problem centers in the person's thinking, that the person is confused. A more correct account is that the challenge involves expression, turning thoughts into followable speech (Beck et al., 2009).

Similar to negative symptoms, these communication challenges are relatable and fall on the end of a continuum of variation in speech clarity that everyone at times experiences. Have you ever taken forever to make a point? Gone off topic? Given an answer irrelevant to the question asked? When are you more likely to speak this way? The answer is likely when you are more stressed or tired. The same is true for somebody who has more significant challenges with communication. But like everyone else, those who experience this challenge more often don't *always* experience it.

In this chapter, we focus on empowerment for communication challenges. We start with the inside view of what it might feel like. This leads us to a useful understanding, which then prompts action. The adaptive mode helps communication efforts in specific ways relating to beliefs and energy. Aspirations take us further into generating more hope, energy, and stronger beliefs. We build empowerment and resilience beliefs along the way to sustain progress. We end the chapter with a few additional considerations.

WHAT IT MIGHT FEEL LIKE

Everything was going fine. The guy seemed to be getting it. But then he wasn't following. What? You can't let him judge you. You are intelligent. He is going to understand. It is important!

You try again. But it doesn't come out right. That is not what you meant to say. Why does this happen? What is wrong with you? Others are looking now. This is really bad. Your heart is racing. You keep thinking, "I am not stupid." This is important. He has to understand. You try yet again. He flinches and begins to move away. The others pull back. This is so frustrating. What you have to say matters. Don't they know?

You give up. Let it go. Walk away. But you keep thinking about it. So bothersome! You are not worthless! You clench your fists. Walk faster. Stupid. Stupid. Stupid. You walk up to another guy. This will make it right. He must understand. You are so angry. Everything is a blur. You speak to him. What is that reaction? Say it louder. Louder!

> **Common beliefs underlying communication challenges include:**
>
> *About the Self*
> ✓ I am mentally defective.
> ✓ I must be broken.
> ✓ I am stupid.
> ✓ I am worthless.
> ✓ I am a failure.
> ✓ I don't belong.
>
> *About Others*
> ✓ Others judge me.
> ✓ Others reject me.
> ✓ Others don't understand me.
>
> *About the Future/World*
> ✓ No one will *ever* understand me.
> ✓ There's no point; the future is hopeless.

HOW TO THINK ABOUT COMMUNICATION CHALLENGES

Combining lived experience accounts with research studies (Beck et al., 2009; Grant & Beck, 2009b) helps enrich our understanding of difficult communication episodes. A large part of the person's vulnerability lies in feeling mentally defective. Despite the complexity of the processes that go into producing speech, it feels effortless. To be unable to successfully communicate with another must mean something bad. The person must be broken and not very smart. Being defective and stupid leads to having no value. Why would others like—let alone love—a *bad apple*? The person feels misunderstood, judged, rejected.

These beliefs make most—if not all—social interactions dangerous. The person is not able to hide their speaking problem unless they remain silent, which can also stand out. There are many sources of pain. Not being understood is frustrating. Being judged hurts. Being rejected can feel devastating.

Anticipating these outcomes with others is stressful. Stress further drains away resources that are vital to mental operations that service successful communication. The person can get caught in a distressing cycle: they want to connect with others to share something important, but they fear failure and judgment, which then makes them more nervous, resulting in speech that is hard to follow. The person reacts to the cycle by either giving up or trying harder. Neither results in the highly desired connection.

Repeated experience of communication difficulty can lead to a profound sense of isolation, of feeling alien, of not belonging. All of this strengthens beliefs about being defective, broken, and different from other people, and, thereby, so alone in the world.

If you listen closely to the person's speech when it is harder to follow, you might find that some of these themes come out. You might hear the person returning to "stupid" or "smart" or "intelligent," which can strengthen your feeling that incapability and defectiveness are present. You might also hear words related to rejection or people not caring: "I'm nobody," "nothing," "fool," "That's not me."

From this understanding we can develop our strategy for empowerment. We want to connect with the person, as this is what they are craving. We want to help them feel that they belong, that others care about what they have to say, and that others can understand. We want them to experience communication success repeatedly. As they connect more, become more active, and develop aspirations, they draw conclusions about making a difference and being a part of something bigger in life. Resilience centers on knowledge that stress can make it hard for them to communicate, but this does not mean they are dumb—everyone experiences stress, it is a part of living.

> The staff at Christine's residence begin thinking about how to connect with her better and help her get more of the life she wants. They note that her speech is frequently hard to follow, especially when she wants to communicate something that matters to her. They find she often talks about children and also about not being herself. Christine likely hits herself because she is trying to make things right. She mentions the sky and stars falling. The staff guess that kids are a great interest of hers. They also suspect that Christine finds herself hopelessly disconnected from everyone and might feel unsafe. They devise an action plan for a staff member to meet with her to genuinely and cheerfully explore her potential interest in children. The challenges section of her Recovery Map is depicted in Figure 10.1.

CHALLENGES	
Current Behaviors/Challenges: • Speech is hard to follow • Hits herself • Talks about the sky falling	**Beliefs Underlying Challenges:** • I am disconnected • I am unsafe • People don't understand me • I'm stupid

FIGURE 10.1. Christine's initial Recovery Map.

WHAT TO DO—EMPOWERMENT

Accessing the Adaptive Mode

Play to the person's strengths and lead with action, rather than verbally focused interventions. Do things together that spark the person's interest:

- *Watch a video:* "Check this out!"
- *Listen to music:* "Here's Michael Jackson!"
- *Do something physical:* "Let's walk around!" or "Here, catch this ball!"

Mutual activity *is* connection. Accessing the adaptive mode in this way will spark positive shared emotion and positive beliefs about you. Stress will go down. Energy and cognitive resources will go up. During the activity, verbal communication may become easier for the person. If this occurs, you can draw their attention to how well you understand them. They will see that you care about what they have to say and that they have successfully communicated with you.

> A staff member goes to Christine's room and Christine begins speaking about kids, future, sky falling, empty, too much. . . . The staff member pulls up a video on her phone and says, "Check out this video! Two kids playing house." Christine says, "They aren't playing, they are learning. Play is a child's work." As the encounter develops, the staff member is impressed by Christine's bright affect, and her impressive knowledge of children. They watch several videos together, laughing and talking.
>
> STAFF MEMBER: This was fun.
> CHRISTINE: Yeah, it was.
> STAFF MEMBER: You know so much about kids.
> CHRISTINE: Thank you.
> STAFF MEMBER: I learned a lot from you.
> CHRISTINE: You did?
> STAFF MEMBER: Yeah. You are pretty knowledgeable, aren't you?
> CHRISTINE: I guess.
> STAFF MEMBER: Should we do this again?
> CHRISTINE: Yeah.
> STAFF MEMBER: What about tomorrow?
> CHRISTINE: Great.
> STAFF MEMBER: Let's put "Talk about kids, Tuesday at 2 P.M." on the whiteboard above your desk.

ACCESSING AND ENERGIZING THE ADAPTIVE MODE	
Interests/Ways to Engage: • Children	**Beliefs Activated while in Adaptive Mode:** • I am connected • I am knowledgeable • It's worth connecting with other people

FIGURE 10.2. Adding interests and beliefs to Christine's Recovery Map.

Since endings can bring a strong sense of disconnection and doubt about when connection will next occur, the staff member is clear to draw conclusions about success and to specifically plan their next time together. The staff member also updates Christine's Recovery Map after this interaction, as pictured in Figure 10.2.

Energize the Adaptive Mode

As you access the adaptive mode more frequently, you will learn more about the person, finding more and more of what they like to do. Since communication is the challenge and disconnection the key vulnerability, your interactions will be filled with good experiences together that can form the basis of a different way to be with others. Each encounter will have capability, success, and belonging in it. Energy will grow. Positive anticipatory emotions will begin to appear prior to your meetings. Looking forward is a form of savoring and energizes the adaptive mode.

During mutual activities, talking will be easier. The person should have more energy and more access to mental resources required for successful communication. Positive beliefs about self and others will be active, lessening stress. In attempting verbal communication, you want to choose topics that excite the person, touching their area of knowledge or expertise. These topics can also lead to future activities. Some promising questions could be about:

TV: "Seen anything good lately?"

Sports: "What do you think of the coach [of the local team]?"

Holidays: "So what's your favorite thing about Thanksgiving?"

Recreational activities: "I am a terrible cook. What should I make tonight?" "Do you like coffee?" "How should I get more fit?"

Family: "Tell me about your [niece, nephew, etc.]."

Helping: "How can I help people more?"

Animals: "What is your favorite pet?"

Religion: "Do you want to go to services?"

You may also find it helpful to use closed-ended questions that allow the person to choose between alternatives. This approach puts less pressure on them to come up with an elaborated response—for example:

"Do you like watching game shows or sports?"

"Winter or summer Olympics?"

"Is the food or being with family the best part?"

"Should I try yoga or weight lifting?"

"Dogs, cats, or neither? Garth Brooks or Billy Ray Cyrus?"

We and others have repeatedly observed that people who have trouble with communicating—confusing speech or not saying much—become much clearer and speak more when the communicating happens during a mutual activity. Talking while *doing* interesting activities together fosters a sense of trust and safety, further lessening the impact of beliefs related to disconnection while also lowering pressure on the person's speech.

Make sure the person notices these benefits during the activity. Several conclusions are useful: doing activities you like makes you feel better and have more energy, doing activities with others is better than doing them alone, talking is easier when you are doing activities with a friendly person.

> After the initial success with Christine, the staff begin to predictably meet with her, doing various activities that interest her. Going for walks, watching videos, drinking coffee, telling stories, and always talking about young kids.
>
>> STAFF MEMBER: It was great going for a walk. I loved hearing all about your ideas for kids. You know so much. How was it for you?
>>
>> CHRISTINE: Good, good.
>>
>> STAFF MEMBER: It's fun, two ladies going for a walk and chatting.
>>
>> CHRISTINE: Yes, fun and easy.
>>
>> STAFF MEMBER: Do you like that?
>>
>> CHRISTINE: Oh yes!
>>
>> STAFF MEMBER: So when you go walking and get to talk, how does that feel?
>>
>> CHRISTINE: Free!
>>
>> STAFF MEMBER: What is the best part of feeling free?
>>
>> CHRISTINE: It all comes out and it's easy to talk.
>>
>> STAFF MEMBER: Yes, I learned a lot.
>>
>> CHRISTINE: Thank you.
>>
>> STAFF MEMBER: Would you like to have more free times?
>>
>> CHRISTINE: Yes. Very much.
>>
>> STAFF MEMBER: If you felt freer, would it make it easier to do things to help kids?
>>
>> CHRISTINE: Yes!
>>
>> STAFF MEMBER: Let's talk more about helping kids next time we get together. This Friday? [*they write this on the whiteboard above Christine's desk*]

You will want to repeat the appealing experiences, drawing the empowering conclusions as a way to build up and energize the person's adaptive mode. This gives you ample opportunities to share your desire to understand, your actual understanding, and to use communication and energy to focus on the life the person wants to be living.

> The staff meet at predictable times each week with Christine. Each starts off by talking about children or watching a video. All notice her excitement, animation, and energy. Christine has a lot to share and pulls from her vast knowledge of development, how infants and toddlers learn, what play means, and so on. When watching a video, she explains her ideas. The staff take care to check that they are "learning correctly" from her. Each time the staff get what she is saying, Christine smiles and appears calmer, more in control. Her speech becomes correspondingly clearer. If Christine begins to struggle with speaking during a visit, the staff focus the discussion—"Do you think this is a song a toddler would like?"—pulling up and playing typical preschool songs on their phone.

> Christine enjoys sharing and the warm feeling of connecting with others. She begins talking with the staff about how to connect with more people. Her sister, who just has given birth, is a natural connection.

Aspirations and Meaning

Energizing the adaptive mode leads to more available resources for activity and speech. It also activates positive beliefs regarding capability and connecting successfully. You want to trade on this and go for the person's aspirations. The person's clearer speech can now be deployed to identify what they want in life. Aspirations will tap into the person's innermost desire to make a difference. Finding the meaning underneath the aspiration will facilitate living this life every day. Developing a powerful image of the aspiration will help the person get through more trying times and develop their strength and resilience.

Discussion of aspirations will also strengthen your relationship. There are few things as exciting as discussing with a friendly person what you most want in life. Even better if you can talk about the best part of the aspiration, what it will feel like, look like, and be like. Hope springs eternal, at least in these conversations. Self-doubt and perceived judgment in the reactions of others is the opposite of hope. This can lead to communication challenges that cut people off from their valued life. To counter this, feel free to repeatedly talk about the aspiration, savoring the best part with the person.

> Every day, Christine experiences her best self. She is doing more with more people. Going on walks and outings. Getting coffee. Sharing her knowledge of children with her sister and with the staff, while they share, in turn, their positive appreciation. Christine draws conclusions about her own capability and other people being terrific collaborators. During a walk Christine appears particularly energized, a staff member decides to ask about her aspirations:
>
> STAFF MEMBER: This is really great, you are sharing with all of us, including your sister. How does that feel?
>
> CHRISTINE: Warm.
>
> STAFF MEMBER: Where do you feel it?
>
> CHRISTINE: I feel it here. [*pointing to her chest*]
>
> STAFF MEMBER: Are there other times you might be able to feel that?
>
> CHRISTINE: Teaching.
>
> STAFF MEMBER: Is that something you want to do?
>
> CHRISTINE: Yes! I want to teach toddlers. They are the best!
>
> STAFF MEMBER: Sounds exciting. What would be the best part about teaching toddlers?
>
> CHRISTINE: They learn from exploring.
>
> STAFF MEMBER: Sounds like you can help them become good people.
>
> CHRISTINE: Yes! From the very first step!
>
> STAFF MEMBER: You totally could! Paint me a picture. What would it look like?
>
> CHRISTINE: I can see myself smiling. They are all playing. I can see their little smiles and colorful outfits.
>
> STAFF MEMBER: That is beautiful.

Aspirations are added to Christine's Recovery Map in Figure 10.3.

Actualizing the Adaptive Mode

When you have an energized adaptive mode, well-developed aspirations, and the meaning the person is going for, you are ready to collaborate on concerted action. Aspirations offer two simultaneous paths to pursue. The first is linked to the underlying meaning. There is activity every day that the person can participate in to successfully experience their values on a regular basis. There are numerous roles that can enable the person's purpose. Roles are a terrific way to make a difference and to belong. Each time the person is successful in their role, they can feel capable—that their efforts matter. During these experiences it is unlikely that the person will feel judged, stressed, or incapable. You can help them notice this and strengthen the beliefs that ease communication and connection.

The second path is to help the person take the steps that move them toward realizing the broader aspiration. It involves a growth of the person's life space, meeting new people, overcoming new challenges, experiencing more success, and living one's capability. The new people in the person's life will have shared interests and provide opportunities for communication success and social success. Acquaintances can become friends. These are huge strides in getting a desired life. You can help the person see this progress all along the way. And you can also help them to take setbacks in stride.

> The staff and Christine talk about the best part of teaching toddlers for a few encounters, each time developing the image and meaning a little bit more. During one of these visits, the staff members ask, "What do you need to do to be able to teach toddlers?" Christine answers, "School." They start a discussion about the steps to get back to school and write out those steps using a tool similar to that in Appendix F, alongside the best parts about being a toddler teacher. They plan action for the next several days. At the same time, they think about ways that Christine can experience the helping feeling now. They hit on volunteering.
>
> Christine's weeks become focused on volunteering at a local nursery school, and systematically working on getting back to school—practicing studying, reading interesting material, looking for schools, and watching teaching videos online. She experiences success in the volunteering, getting positive feedback from the teacher, parents, and the children. And she also makes steady progress toward starting school. This activity puts her in contact with many new people. She worries less and less about rejection, as success compounds success.
>
> Christine begins to dream more about the life she wants, as it starts to seem more and more possible. Among her new aspirations are a home, a rescue dog, and kids of her own.

ASPIRATIONS	
Goals: • Teaching toddlers • Volunteering at local nursery	Meaning of Accomplishing Identified Goal: • I am capable • I am connected • I can trust others • I am knowledgeable

FIGURE 10.3. Adding goals and aspirations to Christine's Recovery Map.

Strengthening the Adaptive Mode and Building Resilience

As individuals realize their desired life, there are many opportunities to strengthen this adaptive mode of living. This work can focus on positive beliefs about capability, belonging, and making a difference. The self is able and strong, others are favorable and worthwhile, and the future is bright and interesting. These will all reduce communication challenges.

The person will still experience setbacks, and they might even have bouts of communication difficulty from time to time. However, you can help the person to not globalize these experiences. It is a part of life to experience stress and to have difficulty talking. It doesn't mean they are defective. And they have developed many ways to be empowered when life gets tough. That means they have resilience.

> With each step of progress, Christine gains more access to her motivation and energy. She feels good much of the time. There are setbacks. Her application to school gets misplaced, she has a day volunteering where her words are hard to control. When talking with the staff at her residence, Christine sees these as experiences she can learn from, ones that make her stronger. Together they conclude that she is always understood by others in the end. And everyone can have difficulty when speaking from time to time. These conclusions help strengthen her drive forward.
>
> After Christine presents her favorite book to the children in the nursery school class, the teacher begins using this presentation as an example to others. When sitting with the staff later, Christine sees that she must have been clear, precise, effective, and enjoyable for the kids—bolstering her confidence. She realizes that she is very capable of teaching toddlers. Even more important than being understood, Christine sees herself as powerfully enabling young lives.

Christine's full Recovery Map is illustrated in Figure 10.4.

ADDITIONAL CONSIDERATIONS

Be Regular, Frequent, Brief, and Jovial

Those who experience a significant challenge with communication may not have much opportunity to successfully talk, let alone connect, with others. In their isolation, they may have concluded that others are not interested in them, and that others don't mean it when they say they want to talk later. Put another way, the person is out of practice talking and may be quick to give up. They might also expect you not to show up when you say you will.

You can counter this demoralization by seeing the person predictably and frequently. Let the person know when you are coming. The encounters do not have to last all that long, just long enough to do something together, show a little interest, and help them experience a success with you. The predictability shows you care. It also counters any worries about when the person will have a chance to try to connect with you again. Think of the person as being thirsty for connection, wanting to share, but feeling very demoralized and protecting themselves at the same time.

The more cheerful or friendly you can be, the lighter your visits will be, and the more the person will grow to look forward to them.

Recovery Map	
ACCESSING AND ENERGIZING THE ADAPTIVE MODE	
Interests/Ways to Engage: • Children	Beliefs Activated while in Adaptive Mode: • I am connected • I am knowledgeable • It's worth connecting with other people
ASPIRATIONS	
Goals: • Teaching toddlers • Volunteering at local nursery • Having a home • Getting a dog • Having a family of her own	Meaning of Accomplishing Identified Goal: • I am capable • I am connected • I can trust others • I am knowledgeable
CHALLENGES	
Current Behaviors/Challenges: • Speech is hard to follow • Hits herself • Talks about sky falling	Beliefs Underlying Challenges: • I am disconnected • I am unsafe • People don't understand me • I'm stupid
POSITIVE ACTION AND EMPOWERMENT	
Current Strategies and Interventions: • Watch videos about children • Walking and talking about ways to help children • Draw conclusions about volunteering	Beliefs/Aspirations/Meanings/Challenges Targeted: • I am helpful • I have purpose • People care about me and understand what matters most to me • I can connect with others

FIGURE 10.4. Christine's completed Recovery Map.

Show You Care and Want to Understand

Many people with communication challenges are keenly sensitive to being judged. So much so, that they anticipate negative evaluation and rejection in each interaction. This can lead them to avoid interactions, give one-word answers, or talk in a difficult-to-follow manner. You can help disarm this defensiveness by taking two related tacks: show a clear desire to understand and then demonstrate that you get what the person is saying when communication is successful.

Be dogged in showing your desire to understand. By showing you want to understand, your actions provide counterevidence for negative expectations. What they have to say matters to you, and you can put the onus on yourself for needing some time to get it right. Use reflection.

Slow down the interaction. Make sure you understand. Be direct that it matters to you that you get what they are saying correctly. The following are useful prompts:

Give your rationale: "It really matters to me what you have to say" and "I want to make sure I'm getting this right."

Summarize what you heard: "So kids are really important to you and you worry about them?"

Test whether your summary is correct: "Is that about right?"

Empathize with the experience if correct: "That must be upsetting."

If you are having particular difficulty following their speech, pay attention to the emotion. You can say, "It looks like you are really frustrated by something" or "Sounds like that is scary." When you check your understanding ("Am I right about that?"), you convey that you do want to understand and that you are communicating together. You both have a role. This can reduce the sense of isolation and being alone that can make speech more challenging for the person. If you are right about how they feel, then they have successfully communicated. If you get it wrong, then they can correct you—again, success. When you empathize, you show that you get what it feels like to be them ("That sounds like it would be upsetting")—this is connection and acceptance, which are the opposite of the rejection the person fears.

Sometimes individuals get emotional and tear up when you say their thoughts back to them accurately. Being heard may be a rare experience for them. This might be especially poignant if they are trying to share something important, such as a life aspiration.

Try Visual Aids

We all benefit from visual aids, such as dry erase boards, electronics, pictures, or even a pad of paper. These make it easier for us to remember things and not have to hold so much in our minds. Using these aids with the person who experiences communication challenges helps them feel less stressed. Mental resources (memory, attention, planning) can focus on important things, like what you want to do and how to do it. Pictures can be an inspiration for one's aspirations—for example, Christine could place pictures of happy toddlers around her room to remind her of her values and to prime the adaptive mode. Positive beliefs and emotions will facilitate ease in communication.

Relax Together

We all also benefit from an activity that reduces our stress level, be it diaphragmatic breathing, progressive muscle relaxation, or mindfulness (Chadwick, 2014; Varvogli, & Darviri, 2011). Because social disconnection is at the heart of communication challenge, doing one of these activities with the person can be effective. Doing it together activates positive beliefs about you, which reduces worry about being evaluated negatively. It also closes the gap between you and the person because we all can use help feeling less stressed. Of course, the activity itself reduces stress. Relaxation activity together can facilitate some very fine communication, which can begin during the relaxation activity and continue well beyond it.

> **WORDS OF WISDOM**
>
> **BOX 10.1. Releasing the Pressure and Kindling Success**
>
> The need to communicate is present throughout the animal kingdom and is a particularly treasured resource among humans. Having difficulty with speech can devastate one's morale and self-confidence, and lead to a profound sense of being disconnected and damaged. Communication efforts can be hard for others to follow, either because of a jump from idea to idea, unique usages, reduced articulation, or one-word answers. Sometimes the clearest part is an explanation for the difficulty the person experiences, such as "They are hacking away at my brain," "My brain is broken," or "My brain is dead."
>
> Many theories have been advanced to account for this communication challenge (McKenna & Oh, 2005), but the therapeutic approach is straightforward. Keep in mind that the individual is trying hard to communicate and feels thwarted and frustrated when unsuccessful. This puts extra pressure on the need to communicate. We want to lessen this pressure and everyone who interacts with the person can do just that: therapist, doctor, team member, family. Start by engaging in an activity that requires little speaking. Take a walk, look at pictures, paint or draw, watch a funny video, throw a ball, sing and dance. Your choice of activity can be guided by the person's interests and your level of comfort. These activities switch on the adaptive mode, bringing along positive beliefs about self and others, and an uptick in energy and positive feelings.
>
> When the person clearly shows brighter emotion and mood, you can bolster effective nonverbal communication with talking. Use your own experience of having a good time to ask the person about it, and move on to other enjoyable activities with others the person is interested in. Your curiosity and explicit sharing that you understand will foster a sense of safety and self-confidence. It may even be the case that historically more stressful topics come up and the person has an easier time expressing them. By playing to the person's strengths and building them up, you will open a whole domain for a sense of achievement and belonging.

SUMMARY

- Negative beliefs about the ability to communicate can prevent individuals from putting themselves in social situations or circumstances where they would need to communicate—this can start a cycle of isolation.
- To access the adaptive mode with individuals who have difficulty communicating, start out with something action based: watch a video, listen to a song, take a walk.
- Displaying empathy and making frequent attempts at understanding can reduce an individual's stress and demonstrate that others care, are interested, and want to connect.
- The key to continually and regularly accessing and energizing an individual's adaptive mode is drawing conclusions about capability, belonging, success, and the benefits of connecting with others.
- Aspirations provide social roles so a person can realize their best self and bolster against disconnection and other factors that make speech difficult.
- Positive beliefs about connection, capability, and belonging can help to build resilience for when challenges—such as stress and things not going right—arise.

CHAPTER 11

Empowering When Trauma, Self-Injury, Aggressive Behavior, or Substance Use Is the Challenge

She didn't want to talk about it. It seemed like everyone else wanted to talk about it. What happened? Who? Why? Where? How often? Who cares! What did it matter? What did she matter? Sometimes she felt nothing. Sometimes everything all at once. Anger, sadness, indifference, disappointment, guilt, shame. Sometimes the feelings built up over time; sometimes they crashed like a wave. There were all sorts of thoughts: Why her? Of course, her. No good. Bad. Stupid. Why not her? Others have it worse. Do people bother others the way they bother her? She tried so many things to show her strength: sometimes being strong against herself, sometimes strong against others, sometimes with what she'd consume. No one else seemed to see this as strong. She didn't want to talk about it. So why does it feel like it's everywhere? Her therapist knew she didn't want to talk about it. But—what *did* she want?

The experience of trauma—whether diagnostically significant or not—can potentially impact an individual's perception of themselves, others, the future, and the world. Reactions to these traumatic experiences may include causing harm to the self, reacting against others, and turning to substances as a solution (Center for Substance Abuse Treatment, 2014). Though these challenges can present independently of trauma, they frequently go together (Beck et al., 2014), and there is considerable overlap in understanding them. In this chapter, we show how we think about trauma and how each stage of recovery-oriented cognitive therapy can be used to address common underlying beliefs. We then consider how to use CT-R to understand and empower individuals who engage in self-injurious behavior, aggression, and substance use.

Given the complexities associated with all of these topics, it is important that we make clear that we are referring to the experience of trauma broadly. For some, the impact of trauma is to meet criteria for posttraumatic stress disorder (PTSD; American Psychiatric Association, 2013). In these circumstances, some individuals may wish to address the trauma head-on through evidence-based PTSD treatment, such as cognitive processing therapy (Resick, Monson, & Chard, 2017) or prolonged exposure (de Bont et al., 2013). Methods for this and other trauma treatments extend beyond the scope of this book.

In this chapter, we first describe a basic cognitive understanding of trauma and how the procedures of CT-R can be used to address some specific challenges. We then focus on the application of CT-R to self-injurious behavior, aggression, and substance use. Our focus is narrow in scope, but we acknowledge the vast and varied approaches used to address these challenges.

HOW TO THINK ABOUT TRAUMA

Many individuals with serious mental health conditions and those who present with complex challenges have had experiences that are perceived as traumatic. Traumatic experiences can range from physical, sexual, and emotional abuses to accidents, hospitalization, poverty, community violence, and so on. Individuals who have experienced one traumatic event have quite likely had multiple such experiences (van den Berg & van der Gaag, 2012). Sometimes you don't always know exactly what happened because, like the woman described at the start, they don't want to talk about it. But you may wonder: Is the behavior I'm seeing because this person has suffered? Whether it is in one way or many ways, one time or repeatedly, you might wonder whether the approach you're taking is trauma informed. Is the impact of the person's experience being considered? In CT-R, a trauma-informed approach is one that considers the ways in which difficult events have impacted how an individual feels, thinks, and interacts with the world. Those ways may make it more difficult to progress toward living a more meaningful life.

Some of the feelings associated with experiences of trauma include fear, shock, sadness, distrust, paranoia, shame, and loneliness. In attempts to understand their experiences, individuals might translate these intense, unpleasant emotions into thoughts about self, others, and the world. Common thoughts revolve around *self-concept* and *worth* (e.g., "It must have been my fault," "I am worthless," "I am weak"), *safety* (e.g., "I am unsafe," "People are dangerous and can't be trusted," "There's nothing I can do to keep myself safe"), *connection* (e.g., "Others don't understand," "Others will take advantage of me"), and *control* (e.g., "The world is unpredictable and unsafe"; "I can't do things I want to do"; "There's no point in trying, I can't get what I want anyway"). If the person believes themselves to be worthless, unsafe, disconnected, and out of control, it's not too big a stretch to see no hope for the future. In response to this way of seeing the world, people attempt to keep themselves safe and regain control over their experiences. They may isolate and stop taking care of themselves, shut down in the presence of conflict, harm themselves, hurt others, engage in sexually expressive behaviors, or engage in frequent reassurance seeking from others (Beck et al., 2014).

For individuals with serious mental health conditions, beliefs rooted in trauma could underlie some of their challenges, such as reduced access to motivation, social withdrawal, reduced expectations

> **Common beliefs resulting from trauma include:**
>
> *Self-Concept*
> ✓ It must have been my fault.
> ✓ I am worthless.
> ✓ I am weak.
>
> *Safety*
> ✓ I am unsafe.
> ✓ People are dangerous and can't be trusted.
> ✓ There's nothing I can do to keep myself safe.
>
> *Connection*
> ✓ Others don't understand.
> ✓ Others will take advantage of me.
>
> *Control*
> ✓ The world is unpredictable and unsafe.
> ✓ I can't do the things I want to do.
> ✓ There's no point in trying; I can't get what I want.

of pleasure, reduced energy, and reduced communication. Voices may repeatedly say things about the traumatic event(s) or the beliefs individuals have developed as a result (Romme & Escher, 1989). Expansive beliefs may be expressed to protect against future harm. Paranoia can reach extremes.

This list is not exhaustive, but each is important to consider as you develop your rich understanding of each individual you serve. How the person perceives and responds to trauma informs your approach to empowerment.

WHAT TO DO ACROSS CHALLENGES

No matter how the challenges present, each stage of CT-R provides opportunities to use guided discovery (see Chapter 6) to strengthen positive beliefs and shift those rooted in trauma in a way that inspires action. In particular, CT-R addresses trauma-based beliefs related to self-concept, safety with others, control, and power.

Accessing and Energizing the Adaptive Mode

Because accessing the adaptive mode (see Chapter 3) evokes strengths, skills, and positive beliefs about capability, it provides a natural opportunity to draw conclusions around self-concept and worth. For individuals who thrive in the expert role, you can ask questions about the self: "What does that say about you that you taught us how to beat this level of your video game?" You can also ask questions about the individual's impact on others: "What does this say about your ability to teach others? You've added a lot of value to our group, what do you think?" To energize the adaptive mode, you can ask, "You've said you feel valuable and like you're contributing when you're playing video games and teaching us. I imagine you might also feel proud, is that right? Would it be worth doing this more often?" The more individuals engage in activities that make them feel proud and important, the more opportunities you have to strengthen those beliefs and counter worthlessness.

Accessing and energizing the adaptive mode can also provide safe experiences with others that help shift beliefs about the dangerousness of others—for example, by engaging in pleasurable activities with others, individuals are experiencing safety in a group. You do not want to draw the conclusion that everyone is safe; rather, "though there may be people who do harm in the world, this is not *always* the case." Perhaps, therefore, "it's worth engaging with others sometimes simply because it can be fun."

Similarly, connection and trust are front and center when accessing and energizing the adaptive mode. If the woman who does not initially want to talk about what she experienced ever decided to address the trauma directly, how would it be possible in the absence of connection and trust? At a more global level, the accessing and energizing procedures can demonstrate that there are, in fact, people who are interested in getting to know them, their interests, their skills, and that others actually *can* and *do* appreciate and understand them. This has great impact even if the individual never wants to talk about the trauma.

Individuals can experience greater control and predictability during this stage. Control comes from selecting preferred activities, deciding when and with whom to do them, and by being in the expert role of teaching others. Predictability can come from interventions, such as positive action scheduling, where the person plans the next positive experience in advance. By choosing to engage in their interests or use their skills, individuals can also draw conclusions that they are in control of their emotional reactions—they can overcome stress, generate their own energy, and bring about positive emotion themselves.

Developing the Adaptive Mode—Aspirations

Aspirations (see Chapter 4) provide hope, and there is great power in achieving the meaning of the aspiration. When individuals share their highly valued aspirations, you gain a perspective on how they want to see themselves and how they hope others will see them. As you collaboratively create vivid and detailed recovery images, you can also collaborate on the narrative the individual hopes to tell to support their self-worth—for example, you can ask, "What would it mean about you to achieve this?" or "What would it say about your value as a person," or "What good can you bring to others if you pursue this dream?" This can inform how you use guided discovery as the individual takes steps toward achievement in the next stage.

When individuals share their aspirations with you, it can enhance mutual connection and trust. It takes a fair amount of trust to reveal one's meaningful desires in the first place, but even more so when trauma has impacted a person's beliefs about others as uncaring, hurtful, or dangerous. Enriching aspirations through imagery and eliciting the positive emotions that are connected to the aspiration invites the person to be even more vulnerable. Successfully sharing this provides further opportunity to strengthen beliefs like "Others care about what I want," "Others can understand me and what's important to me," and "It's worth sharing with others."

Linked with this are beliefs around safety—having the experience of being safe emotionally to share deep meaningful desires with someone and have these be respected. To draw the person's attention to this, you can say, "How was it sharing that with me just now? It looked like just talking about it got you excited! I'm excited to work together with you toward getting you there! I wonder if that went better than you expected?"

Developing aspirations can also shift beliefs about power and control, because the individual is the one who makes the determination about what missions they would like to pursue. This puts the individual in the position of a leader and expert in their own recovery, and you in the position of collaborative partner. In the leader role, the person can guide the interaction and their future—for example, you can draw the individual's attention to this by saying, "No one knows what you want for the future better than you. I just know some ways other people have gotten to reach their aspirations. So together, I think we could be a pretty good team. What do you think?" If individuals change their minds about what they would like in the future, you have another opportunity to emphasize the control they have. Asking about aspirations focuses attention on something a person wants or hopes for. It puts trauma into perspective and inspires the idea that the trauma a person may have experienced does not define them or their life.

Specific interventions for developing and enriching aspirations across challenges include techniques for recalling the aspirations(s) and associated imagery, such as using empowerment cards or vision boards. When doubts or fear arise, the individual can use these tools to refocus their attention on their aspirations and the respective meanings.

Actualizing the Adaptive Mode

Break aspirations down into steps and take action toward them or their meanings (see Chapter 5). This will provide some of the best opportunities to strengthen empowering beliefs and counter those developed as a result of trauma. You might say, "When we first started, you weren't sure you were capable of taking even small steps toward your goals. Now you're accomplishing something each day. What does that say about you?" For individuals who held beliefs about not deserving good things or not being worthy of living a meaningful life, you might say, "What does achieving this step mean about your ability to achieve your dream?" or "You said you feel good and strong to have taken steps that get you closer to your aspiration. You had the dream; you took the steps, and you reaped the rewards. It seems like you might deserve better than you even realized. What do you think about that?"

The collaborative pursuit of aspirations provides opportunities for individuals to see that not all people are bad or dangerous, neutralizing beliefs about safety. Beliefs about connection can also be strengthened, as you are working together toward a common goal. Taking steps toward aspirations can be scary or intimidating—taking active steps with someone who understands can ease that tension and strengthen the conclusions that it's worth doing things with others.

Actualizing the adaptive mode can also counter defeatist beliefs and increase an individual's sense of control about the future. Individuals can strengthen beliefs such as "I am the one who took these steps, so I'm taking control over my success." Successful pursuit of aspirations can also help individuals to feel in control despite the trauma: "I can live well despite what happened to me. By reaching for the things that matter to me, I am not a victim." Positive experiences feel more predictable because they are planned. Success and action are more consistent, which can strengthen both control and safety beliefs.

It is during the actualizing stage that you can actively work together with individuals to overcome challenges. This provides the context for developing empowerment beliefs specifically related to whatever it is that might be impacting movement toward aspirations—for example, some may draw conclusions like "I am strong and have the ability to keep myself safe by being assertive, which will ultimately get me closer to my goals" or "The person who has the most control in the situation is the one who doesn't react with hostility. Refocusing on what I care about gives me power and gets me closer to where I want to be."

As one individual shared with us: "One of my favorite things about CT-R is that it didn't focus on what happened to me as much as it focused on how what happened to me impacts my life now." What you might find is that going through the CT-R steps sufficiently helps a person move forward, navigate their life, and build resiliency without digging into the details. For others, the CT-R process moves them forward enough so that they then decide they are ready for deeper-level processing of their trauma. In both situations, the mission remains their pursuit of aspirations and living the meaningful life of their choosing. They are ultimately in control of their story.

Taken in sum, the strategies and techniques of CT-R are inherently trauma informed. Therefore, when challenges such as self-injury, aggression, or substance use are the issue, beliefs tied to trauma are readily built into the formulation. The following sections address the nuances of how to understand these particular challenges and what you can do to facilitate empowerment.

HOW TO THINK ABOUT SELF-INJURIOUS BEHAVIOR

Self-injurious behaviors include actions done to oneself, such as cutting, burning, swallowing objects, inserting objects into the body, head banging, and so on. In this section, we are explicitly referring to nonsuicidal self-injury (Nock, 2009), meaning that individuals are not engaging in self-harm with the intention or hope of killing themselves. This does not mean that the behaviors are superficial—in fact, many acts of self-harm have the potential for unintended serious outcomes (Hooley & Franklin, 2017), making them all the more important to understand. It may seem as though these behaviors occur randomly or unpredictably, but using a CT-R approach can help you understand what a person might be experiencing that leads to self-injury. Our understanding of self-injurious behavior (see Figure 11.1) begins with individuals' basic vulnerabilities: beliefs they have about themselves, others, and the world. Common beliefs associated with self-injury include being worthless, having no control, deserving hurt or pain, and being uncared for by others. There may be an expectation that others will reject them and that the future is hopeless (Beck et al., 2014).

Given these negative expectations, individuals can become hypervigilant—meaning they may seek out evidence that reinforces their beliefs and expectations. Examples of this might be determining that a family member not answering a phone call is intentional and personal, or that a staff member asking the individual to wait a minute before answering a question is a rejection. When these perceived slights occur, individuals may feel diminished, devalued, vulnerable, and powerless. Sometimes individuals are correctly assessing the situation, but sometimes it is a misinterpretation based on how they expect things to be.

> **Common beliefs underlying nonsuicidal self-injury include:**
>
> *Beliefs about Self*
> ✓ I am worthless.
> ✓ I have no control.
> ✓ I deserve hurt or pain.
>
> *Beliefs about Others*
> ✓ No one cares about me.
> ✓ Others will reject me.
>
> *Belief about the Future*
> ✓ The future is hopeless.
>
> *Beliefs about the Self-Injury*
> ✓ Nothing else comforts me.
> ✓ If I act, the urge will stop.

In either case, when an event occurs that triggers these vulnerabilities, two things happen: the person experiences an urge to hurt themselves and another set of beliefs specifically related to the self-injury is activated (e.g., "It's never going to get better"; "This is the only thing that works"; "I can't stand this [the intense emotions, the rejection]"; "Nothing else comforts me"; or "If I act now, the urge will stop"). The individual then acts.

In the moment, self-injury provides relief from the urge and from distress and can take the person's attention off of the immediate event. It can also give the individual the experience of control—control over the urge, and control over others. People in the individual's life often respond to an act of self-harm in very predictable ways (e.g., people run to the individual's side, and depending on the severity,

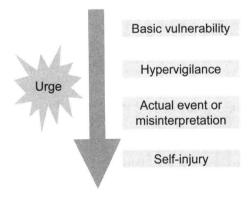

FIGURE 11.1. The self-injury model.

the person receives care in a hospital). However, these benefits are short-lived. The temporary relief is sometimes completely eclipsed by feelings of shame, disappointment, sadness, disconnection, and other emotions that can retrigger the vulnerabilities, leading to a cycle of repeated self-injury. The urge can resurface at any point of the cycle, making the experience all the more intense.

WHAT TO DO—EMPOWERMENT FOR SELF-INJURIOUS BEHAVIOR

The basic vulnerabilities are important clinical targets for intervention. Experiences that enhance connection, control, and hope can be incredibly empowering and lead to new perspectives.

Accessing and Energizing the Adaptive Mode

Because a major root of self-injury is perceived disconnection and rejection, methods for accessing the adaptive mode are very important. These methods unite people, show that you and the individual have more in common than they may have thought, and can put the individual in an expert role. They can then experience control over how interactions with others will go. Being in the adaptive mode also involves experiencing energy and positive emotions that can be used to reduce the intensity of self-harm urges or ward them off altogether. Energizing the adaptive mode by planning continued engagement in pleasurable, connecting activities further increases control by creating greater predictability about the future. For most individuals, having sporadic positive experiences is insufficient, and can even lead to feeling like the future is even more unpredictable. Individuals might not be sure when they will experience positive relief again, and they therefore continue turning to self-injury. Energizing the adaptive mode, however, provides assurance that the good will happen again. By planning to engage in these positive experiences on a regular basis, it is the individual who is in control. Providing as many opportunities as possible for individuals to choose what they will do and how it will look is an important element. Having choices is a form of having greater control.

Techniques for accessing the adaptive mode should be used to start every interaction with an individual. This should be the case even if an incident of injury has recently occurred—perhaps it is even more important in this circumstance. Opening a session or meeting with an individual by asking about the latest celebrity gossip or asking whether they have any new jokes to share demonstrates that the interests of the individual and the connection you share are most important. It can shift expectations about rejection, from beliefs such as "If I hurt myself, even my therapist will abandon me" to "Even though I hurt myself, people still care about me as a whole person." Opening with these strategies can help those who've recently been in crisis or are feeling hopeless build enough energy and cognitive resources to talk about what happened leading up to the injury.

In inpatient settings, people may be put on close observation or have staff within arm's length at all times following an incident of serious self-injury. Direct care staff can keep individuals in the adaptive mode during these shifts through engagement in activities (e.g., playing cards, creating art, listening to music) or creating action plans for when the individual will pursue their interests next. Together, the individual and the staff do not talk about trauma or the self-harm incident but rather focus on keeping the connection alive.

Developing the Adaptive Mode—Aspirations

A key to lasting change is having a sense of purpose and a powerful, motivating reason to do something other than self-harm. The aspirations provide this drive.

Developing a vivid image of future desires is an important technique. Individuals can use these images when situations come up that might otherwise lead to self-injury. The image of what the individual wants to do or get in the future is best when really well developed. What would the future look like? What could they do? Who would they be with? Can they imagine how they would feel? The person might imagine feeling happy, loved, worthy, and in control. This should be an image that, when they think of it, provides a sense of relief, joy, and hope in the moment. For this reason, recovery images can help individuals push through urges and experience greater control and power over negative emotions.

If a person is able to successfully use this approach, you can help them draw conclusions about their capability and how it is worthwhile to focus on the future. With repeated successes, individuals can draw even more conclusions about their own resilience in the face of stress.

Aspirations can also provide context for using problem-solving, relaxation, grounding, or other skills that help individuals overcome urges. Sometimes, individuals will have learned these different mind–body skills in therapy or through reading. However, when the urge comes up, it is not always apparent to the individual why it is worth using the skill over hurting themselves. Aspirations are personal and meaningful, so for many, they may be the reason why it is worth it to use the skills they have. Then, once individuals have used a skill to push through or detract from the urge, the aspirations are compelling targets for refocusing energy. An individual can use the energy they had been putting into negative thoughts and emotions and instead use it toward pursing aspiration-driven actions.

Actualizing the Adaptive Mode

Refocusing on aspirations involves planning and taking steps toward them. Taking action toward aspirations brings a sense of purpose to life. Individuals do not have to just imagine what it would be like to be valuable, worthy, strong, or connected, because they can experience it with every step forward. Techniques that are particularly helpful for individuals who self-harm are positive action scheduling and establishing a meaningful role in the treatment setting, in the community, or with family.

Both techniques involve a person taking control and finding ways in which to belong without the connection being based on the injury. As individuals encounter difficult experiences (e.g., rejection from a family member, the stress of applying to college), techniques such as role-playing can be useful in coming up with different options for responding. If an individual responds to stress using self-injury during this process, you can use a chain analysis (see Chapter 6) to better understand what led to it, thereby improving or confirming your understanding.

Strengthening the Adaptive Mode

Conclusions that can be drawn throughout your collaboration with individuals include:

- "I can have more control than I thought."
- "It can be worthwhile to do things with and for others."

- "Sometimes people might reject you, but that doesn't mean everyone will. And it doesn't mean I'm a complete failure."

At every step, you can ask individuals what it says about them that they were able to take steps toward aspirations. As hardships or stress arise and individuals use new or different methods of resilience, you can ask, "What was it like to do something differently? Did it go better or worse than you thought it might?" and "What does it say about you that you were able to do that instead of hurt yourself?" As people have longer periods of success, you can draw their attention to the difference from when you started to where they are: "What is it that you're experiencing now that you didn't have before?" You can then reflect back the value that individuals put on their experiences of control, purpose, connection, or whatever else they attribute to their achievements. Of these, we have seen purpose be especially effective to help individuals move beyond the cycle of self-injury and on to the life they have always wanted but felt they could never get.

HOW TO THINK ABOUT AGGRESSION

Aggressive behavior is another difficult challenge for individuals, families, and professionals. Individuals may threaten others, cause physical harm to others, damage property, and so on. Like self-injury, acts of aggression can feel unpredictable, happening with no warning.

However, there are ways to understand why it is that someone acts with aggression (see Figure 11.2). The progression from beliefs and vulnerability to aggression follows a path similar to that of self-injury—however, there are additional considerations for what the driving beliefs might be. Individuals may become aggressive when they feel afraid, threatened, or susceptible to danger from others. It might also occur when individuals are frustrated or feel blocked from a goal or having a need met. Disrespect and feeling devalued can be another trigger. Beliefs around powerlessness, having no control, weakness, or being vulnerable may also be involved. Individuals may experience others as controlling, dismissive, and rejecting. This can lead to safety and protection-based beliefs such as "You need to get people before they get you," and "It's better to push people away than to be vulnerable to getting hurt."

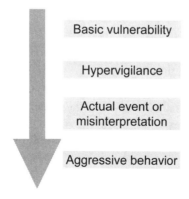

FIGURE 11.2. The aggression model.

> **Common drivers and beliefs underlying aggression include:**
>
> *Drivers for Aggression*
> ✓ Being afraid, threatened, or in danger from others.
> ✓ Feeling frustrated; blocked from a goal.
> ✓ Feeling blocked from having a need met.
> ✓ Feeling disrespected and devalued.
>
> *Beliefs about the Self*
> ✓ I am powerless.
> ✓ I have no control.
> ✓ I am weak and vulnerable.
>
> *Beliefs about Others*
> ✓ You need to get people before they get you.
> ✓ It's better to push people away than to be hurt.
> ✓ Other people take advantage or hurt you.
>
> *Beliefs about the Future/World*
> ✓ The world is dangerous.
> ✓ If I don't fight, I'll undoubtedly be harmed.

In response to these beliefs, individuals may mentally prepare for them to happen—collecting in their mind examples of real or perceived threats, or repeatedly reviewing old threats or rejections in their mind. Individuals may, in effect, become hypersensitive to rejection or threat, seeing it where it may not actually exist (Beck, 1999).

WHAT TO DO—EMPOWERMENT FOR AGGRESSION

Interventions that provide an opposite experience of what the individual expects can ward off triggers to aggression. This involves repeated experiences of connection versus rejection and having control versus being overpowered. Refocusing on the individual's desired life provides the sustaining motivation for responding differently.

Accessing and Energizing the Adaptive Mode

The starting point and driving spirit of CT-R is connection, and the desire to connect is no different in those who respond with aggression from those who experience other challenges. This presents an interesting puzzle. These individuals may desire to connect but they expect that they will be rejected, and aggressive behaviors often have the effect of pushing people away or keeping others at a distance. This creates a cycle of verifying the individual's expectation that they will be rejected or alone, resulting in continued aggressing and withdrawing from others.

Techniques that activate the adaptive mode create the contrary experience. Genuine connection through shared interests or inviting the individual to teach you allows the person to experience inclusion and respect. Individuals feel understood for their strengths and interests, rather than just on the challenges they experience or the behaviors they exhibit. This counters beliefs that no one cares or that they're not good enough.

You need to draw the individual's attention to these moments every time: "This is fun! If it weren't for you, I'd never know how to do this. What do you think about that?" and "Thanks for helping me, you really are a good teacher, don't you think?" Other beliefs you can strengthen include:

- "I am not alone."
- "I have something in common with other people."

Trauma, Self-Injury, Aggressive Behavior, and Substance Use

- "Other people will listen to me."
- "Other people respect my opinion."
- "I can be part of a team."

As the individual experiences connection, it is especially important to make it a more consistent and predictable occurrence. This becomes a powerful contrast to the expectation that the world is unpredictable—for example:

INDIVIDUAL: Everybody loves my sweet potato pie!

PROVIDER: Really? Do you mind me asking what the recipe is or is it a secret?

INDIVIDUAL: [*laughs*] No, it's not a secret, do you really think you can do it?

PROVIDER: I don't know, I hope so!

INDIVIDUAL: Okay. [*Individual and provider go through the recipe; provider writes down the steps.*]

PROVIDER: Oh my goodness! When I make this, can I take a picture of it and show you?

INDIVIDUAL: Sure! That'd be fun.

PROVIDER: This was really fun doing this together. Did you have a good time, too?

INDIVIDUAL: Definitely.

PROVIDER: Do you think we should do this again another time—go through different recipes you know?

INDIVIDUAL: I would love that.

PROVIDER: Are there other people you think might also enjoy talking cooking with you? I wonder if there's anyone you can do this with before I see you next.

Planning future connection increases its predictability; having the individual come up with the type of connection (e.g., sharing recipes) increases control. Suggesting that there may be more people who want to connect in this way introduces the possibility of broadening connection and relationships.

You might be concerned that using accessing and energizing techniques reinforces aggressive behavior. Activities that activate and energize the adaptive mode are enjoyable, but it is important that they not be seen as rewards for "good" behavior—rather, they have an intentional therapeutic value and provide the foundation for future work together. In fact, predictable and consistent connection can prevent aggressive behaviors from happening in the first place.

Developing the Adaptive Mode—Aspirations

Focusing attention on hopes and desires that can be pursued *together* with others reduces beliefs about having no control or being blocked by others. The individual is in the driver's seat because it is *their* aspiration. Your curiosity about the aspiration and help in taking action steps makes for a great team. The more vivid the recovery image, the more powerful and effective it will be at motivating positive change. You might use the image in the following way:

PROVIDER: When you are sitting in the dayroom, feeling really angry about what your brother said to you on the phone, what can you do instead of hitting the wall or getting into a fight?

INDIVIDUAL: I can picture myself in the apartment. Having my cousin over. Playing music. Decorating the walls with pictures of my cat.

PROVIDER: That sounds really great. What will be the best part of thinking about the apartment decorated with cat pictures?

INDIVIDUAL: Reminds me that the other stuff isn't worth it. My brother isn't going to get me to my apartment. I am. Getting put on observation doesn't get me any closer either.

Successfully using the recovery image in this way helps shift beliefs about power and control. The strongest person is the one who doesn't act and stays in control.

Developing and enriching aspirations also provides individuals with experiences of receiving respect. You are demonstrating that their desires matter and that it can be safe to share desires with others. You can guide individuals to notice that they are valued, and that others are not out to get them.

Actualizing the Adaptive Mode

For individuals who expect rejection and dismissal from others, successful pursuit of aspirations can broaden social connections, strengthen existing relationships, or build new ones. Planning and taking action also continues the theme of the individual taking control over their future. It is in this context that you can introduce methods of stress reduction (Varvogli & Darviri, 2011), assertive communication (Bellack, Mueser, Gingerich, & Agresta, 2013), or other approaches to navigating stress better. It is worth using a technique such as progressive muscle relaxation (Jacobson, 1938) when, for example, the individual's parents are in an argument. Another technique is to write out and prepare for a difficult conversation, such as one the person wants to have with their boss.

As people begin making progress toward their goals, challenges are more likely to come up. It is very important to demonstrate genuine empathy and understanding, reiterate the value of connection, and give the individual the opportunity to take control over their story. Two methods for this are (1) summarize, test, empathize, empower and refocus (STEER) and (2) chain analysis.

Summarize, Test, Empathize, Empower and Refocus

Reflective listening is an important intervention, and STEER is especially useful when an individual is particularly upset. You first *summarize* back what the person has said ("I hear you saying that everyone is out to get you and that no one cares." Next, you *test it out* to make sure you are understanding the person correctly ("Have I got that right?"). You then *empathize*, making a statement reflecting how you imagine they might feel, and suggest that you might feel that way yourself in their same circumstance ("I imagine that must feel really lonely and frustrating. I think I might feel the same, given what you said"). This communicates to the individual that you are trying to understand things from their perspective. They are in control of this understanding, by being given a chance to correct what you said. Empathizing is not saying whether or not you think the person is correct or that their actions are right—rather, it is that you can understand why the person might experience things as they do. You can repeat these steps in the process as many times as necessary for an individual to feel heard and let you know that you've got it right. You can often tell this is happening when the individual's posture relaxes, tone of voice is reduced, there's an increase in eye contact, and pacing slows or stops.

After the individual feels heard, you can shift to interventions that *empower*, guiding a person to *refocus* on aspiration-driven action—for example, "Could we try something together to start feeling a bit better?" Bringing each step together, you might say something like "I hear you saying no one cares, have I got that right? I imagine that has to feel very lonely and upsetting. I also know that having that amazing apartment covered with cat pictures is so incredibly important to you. Could we go look at some pictures right now and maybe draw out where they could go in your place?" (STEER steps are illustrated in Figure 11.3; see Figure 11.4 for a clinical example of the process.)

Chain Analysis

You can also use a chain analysis (Beck et al., 2014) to better understand situations that come up (see Chapter 6 for elaboration). Working through what leads up to aggressive incidents can help determine additional points for intervention, such as when it would be good to use relaxation strategies—for example, if a person indicates that treatment team meetings are times when a person feels weak and needs to show strength and power, suggest practicing stress reduction or rehearsing what to say before the next meeting. These interventions now fit into a broader

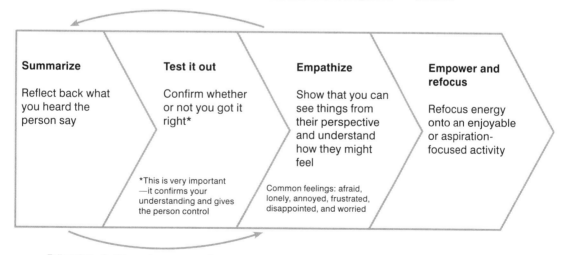

FIGURE 11.3. The steps of the STEER process.

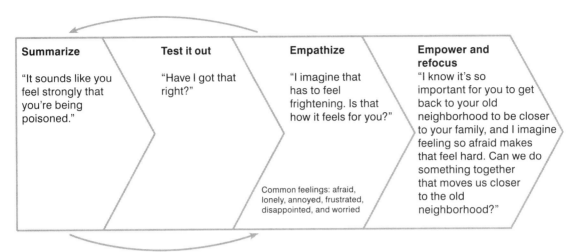

FIGURE 11.4. A clinical example of the STEER process.

context. Getting through a treatment team meeting without becoming aggressive gets the person closer to their aspirations and gives them control and strength in a situation where they previously viewed themselves as vulnerable.

Strengthening the Adaptive Mode

Strengthening positive beliefs about safety, connection, strength, and control are paramount for individuals who respond to situations with aggression. Resiliency beliefs can also be more fully developed, such as "Others may expect me to react, but I can show how strong I am by living a great life" or "Just because something didn't go how I wanted it to, doesn't mean I don't have a lot I want to try and do." Beliefs such as these and the others highlighted throughout the different stages of CT-R can refocus energy away from the target of frustration and toward the future.

HOW TO THINK ABOUT SUBSTANCE USE

There are people who have spent years and decades in a daily cycle of using. Their drug of choice may be alcohol. It might be prescription medications, such as Oxycontin. It could be street drugs, such as crack cocaine, heroin, or K2. Some are homeless on the street, or in the woods. Others live in group homes or in their own apartment but reject most case management. They may not be help seeking at all. They often have other challenges, some mental health, some physical, frequently related to years of using.

Despite what might seem like cultural ambivalence (some substances are legal, some not), there is considerable stigma for use (Birtel, Wood, & Kempa, 2017). The person who uses substances can see themselves in these terms: weak, incapable, dependent, inferior, and without hope. Judgment of one's self can be harsh; the judgment of others—both experienced and anticipated—can be witheringly severe. For some people, disconnection may be at the heart of continuous substance use or frequent relapse. The person may feel ashamed. They may not trust others. They may feel isolated. They may feel that others are capable, while they are not. Their beliefs might include "Something is wrong with me," "Others are out there to hurt me," or "It is not worth being around other people."

A counterweight to these beliefs is the good that the person perceives comes from each act of using. You will want to know what the person is getting out of using. What is the best part about it? Does using make them feel good? Does it give them temporary relief from trauma-related images, ideas, or other unpleasant thoughts and feelings? Is the act of using the only chance they have to be social? To feel connected? To be one of the group? Is using a source of control? A way to make an uncertain life predictable for a short time?

Another consideration is the urge to use; the person feels compelled. The urge is experienced as overwhelming, unendurable, awful. The person may believe they cannot stand it any longer and give in to the urge: "I couldn't help it. The feeling was too strong." The person may not want to continue; they may be tired of it but feel stuck and out of control. And using feels good. Afterward, they may feel worse about themselves, more alone, more ashamed, and more defective (Beck, Wright, Newman, & Liese, 1993).

It is hard work to stop the cycle of using substances. Individuals may have tried and not succeeded multiple times. They may have found that others minimize how tough it is, further demoralizing them, as well as enhancing the stark sense of disconnection. In order for them to have a better chance of success, you need to be mindful of the negative beliefs they have about their own incapability, as well as their lack of trust in you. You need to help them activate different beliefs, building up the adaptive mode and trusting relationships. You need to collaborate to develop a vision of life that realizes their values. Achieving the meanings of their aspirations provides the countervailing power to the urge. They can refocus their energy away from using and toward activities that help them feel connected and purposeful in some way. They can go from feeling weak to feeling strong. They can come to experience empowerment for having a life they have never thought possible.

Common beliefs underlying substance use include:

Beliefs about the Self
- ✓ I am weak.
- ✓ I am incapable.
- ✓ I am an addict.
- ✓ I'm dependent.
- ✓ I'm inferior.
- ✓ I'm disconnected.

Beliefs about Others
- ✓ Others are out there to hurt me.
- ✓ It is not worth being around other people.
- ✓ Others are capable, I'm not.
- ✓ No one understands why I need this.

Belief about the Future
- ✓ The future is hopeless.

Beliefs about Substance Use
- ✓ I couldn't help it; the feeling was too strong.
- ✓ This is the only way I belong/am connected to others.

WHAT TO DO—EMPOWERMENT FOR SUBSTANCE USE

Accessing the Adaptive Mode

Getting started requires care and patience. You want to access their best self. However, they may not be thrilled to see you. Experience may suggest to them that they cannot trust you, that meeting with you is not worth it, or that something bad could happen that is out of their control. Conversations about their using are likely to fire up all of the negative beliefs.

You have to go to them, put the energy in. Finding the hook may take persistence and repeated visits. Putting them one up as the expert is a good lead move. You are looking for interests, activities, and conversations that will connect you. You might be surprised by what works: puzzles, pets, reading, being in nature, fishing, music, art. Consider the following:

> Two members of Joe's case management team approach him while he is lying on a street grate, appearing tired. Joe has drunk a fifth of vodka a day for 40 years.
>
> PROVIDER: Hi, Joe! I have this great job. I get to talk with people about what they want.
> JOE: Okay. Leave me alone.
> PROVIDER: Sure. But I need your help. Can you tell me what song this is?
> JOE: [*bopping head a bit while listening*] Ike and Tina Turner.
> PROVIDER: Yes!
> JOE: Proud Mary.
> PROVIDER: Right!
> JOE: [*beginning to move more*] A good one. I like the fast part.
> PROVIDER: [*beginning to dance*] Me too! This is fun.
> JOE: Yeah, not bad.
> PROVIDER: Want to listen to another?
> JOE: Not sure.
> PROVIDER: What is this?
> JOE: [*smiling*] Brick House. [*gets up*]
> PROVIDER: [*after they both dance to the song for a bit*] You seem to know a lot about music.
> JOE: I do.
> PROVIDER: I am going to come back on Friday. Maybe you can help me learn more about good music. What should I know?
> JOE: I don't know about that.

Energizing the Adaptive Mode

It is important to not hurry things. You have found one hook. You will look for many. Trust is not easily developed—the person has a lifetime of experience of disappointment that your work together will counter. You will do well to spend a good amount of time on the top box of the Recovery Map. Doing things together can lead to other activities that energize the adaptive mode and strengthen the connection. You can begin to think about what beliefs might be active when you are doing activities—Is it fun being with others? Belonging? Being a helping person?

> JOE: [*as the team member approaches*] You need to know Peter Frampton.
> PROVIDER: Peter who?

Trauma, Self-Injury, Aggressive Behavior, and Substance Use

> JOE: Get out! Frampton!
>
> PROVIDER: Never heard of him. [*pulls name up on phone*]
>
> JOE: That's it. [*bobbing his head*]
>
> PROVIDER: [*bobbing too*] This is great. You are teaching me about music.
>
> JOE: Good music.
>
> PROVIDER: Right.
>
> JOE: I used to go see live music—long time back.
>
> PROVIDER: Wow—Is that something you want to do?
>
> JOE: Yeah. [*smiling*] Do you know Boz Scaggs?

As you have a consistent and safe connection, aspirations will begin to emerge.

Aspirations and Meaning

Similar to the other challenges in this chapter, empowerment is hard work with substance use. The urges are strong. The person feels weak. It is easy for them to give in. Finding the person's mission is critical. Aspirations are at the heart of this process. Getting that meaning into life makes the hard work more palatable and more possible. The effort has to be worth it. The bigger things in life are the fulcrum.

> PROVIDER: [*after listening to some new music together*] This is fun. How are you feeling?
>
> JOE: I like this music thing we do. But I am tired of living this way. The street. The booze. [*shaking head*]
>
> PROVIDER: I hear you. If you weren't living this like this, what would you want to be doing?
>
> JOE: [*shrugs*] I am not sure. [*pause*]
>
> JOE: Is there something with music? Something you used to like or want?
>
> JOE: Fishing. . . . Playing in a band. . . . I used to do both. [*smiling*]
>
> PROVIDER: Those sound great.
>
> JOE: Yeah. [*smiling more broadly*]
>
> PROVIDER: What would be the best part?
>
> JOE: Doing bigger things together. Making something beautiful. Being close to nature.
>
> PROVIDER: Sounds wonderful. Paint me a picture. . . .

Talking about aspirations produces hope, enhances access to energy, and strengthens your relationship. The image is a powerful counter to the craving the person experiences. And the conversation can lead to developing an action plan. You can have the person focus on the emotion they will feel when achieving the aspiration.

The Pie Technique

A variation you can consider in developing aspirations is the "pie technique" (Beck, 2020). Start by talking about what the person cares about. What are potential sources of satisfaction for them: other people (family, friends), recreation (hobbies, sports, art), using their special talents (teaching, volunteering)? Discuss the significance of each source until you see that the individual experiences emotion. This part can create energy and access to motivation regarding getting these activities into everyday life more. Now draw a circle and put each of the activities in, one by one, asking how much satisfaction the person has in each area and how much time and energy they are putting into those currently. See Figure 11.5 for an example of how this might look.

You can then compare how much time and energy the person is spending on their substance use behaviors, as a way to develop resolve to get through tough feelings. Draw a circle and ask what proportion of this pie is invested in addiction-related activities. You can compare this to the satisfaction pie. The individual may see that the more desired items are being crowded out by the substance use. This recognition can help marshal the person toward empowerment:

> PROVIDER: All of these things seem really important to you and I know you are really upset with the care you've gotten thus far. I can't promise you'll feel better or find the care any better tomorrow, but will using more get you closer to those important things or get you further away?

Actualizing—Positive Action

The person's strength will become obvious to them and others as they are able to bring about their most desired life, experiencing deeper meaning and satisfaction daily. You can help the person to see this strength. They are capable, not incompetent. They are valuable, not valueless. They have control, rather than being helpless. They are strong, not weak.

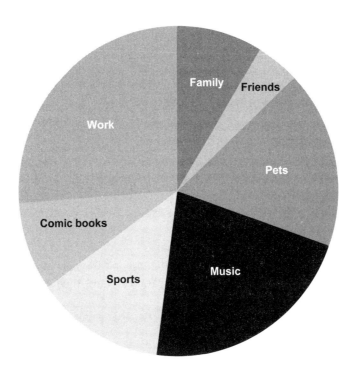

FIGURE 11.5. Using the pie technique for finding values.

As the person begins to stretch themselves, the stress of daily life comes up and substance use cravings will likely get stronger. You can trade on your good relationship. Determining the role the use plays for the person can be especially helpful. Together you can think of other ways to meet the same need:

PROVIDER: So when you drink you get some peace?

JOE: Yeah.

PROVIDER: What if we worked together to get the peace without having to drink, would you like that? Then you have options?

JOE: What do you mean?

PROVIDER: You have lots of ways to get peace. Drinking might be one, but you also would have others. Would it be worth trying to find some of those?

JOE: We can try.

PROVIDER: Then if you have more peace, would that make it easier or harder to find members to form your music band?

Your aim is to help the person achieve their aspirations. These meaningful pursuits have a gravitational pull. Empowerment comes as they refocus away from cravings and toward the positive values that are represented in active pursuit of aspirations.

Strengthening

Throughout this empowering process you are drawing the person's attention to important experiences that strengthen their best self. Resilience resides in the realization that the urge to use will pass. As painful and unpleasant as it is, as easy as it would be to give in, the person can ride out the urge. This conclusion can be drawn repeatedly.

Further, there are things the person can do to not focus on the urge. These include doing activities that matter, often with others. This refocusing involves the person's sense of agency. You can gently draw the person's attention to this. Who chose to play the piano? Who went to volunteer? Who went fishing? What does that say about you?

Resilience is important when individuals experience a setback. The key move is to collaborate with them to put a flare-up of use in context. It is not a catastrophe. All of the gains are not washed away. We learn from every experience. We are all fallible and strong at the same time. A slip is just that. We all have them. It is part of being human. What does the person really care about? Can they still do that? Of course they can. As you help them work toward doing it, you can also investigate what led to the slip. How can they deal with it better next time?

ADDITIONAL CONSIDERATIONS

Behavior Change Can Take Time

Initiating and moving through the stages of CT-R does not mean immediate alleviation of the challenge. People will likely continue to hurt themselves, respond with aggression, and use substances while you begin working through the steps. Abstinence from harm or use should never be used as a prerequisite for therapy. Part of your mission will be to find ways of connecting in spite of the challenge, to uncover the meaning of the behavior, and to focus intervention around desires for the future. It is likely that these behaviors will continue until a person begins experiencing and noticing their successes.

Relapse Happens

Even if someone has had an extensive period of refraining from risky behaviors, relapse happens. When it does, you can work collaboratively with the person to understand what happened. Was a vulnerability triggered? Were they afraid they would ultimately fail and acted to make it so? Whatever the case may be, connection and aspirations will continue to be the center around which these more difficult conversations happen.

Continuing to focus energy on the aspirations provides the opportunity to de-catastrophize relapse. You can give the person an opportunity to think through what happened, but it is not automatically the central focus—for example, you can say, "What might be the best use of our time today? Should we go through the day leading up to the incident and figure it out, or should we do something related to your aspiration and come back later to figuring this out?" The person has control through choice in the situation, and you demonstrate again that the most important thing is the life they are working toward.

You will also want to be sure that you are using guided discovery questions that align with strengthening the most significant positive beliefs, and countering those that underlie the relapse. Figure 11.6 shows how each of the steps of CT-R help a person get through these setbacks.

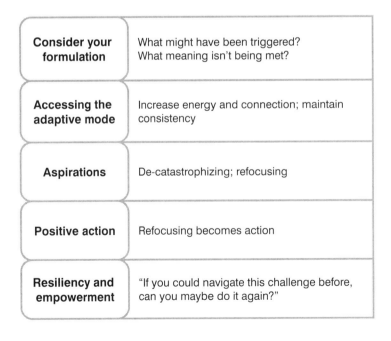

FIGURE 11.6. Getting through setbacks.

Provider Safety and Risk of Aggression

You may be concerned that attempting to connect with individuals with a history of aggression will put you at an increased risk of harm. This is where a CT-R understanding can be incredibly helpful. How do you understand what fuels the aggression? For many people, rejection is at the core of aggression. Avoidance and disconnection should increase the likelihood of an aggressive incident. Accessing the adaptive mode, which embodies connection and trust, should, therefore, put you in a position of being safer.

In the Heat of a Crisis

Sometimes you may find that you are actively in a crisis situation. Someone is tearing things off the wall, running after someone, or trying to harm themselves. In those times, you may have very specific protocols to follow for your place of work and CT-R in no way replaces that.

However, in CT-R the aim is connection during these turbulent moments, which can be effective at deescalating an intense situation and also in helping people rebound after an event has occurred.

With deescalation, it is especially important to use your understanding of the individual to reflect genuine empathy and understanding: "I can see how angry you are—help me understand what happened" or "I know we've talked about how sometimes everything feels so hopeless; I also know we've said sometimes it's not. Can we do something together to get us there right now?" You can also reference aspirations: "I hear you; you're disappointed and frustrated and it seems like everyone is against you. Is that right? I also know that you are doing everything you can to be the best aunt in the world for your nephew. I'm wondering if we can channel this energy into working on something to make for him. At least to see if we can take the edge off. What do you think? Is it worth a try?" You can use the STEER technique as well.

After an act of aggression, self-injury, or substance use has occurred, you can use the same approach to demonstrate to the person that even though this happened, you still care, are interested in them, and that it does not mean the person has lost any progress made—for instance, you still start off a session with a joke, with music, or by asking about the recent football game. Connection and getting in the adaptive mode fortify your relationship, making it easier to move into talking about the incident itself.

Consideration for Different Provider Roles

Everyone working with an individual can have a meaningful role in helping them overcome challenges related to trauma, including self-injury, aggression, and substance use. There are some situations to address that may extend beyond the specific provider's role or training. In the case of an individual provider, you will likely find it helpful to have a network of colleagues to consult with or potentially refer the individual to should they build the desire to engage in other evidence-based approaches—for example, to address their trauma. In multidisciplinary teams, each team member plays a valuable role in collaborating with individuals to achieve their aspirations and can reinforce these pursuits to ensure that each member's contribution fits their role.

> **WORDS OF WISDOM**
>
> **BOX 11.1. How to Refocus on Positive Action**
>
> When it comes to feeling better, nothing succeeds like action. Aggressive behavior, self-injury, and substance use are difficult. Part of what makes these matters difficult is that each involves action that is successful in the short term. Hitting, yelling, swallowing objects, drinking, using—all lead to the person feeling better temporarily. However, each of these actions fails to sustain the desired feeling and, oddly enough, produces the opposite feeling: out of control, distressed, broken, and disconnected. Individuals get caught in a cycle that can be quite destructive for their long-term plans.
>
> Our aim in CT-R is to turn this action orientation to the person's advantage. Aspirations drive sustained positive action. They bring important value into everyday life, and help refocus away from urges, impulses, and beliefs that could lead to self-harm, aggressive behavior, and using. When calling up the image of achieving their aspirations, individuals experience a shift of attention toward the future, activating hope, positive beliefs, and emotions of the adaptive mode. They shift investment away from alleviating the dysphoria and toward satisfying their basic needs, such as connection, control, competence, and purpose.
>
> In order to create and maintain a pathway toward achievement of the aspiration or its meaning, you will need to provide opportunities for fulfillment of these basic needs, as well as to collaboratively solve the problems that crop up in striving for the target. Action will produce success, satisfaction, and improve self-image as belonging, competent, having control, and making a difference. You can draw the person's attention to their inner power as they refocus away from the distress and toward value and purpose. Setbacks are framed as learning experiences that enhance one's power.

SUMMARY

- CT-R takes a trauma-informed approach to understand how traumatic experiences could influence an individual's thoughts about themselves, others, and the future.
- Beliefs about the self, others, and the future can be rooted in trauma and can underlie challenges such as reduced access to motivation, social withdrawal, reduced expectations of pleasure, reduced energy, and reduced communication.
- In response to these negative beliefs, individuals can engage in behaviors that they feel will keep them safe and give them control. They can isolate, stop taking care of themselves, shut down in situations of conflict, harm themselves or others, or engage in substance use.
- Drawing conclusions together about positive beliefs regarding an individual's self-worth, safety, control, and the worthwhileness of connecting with others are key to countering negative beliefs that can underlie challenges associated with trauma.
- The interventions used across challenges may be the same but will be effective only if they address the target beliefs (e.g., strengthening the positive beliefs that negate the negative belief underlying the challenges).
- Aspirations provide action that the person can take instead of the action of self-injury, aggression, or using. Refocusing on and noticing the meaning inherent in these actions sustains empowerment long term.
- Providers in all roles can help individuals address challenges as they come up.

PART III
CT-R CONTEXTS

You will likely be using CT-R in a variety of settings and will be collaborating with a variety of people. This section describes the CT-R approach in these contexts:

CHAPTER 12. Individual CT-R for the Sole Provider 179
How you transform lives one-on-one as a sole provider, using the example of a veteran with lived experience

CHAPTER 13. The CT-R Inpatient Service 193
How you can energize treatment milieus to energize recovery

CHAPTER 14. CT-R Group Therapy 211
How you can apply the principles of CT-R to group therapy

CHAPTER 15. Families as Facilitators of Empowerment 222
How families and providers can connect and collaborate

CHAPTER 12
Individual CT-R for the Sole Provider

David was given a diagnosis of schizophrenia during his military service and had been medically and honorably discharged. After a 1-year period of being in and out of the hospital, David started doing better, met a woman, and fathered a child with her. They talked about getting married. David's mother lived in the same town, about 20 minutes from his apartment, where he would visit her from time to time.

David continued to have fluctuations in experiencing the challenges that impacted his military service. During one particularly stressful episode, he became so fearful that he barricaded himself in the basement for several days. The woman then obtained primary physical custody of their son and moved several hours away. David became homeless for a while, but he eventually connected with the U.S. Department of Veterans Affairs (VA), where he obtained housing and started seeing a psychiatrist and taking medication.

According to medical records, David believed that men gave him aggressive looks and tried to convey to him that he was weak and that they were superior to him. He heard a male voice saying insults like "useless."

David was referred to the outpatient clinic at the VA by his psychiatrist after a recent hospitalization for paranoia and auditory hallucinations that were significantly interfering with his life. The hospitalization occurred when David nearly had an altercation with another man inside a convenience store, prompting the clerk to call the police. David seemed confused and was having difficulty communicating when the police arrived. His psychiatrist suggested that David go to the clinic to get therapy for his paranoia and voices upon discharge.

Many individuals given a serious mental health condition diagnosis, especially those who find themselves stuck in the throes of the challenges, receive support from agencies such as civil and forensic hospitals, assertive community treatment or patient-aligned care teams, programmatic residences, multidisciplinary outpatient clinics, or some combination of these services. However, some people are also served in outpatient settings, such as community mental health centers, university medical centers, VA hospital outpatient clinics, and private practice. In these settings, they are treated with individual therapy, usually by a sole provider who may not be part of an interdisciplinary team.

> **BOX 12.1. Be Flexible with Resources**
>
> You need to be flexible and make the most of what is available in your work settings when practicing CT-R. Making full use of the limited session time becomes especially important. You can involve families and other social connections (e.g., friends, clergy) as partners to promote the empowerment of individuals. You might also consider complementary therapies and services, such as groups or clubs, wellness classes, supported employment and education, and peer support.

Like team-based services, it is sometimes the case that individual therapy settings have administrative and logistical challenges to navigate: a high volume of clients, time-limited sessions, and so on. Since engaging in activities with individuals is an important vehicle of change in recovery-oriented cognitive therapy, this chapter illustrates how to succeed at this in individual therapy as a sole provider.

ACCESSING AND ENERGIZING THE ADAPTIVE MODE

The first step in CT-R is to access and activate each individual's adaptive mode by discovering what interests them through action (see Chapter 3). Coming to a clinical office (especially if it is on the grounds of an institutional setting, like a hospital) to have a one-on-one conversation with a therapist can be a powerful trigger of the "patient" mode, so this first step is critical to your success. Having sessions outside of the office, such as taking a walk outside or visiting the clinic gym or art room, can be extremely beneficial, especially if the individual seems anxious, suspicious, or is stuck in the "patient" mode. Reviewing medical records prior to meeting with the individual and making keen observations during the session can help.

The main goal in the first sessions is for the individual to see the benefit of therapy and return to it. You energize the adaptive mode whenever possible in each session and aim to inspire the individual to continue this work between sessions. This is done through strengthening beliefs about the session's activities being worthwhile and drawing conclusions about benefits provided in the moment (see Chapter 6).

> Importance of the adaptive mode: Accessing and activating the adaptive mode quickly is key. Use the time in-session to energize the adaptive mode whenever possible and encourage the individual to continue this work between sessions.

When David arrived at his first session at the clinic, he seemed tense. His eyes darted around the room. He provided vague, short responses to the therapist's questions. After providing a brief introduction to the clinic, the therapist steered the conversation to a topic of mutual interest in order to start activating David's adaptive mode:

THERAPIST: Hi, David, it's good to meet you! What do you know about our clinic here?

DAVID: I came here because my doctor told me to. That maybe this can help me get a job.

THERAPIST: Well, I'm glad you're here. Let me tell you a little about what we do. We partner with veterans to figure out what they want to be doing or getting in their lives, like working, so that they can feel better and happier. A lot of times our veterans are having a tough

Individual CT-R for the Sole Provider

time with certain challenges that make it trickier to get the life they want, so we also work together to find ways to deal with those things.

DAVID: Well, I just got out of the hospital because people were following me, trying to mess with me. Nobody was believing me; I was so stressed out! You must think I'm crazy, too.

THERAPIST: I am so sorry you experienced that; that sounds very scary. And no, I don't think that. A lot of the Vets we see here have had a similar experience. I'd like to hear more about what it is like for you later on. But today I'd like for us to just get to know each other better, is that okay?

DAVID: I guess.

THERAPIST: Great. I'm a big music lover myself. Do you like music?

DAVID: Yeah.

THERAPIST: What's your favorite?

DAVID: I like electronic dance music.

THERAPIST: Nice! That's actually my favorite, too.

DAVID: No way! I like house and progressive mostly.

THERAPIST: Ah, yes, that's good stuff. I like trance a lot, too. What's one of your favorite tracks? Let's look it up on YouTube. [*pulls up a song; they listen and watch the video*] That was fun! It's nice to see you smiling. How are you doing?

DAVID: Yeah, that song makes me feel good.

THERAPIST: It's pretty cool to share that, I think, and neat that we both feel good now. Would it be worth watching some music together again?

DAVID: Yeah, maybe.

The therapist noticed David seemed more at ease as they discussed music and watched the video together. He spoke more and with more ease and he seemed less nervous. One of the videos was from a live performance in Mexico City. The therapist says he has always wanted to go there. David, who is Mexican American, tells him about what it's like, and the therapist asks for his suggestions on where to go. David says that he likes traveling and that was one of the main draws of the military, but expresses guilt about serving only 2 years, saying, "I screwed that up."

In an ensuing session, David commented on all of the books on the therapist's shelves and asked about what it was like to go to school to become a psychologist. This conversation led to the discovery of another important and related belief:

DAVID: Wow, that is a lot of school.

THERAPIST: Yes, it felt like it took forever!

DAVID: I like listening to podcasts sometimes about the brain. It's amazing what it is capable of. It's too bad I screwed mine up by drinking so much in the military. I made myself mentally handicapped with all that drinking.

THERAPIST: What makes you say that?

DAVID: Well, alcohol ruins your brain. These voices I hear now, I caused them.

Despite energizing David's adaptive mode, he seemed tense in some sessions and talked quite a bit about people from the past he believed had persecuted him. The therapist noticed that David had previously brought a coffee to a session, so he asked, "You know what, I can really use a coffee right now, how about we take a walk to the coffee cart downstairs?" David agreed and he seemed clearer and more relaxed outside, so they walked to a quiet area outside of the hospital, sat on a bench, and had the rest of the session there, while enjoying coffee together.

David commented on some landscaping that needed tending. Turns out, he likes working with plants. The therapist said, "Oh, so you have a green thumb! I could use your help. I have a plant in my office that seems to be dying, and I don't know what I'm doing wrong." They stop by the office and David tells him that he is overwatering the plant and suggests a special fertilizer.

As they wrap up, the therapist says, "That was great—I needed to get out of the building, thank you. And maybe I won't kill this plant after all, thanks to your skills! You seemed more relaxed, too, did you notice that?" David smiled, "Yeah, it was cool to do something normal, thanks doc." David agreed with the therapist's suggestion to go out for coffee once on his own and pick out a nice plant for his place before the next session. Figure 12.1 shows David's Recovery Map for the adaptive mode and challenges.

DEVELOPING THE ADAPTIVE MODE

The process of developing the adaptive mode consists of eliciting the individual's aspirations and enriching them through imagery, focusing on the positive emotions that would come about by achieving the aspiration, and uncovering the deeper meanings or beliefs that are associated with the aspiration (see Chapter 4). You should not move to aspirations until having established a solid relationship of connection and trust with the individual. You should also make sure that they are currently in the adaptive mode.

You might find this a challenge if your organization limits the duration of individual therapy, leaving you very little time to form this important relationship. Your settings may also require that treatment *begins* with a documented list of the individual's recovery goals. Here, it is best to start off with a preliminary list of aspirations and repeatedly return to it

ACCESSING AND ENERGIZING THE ADAPTIVE MODE	
Interests/Ways to Engage: • Music • Travel • The brain • Plants	**Beliefs Activated while in Adaptive Mode:** • I am a regular guy • I am intelligent • I am capable • I have something to offer
CHALLENGES	
Current Behaviors/Challenges: • Believes men are giving him aggressive looks, messing with him, think they're better than him • Sometimes acts aggressively to people he thinks are judging him • Voices saying "useless" • Believing that he caused his voices by drinking • Guilt about being medically discharged from military • Isolating	**Beliefs Underlying Challenges:** • I am inferior to other men • I am weak • I am in danger • Others can't be trusted • I am useless • I am not normal • I am defective • It's my fault I have schizophrenia • I am a failure

FIGURE 12.1. David's initial Recovery Map.

and flesh it out as the relationship strengthens and the individual spends more time in the adaptive mode.

> The therapist had to follow hospital policy by starting treatment with a documented recovery plan that includes the veteran's goals and specific objectives in their own words. The therapist documented David's goal of finding a job on his preliminary Recovery Map.
>
> As their relationship strengthened and David seemed more at ease, the therapist asked him questions to develop his aspirations, such as "What would be the best thing about working?" He replied, "It would mean I'm a good dad, a provider for my son, like I should be, not like how my dad was with me." He explained how important family was in Mexican culture. Turns out, he wanted to get joint physical custody of his son but was pessimistic. "How can I hold down a job with the way I am? My brain is fried."
>
> David noticed a stuffed toy cat on the therapist's shelf and said, "Luis really loves cats." The therapist handed it to him to hold and asked him to tell him more about his son, Luis. "What would he think about this stuffed animal?"; "What is he like?"; "In what ways is he like you?"; "What kinds of things would you want to do with Luis?" David smiled as he described a fond memory of having gone to the park together once and imagined taking him to the toy store. David brightened, pulling out his phone, and eagerly showed pictures of his son.
>
> The therapist drew attention to how even just imagining doing things with his son shifted David's whole mood. The therapist wondered whether it would help to put the son's picture as the wallpaper of his phone, to remind David of what he's working toward. David liked the idea but didn't know how to do that, so the therapist showed him.
>
> "What can you do in the coming week to feel like a good dad?" the therapist asked. "I can try FaceTiming with him; I haven't talked to him in a couple of weeks," David replied. They then programmed a reminder to call his son into his phone. The aspirations portion of David's Recovery Map is shown in Figure 12.2.

Aspirations are critical to progress. The goal of your collaboration with the individual is to set the most effective targets and get the most out of each in terms of action and conclusions. One way of describing this to individuals is to think of it as the mission you are on together. The concept of having a mission and working as a team may be especially useful for veterans who express values of camaraderie and working together toward a bigger purpose.

ACTUALIZING AND STRENGTHENING THE ADAPTIVE MODE

Since your number of contacts may be limited, take full advantage of your time with the individual in session to jumpstart positive action. You might also involve loved ones, other providers or services, or electronic reminders to boost positive action between therapy sessions. Both in-session and between-session action is ideal for you to draw attention to positive meanings and

ASPIRATIONS	
Goals: • Get a job • Get joint custody of son	Meaning of Accomplishing Identified Goal: • Capability and responsibility • Good father

FIGURE 12.2. Adding goals and aspirations to David's Recovery Map.

beliefs, as well as to develop their resiliency beliefs. In this way, you strengthen their adaptive mode.

> David's aspirations were to work and be a good father to his son. He and his therapist broke these aims down into smaller steps:
>
> - David said he didn't even know where to start with working. He had a few ideas but wasn't sure what would be the best job for him. He had major doubts about his ability to work because people were against him and he was sure that would happen at work, too. In short, he didn't feel safe. He spent a lot of his time alone at home. His sleep schedule was erratic, he didn't have a routine, and he wasn't happy with his weight.
> - For his aspiration about his son, David said he would have to have "stability," a good income, and a safer place to live. He would also need to "stop the chaos," which meant to feel emotionally stable and less bothered by people and the voices.
>
> The therapist suggested that doing things that brought David consistency and routine might be a good place to start, since that would help with both getting ready to work and to have his son in his life. They talked about simple ways to try this out and came up with going to bed and waking up at the same time every day and doing at least one activity that would make him feel good every day.
>
> David's mother came to a session and talked about how worried she was for him being alone so much. She had some plants that needed his special touch, and he agreed to visit weekly and help her out with them.

You can gradually incorporate aspiration- and meaning-driven action between sessions. This provides opportunities for incremental success—for example, the person can see that they are more capable than they realize. While taking these action steps though, it is also likely that the individual will be confronted with stressors or situations that bring about their challenges. When this happens, you can develop an understanding of why it might be so and include additional actions or problem-solving strategies to empower them.

> One challenge that repeatedly came up was David's perception of others judging him and provoking him. The therapist used chain analyses (see Chapter 6) to review some of these recent incidents. They discovered together a common theme: David would become suspicious of other men when feeling insecure about himself (e.g., if the man looked more muscular, wealthier, or more successful than him or if they had a strong swagger about them). In these situations, David felt weak and inferior. He talked about how this was very offensive to him because of his sense of machismo as a Mexican man.
>
> The therapist asked David whether there were ever times that he felt strong and capable. The only example he could think of was when he used to exercise, but he had not done that in quite a while. The therapist asked David whether he could teach him a favorite exercise. David taught him to do a squat with proper form. Noting this successful demonstration of capability, the therapist asked David whether he might want to exercise more often. David agreed that he'd like to.
>
> The therapist then floated the idea that if David got back into exercising, is it possible that the physical feeling of strength could also make him feel mentally strong, which might make him feel more comfortable, less intimidated by other men, and more confident about working toward his aspirations. David agreed to try going to the gym two times in the coming week and make note of how strong he felt before and after.
>
> David went to the gym twice but unfortunately, he became angry at some of the men in the gym because they had what appeared to be "aggressive looks" on their faces as they were working out,

which he interpreted as them posturing and asserting their superiority over him. He yelled at one of them to stop it, which caused a scene. The therapist attempted to encourage him to reconsider these interpretations (e.g., "Could there have been another explanation for the looks on their faces?"), but David was totally convinced and seemed irritated that the therapist questioned him.

The therapist then suggested that David instead consider building his strength through a free Tai Chi class for veterans in the community that he had found, speculating that David might be less likely to see aggressive-looking faces in this setting and that Tai Chi might also give him some relief from the "chaos." With the therapist's help, David put reminders for the classes in his phone and added messages that linked the activity to his valued aspiration "for my stability and Luis."

David and the therapist continued to periodically have sessions outside. The therapist would recommend this whenever noticing that David seemed uneasy, distracted, or would otherwise slip into the "patient" mode. David would be somewhat nervous outside, especially when men walked by. The therapist taught David some refocusing techniques, including simple mindfulness and the Look-Point-Name game (see Chapter 9), to lessen his stress about being victimized and to take power away from his voices.

One day when David was particularly struggling with his voices, they walked and took turns practicing the Look-Point-Name game. Another time, they walked outside and both practiced mindfulness by walking silently for 10 minutes while keenly trying to observe as much as possible in their surroundings, and then sharing with each other what they saw—they shared a laugh over some of their funny discoveries, like a dirty sock along the edge of the road.

As certain challenges begin to resolve, others may come more to the forefront. Your approach remains the same: energize the adaptive mode and link positive action to aspirations. Broadening social connections, especially in the community, is a natural extension of this work. Part of the mission is the relationships with others, doing things together that are fun and have purpose, and bringing about the person's valued meanings more and more often.

David slowly started to feel more confident about himself. He spoke less about being persecuted by others, and was a little less bothered by his voices, but he still struggled with isolation and loneliness. The therapist suggested that he try joining a new club at the clinic. The purpose of this weekly gathering was to design cards with hopeful and inspiring messages. The group mailed these colorful materials to bolster other veterans who had suicidal thoughts and had recently discharged from the inpatient unit. David was intrigued by the club because he once was suicidal, and he liked the idea of helping other veterans. He went and seemed to enjoy it. Some of the veterans told him that they get together at a diner down the street after the meeting for a bite to eat and invited him to join, and he did. Another clinic at the VA had heard about the club and wanted to launch it there, too, but needed help. The facilitator of the club and the veterans were planning on going to the clinic to teach them how to run it. David offered to be responsible for telling them about the best kind of music to play during it, to help people concentrate and be creative:

> THERAPIST: I walked by the Caring Cards Club the other day. You looked like you were having fun!
>
> DAVID: Yeah, it's a pretty cool time. We just draw and write, listen to music, and talk about random stuff.
>
> THERAPIST: And you're with a bunch of other veterans, mostly guys. Have you felt intimidated by them at all?
>
> DAVID: Not really, these guys are cool. They get me. They've gone through some stuff themselves, like I have. We're all there to help other veterans.

> THERAPIST: That's so good to hear. What does it mean that you're able to enjoy your time with these guys and feel safe around them?
>
> DAVID: I guess not everyone has it in for me. There are good people still around.

> David said he was starting to feel some of the stability he had wanted, but he was still troubled by his voices. The Look-Point-Name game and other refocusing techniques helped a bit, but he was still hearing the insults, especially when he was alone, and they really bothered him.

As you develop trust, certain experiences that they had been guarded against addressing earlier, such as trauma, may feel safer to discuss and work through. This speaks to the importance of connection and the development of trust in CT-R. You do not have to focus on such topics or resolve them first for the individual to pursue aspirations or build up a meaningful life. It's the thirst for even more of this desired life that makes the most difficult challenges worth working on.

> Although David had completed an intake assessment before he started in the clinic, he seemed more comfortable sharing about his traumatic experiences now, so the therapist reassessed him for PTSD. David reported some symptoms like occasional nightmares of his father's abuse and avoidance of those memories and had an elevated score on a PTSD measure but did not meet the full criteria for PTSD. However, he was clearly struggling with posttraumatic symptoms that seemed directly related to his voices and probably his feelings of persecution as well. David grew up hearing that he was inadequate from his father and now believes other men view him that way, too.
>
> The therapist asked David whether he thought that trauma was getting in the way of his aspirations to work and having a better relationship with his son. David agreed that it was. The therapist asked whether David would be willing to talk with a peer specialist about the experience of trauma therapy. David agreed. He later said this was helpful and he eventually decided to participate in trauma treatment. The therapist then integrated a course of cognitive processing therapy for PTSD (Resick et al., 2017) into their sessions. David's PTSD scores went down.
>
> A significant breakthrough was realizing that his father, a veteran himself who had experienced combat, abused alcohol heavily and likely had undiagnosed PTSD. This helped David to dismiss his father's hurtful messages:

> THERAPIST: David, you haven't said much about the voices lately. How's it going with that?
>
> DAVID: I still hear them here and there, but they don't bother me as much. I see them now as parts of my past.
>
> THERAPIST: That is a big change.
>
> DAVID: Yeah, I see now that my dad had a lot of his own crap going on. When he would say those things, that wasn't really about me. He was going through a lot.
>
> THERAPIST: He really was. It took a lot of courage to talk about that painful part of your life. What does it say about you that you got through that?
>
> DAVID: I guess I am a survivor.
>
> THERAPIST: Absolutely. I also wonder if you're stronger and more capable than you sometimes realize.
>
> DAVID: That's true.

> They created empowerment cards that contained these new conclusions. The positive action and empowerment section of David's Recovery Map is shown in Figure 12.3.

POSITIVE ACTION AND EMPOWERMENT	
Current Strategies and Interventions: <ul><li>Identify ways to activate the adaptive mode<ul><li>Watch music videos</li><li>Talk about places traveled</li><li>Ask for advice about plants</li><li>Have sessions outside</li></ul></li><li>Create recovery image of being a good dad</li><li>FaceTime with son weekly</li><li>Stick to consistent daily routine</li><li>Help mom with plants</li><li>Go to Tai Chi class for veterans</li><li>Use refocusing techniques (Look-Point-Name game, mindfulness)</li><li>Go to card group, hang out with veterans' group, teach other veterans how to run a group</li><li>Trauma therapy</li><li>Supported employment</li></ul>	**Beliefs/Aspirations/Meanings/Challenge Targeted:** <ul><li>Beliefs about being able to connect with others</li><li>I am responsible</li><li>I am a good father</li><li>I am strong and capable</li><li>Stability</li><li>I am useful</li><li>Get ready to have my son in my life</li><li>Believing what the voices say is true</li><li>People accept and like me</li><li>Helping other veterans</li><li>Reduce posttraumatic symptoms (nightmares, avoidance) and belief about being "useless" that fuels voices and paranoia</li></ul>

FIGURE 12.3. Adding strategies and targets to David's Recovery Map.

ENDING INDIVIDUAL THERAPY

The process of ending therapy with individuals with serious mental health challenges, particularly a recovery-oriented one like CT-R, may appear difficult. The spirit of CT-R is to empower individuals to live the life they desire on their own with their friends and loved ones. So, when does therapy end? In some health care settings, the duration of therapy is limited by policies designed to control costs or facilitate access to new people seeking care. When these limits do not exist, ideally the therapist and the individual together decide when it is time to bring their relationship to a close.

Since CT-R is a therapy in which a strong attachment is often made to the therapist, ending it can bring up difficult feelings for the individual. The essential elements of successful therapy termination include (1) celebrating successes and boosting confidence through strengthening positive and resilience beliefs, (2) planning for the future, (3) recruiting friends and loved ones, and (4) making appropriate referrals.

> David was feeling more and more in control of his life and more driven by a sense of purpose, as his positive self-concept evolved. He still believed that men would sometimes intimidate him, but this was happening less often and it did not bother him as much. The voices were less bothersome, too. David saw he had more control over the previously incapacitating experiences. What he heard was not credible or worth listening to.
>
> He was consistently FaceTiming with his son. David practiced communication skills in therapy and between sessions to improve his relationship with his son's mother. He hoped she would become more comfortable granting him greater amounts of time with Luis. David planned a trip to visit him soon, for the first time in a year.
>
> David had repeatedly declined his therapist's suggestion to see the clinic's vocational rehabilitation counselor in the past. Now, he felt ready for work. He met with the counselor and enrolled in the supported employment program. With time, he found a job as a security guard.

Still, David was nervous about ending therapy; he worried about ending up back in the hospital or homeless again. Together, David and his therapist reviewed all of the successes he had accomplished along the way and they wrote these down for him to read whenever he started to worry. They specifically planned for ways David could be his own life coach should difficulties arise (e.g., do Tai Chi when feeling stressed out, watch a music video or practice Look-Point-Name when getting bothered by the voices, call and hang out with the friends he made in the Caring Cards Club, attend a support group in the community).

They created a list of everything he would be taking away from the therapy (e.g., resilience beliefs). David titled this compendium "Moving Forward." It included "I am a survivor," "I am strong," "I am capable," "Not everyone has it in for me," "There are still good people around," and "I am on my way to being a good dad for Luis."

David's mother came in for a session to help with the planning. The plants were looking good thanks to David, and she looked forward to having her grandson back in her life. The therapist and David tapered the therapy from weekly to every 2 weeks, and then monthly before drawing to a close. He invited David to call him if he needed booster sessions in the future.

In their final session, the therapist gave David a polished stone as a symbol of the strength and stability he had developed, and as something to remember the therapist and their good work together during challenging times. Figure 12.4 shows David's full Recovery Map.

ADDITIONAL CONSIDERATIONS

The Structure of Each Individual Therapy Session

The structure of each individual therapy session matches the structure of any CT-R interaction (see Chapter 1), including group therapy (see Chapter 14). The key parts are accessing and energizing the adaptive mode, bridging between sessions, eliciting and developing aspirations, problem solving in the context of aspirations, and developing an action plan.

Accessing and Energizing the Adaptive Mode

Each session should begin with attempts at *accessing the adaptive mode*. This generates energy, puts connection upfront, emphasizes the value of pleasurable activity, and reflects that it is as important to do the good stuff as it is to work on the challenges—it's humanizing.

Mission—Bridging between Sessions

When the individual is in the adaptive mode, you will *bridge* between your previous session and the current one, much as you do in traditional cognitive therapy (Beck, 2020). In this bridge you will ask about any action steps they did between sessions. You can also do an energy level, mood, or symptom check if that's an area being targeted (e.g., "How's your energy been this week overall?"). Most important in a CT-R bridge is establishing a sort of mission for the sessions, which tend to revolve around the aspirations, once known. Referred to as a *recovery check*, you use time early in the session to ensure you and the individual are working toward the same targets—for example, you might say, "So we've been working together on getting back to work so you can be a provider in your family, is that still our mission?" or "Is that still most important to you?" The recovery check reinforces the purpose for involvement in therapy, and also gives the individual the opportunity to prioritize aspirations or other targets. Based on the

Recovery Map
ACCESSING AND ENERGIZING THE ADAPTIVE MODE

Interests/Ways to Engage:	Beliefs Activated while in Adaptive Mode:
• Music • Travel • The brain • Plants	• I am a regular guy • I am intelligent • I am capable • I have something to offer

ASPIRATIONS	
Goals: • Get a job • Get joint custody of son	**Meaning of Accomplishing Identified Goal:** • Capability and responsibility • Good father

CHALLENGES	
Current Behaviors/Challenges: • Believes men are giving him aggressive looks, messing with him, think they're better than him • Sometimes acts aggressively to people he thinks are judging him • Voices saying "useless" • Believing that he caused his voices by drinking • Guilt about being medically discharged from military • Isolating	**Beliefs Underlying Challenges:** • I am inferior to other men • I am weak • I am in danger • Others can't be trusted • I am useless • I am not normal • I am defective • It's my fault I have schizophrenia • I am a failure

POSITIVE ACTION AND EMPOWERMENT	

Current Strategies and Interventions:
• Identify ways to activate the adaptive mode
   ◦ Watch music videos
   ◦ Talk about places traveled
   ◦ Ask for advice about plants
   ◦ Have sessions outside
• Create recovery image of being a good dad
• FaceTime with son weekly
• Stick to consistent daily routine
• Help mom with plants
• Go to Tai Chi class for veterans
• Use refocusing techniques (Look-Point-Name game, mindfulness)
• Go to card group, hang out with veterans' group, teach other veterans how to run a group
• Trauma therapy
• Supported employment
	Beliefs/Aspirations/Meanings/Challenge Targeted:
	• Beliefs about being able to connect with others
	• I am responsible
	• I am a good father
	• I am strong and capable
	• Stability
	• I am useful
	• Get ready to have my son in my life
	• Believing what the voices say is true
	• People accept and like me
	• Helping other veterans
	• Reduce posttraumatic symptoms (nightmares, avoidance) and belief about being "useless" that fuels voices and paranoia

FIGURE 12.4. David's completed Recovery Map.

session mission, you can establish goals for the session: "Based on this, what might be the best use of our time today—should we keep finding ways to get our energy up, or work on our project?" If individuals are less verbal, you can move right into the action of the day, such as asking for help or playing music.

Eliciting and Developing Aspirations

If *aspirations* are not known, the next step in session is to identify and enrich them. Once you have these, though, this step is incorporated into the bridge—checking in regularly that they are still important and emphasizing the meaning. With a routine established, the first three steps (accessing the adaptive mode, bridge, and aspirations) can be done in the first 5–10 minutes of a session.

Challenges—Problem Solving in the Context of Aspirations

Challenges are addressed in individual therapy if they are impacting the person's pursuit of their aspirations. Sessions can be used to problem solve such challenges using whatever interventions may be effective. Problem solving may also look like experiential activities that bring about strong positive emotion and access to positive beliefs. In either case, you are using this time to draw conclusions about how these tools empower a person and get them closer to their aspirations.

Developing an Action Plan

The end of each session should have an *action plan*. Action plans bring the successes of sessions into daily life. You can ask the person, "Based on what we did together today, what might be something you want to do between sessions?" This might be doing a preferred activity, practicing a voice control strategy, or taking an action step toward an aspiration. The plan should be

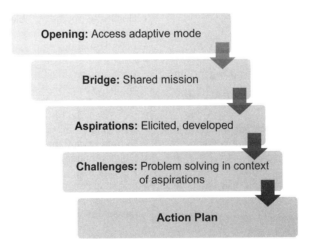

FIGURE 12.5. Structure of a CT-R session.

developed collaboratively but feel comfortable to make clear suggestions if the ideas developed are not linked to the events of the session or broader mission. You will also want to have a way for the individual to remember the action plan—for example, ask whether they'd like to write it down, put a reminder in their phone, or use a planner.

Early in therapy, sessions might focus solely on accessing the adaptive mode, concluding with action plans to do these activities between sessions. Sessions might be oriented around identifying and enriching aspirations for several meetings. Meet the individual where they are and be flexible. Figure 12.5 illustrates the overall structure of a CT-R session.

Collaborating with Other Providers

Sometimes it is appropriate to bring other service providers into the mix. This can be when a specific modality appears warranted, such as the case with David and peer specialist and vocational services. If you do not have specific expertise with certain areas of practice, collaborating with colleagues can be a great help. You can still use the CT-R framework in these collaborations. The Recovery Map is a useful document to share. It can also be used to capture feedback or information gained by the other provider. A one-page synopsis, the Recovery Map can also help jumpstart connection with an added provider by putting interests and ways to engage up-front. Sharing aspirations and positive action targets keeps everyone united along the desired life of the individual, reducing the risk of disjointed care.

WORDS OF WISDOM

BOX 12.2. Aspire to Be Fired

We have high hopes for treatment. Our aim is to collaborate on building a desired life. We do this through the bond we establish. Doing activities together. Earning trust. Dreaming big. Realizing the dream. Living it every day. Drawing conclusions. Strengthening a best self.

At the start, an individual may be profoundly isolated. Our actions reverse this, and we become important to them, possibly the only positive relationship they can think of. As you do more together, over time, they begin to do more in between the times they see you. Wherever their interests and aspirations take them, there are other people.

Your relationship has whetted their appetite for more life, more purpose, more connection. You help them see this progress, recognize their inner power to handle difficult situations, like loss, or things not working out.

There will be a first time they let you know they are too busy to see you. Each time this happens, you can smile. This is by design. Life is happening—in a good way.

Life doesn't revolve around therapy. Therapy should fit into life.

There should be a built-in obsolescence. The person closes the distance between themselves and everyone else—their life space gets fuller and fuller.

At some point they do not have time for you. This is the best result. The person has too much to do. They fire you.

In CT-R, aspire to be fired. You never lose the connection and the great work you did together.

Time and Location Limitations

If you feel constricted by reduced session times or if your location makes it difficult to take sessions out of the office, there are many ways to still create an engaging and active session. If you can only see someone for a brief time, you can activate the adaptive mode more quickly by inviting the individual to teach you a quick tip on their favorite activity, such as teaching you one chess move a week or a new word they learned in a foreign language class. Consider office-based ways for the individual to help you: Can they give suggestions on how to improve your office decor? Can you stretch or do exercises in the small space? Can you still listen to music or be taught a game of cards? Activities can also be done over web-based telehealth programs (see online Appendices J and K). Be creative!

SUMMARY

- CT-R can be successfully delivered in outpatient individual therapy settings, using the same recovery mapping and following the same structure used in other settings.
- Given the limited contact with the individual, accessing the adaptive mode quickly is key. This can be facilitated by having sessions outside of the clinical office (especially if the individual is anxious, suspicious, or stuck in the "patient" mode) and doing enjoyable activities together.
- The therapist should use the session time to jumpstart positive action and take advantage of any connections or resources that are available to the individual (e.g., loved ones, other providers or services, electronic reminders) to encourage positive action between sessions.
- The benefit of therapy can be enhanced by connecting the individual to complementary therapies and services, including group therapies or clubs, wellness classes, supported employment, education, and peer support services.
- Therapy is successfully terminated by celebrating successes and boosting confidence, planning for the future, recruiting friends and loved ones, and making appropriate referrals. It can be helpful to titrate the individual off of therapy gradually and offer booster sessions as needed.

CHAPTER 13
The CT-R Inpatient Service

A new staff member arrives on an inpatient unit and observes the scene: While a select few individuals are in therapy groups, more than half remain on the unit. Several are in their bedrooms. Others are sleeping in hard plastic chairs along the perimeter of the dayroom, which is quiet—except for the white noise of television infomercials and faint snores. When the others return after group, two go to the chairs and put coats over their heads. Soon, something changes. A mental health worker invites an individual to play cards. As they play a game of Rummy, the individual begins to hum a popular song from the 1960s. The staff recognizes it and starts to sing, pulling the music up on the unit tablet. Hearing this, two other individuals go to the table. They are asked what music they like. Next thing you know, all four are singing '90s hip-hop together. Others in their chairs look over. Someone shouts a song request from across the room. The staff member jots down the start of a unit playlist and the energy becomes palpable. It's a stark contrast to the previously sleepy unit.

This example is a snapshot of a common dichotomy on inpatient units: shifts between inactivity and interaction. Jumpstarting energy on an otherwise sleepy unit can sometimes be a challenge, as low-stimulation environments can inadvertently maintain challenges, such as reduced access to energy and initiative, and increased attention to voices (Curson, Pantelis, Ward, & Barnes, 1992; Oshima, Mino, & Inomata, 2003, 2005; Wing & Brown, 1970; Zarlock, 1966). When there's more action and connection on the milieu, there are more opportunities for people to access their adaptive mode and imagine possibilities of what they'd like and want for the future. The challenges also become less prominent. This chapter addresses how to apply recovery-oriented cognitive therapy on an inpatient milieu. You'll learn how to create an environment that propels individuals toward recovery, how to increase energy and opportunities to shift beliefs and help individuals take action toward aspirations, and how to implement strategies for continuity within treatment teams. You will also be introduced to a self-assessment tool for evaluating and sustaining CT-R practices within organizations: the CT-R Benchmarks (see Appendix H). Of note, this chapter refers to inpatient milieus and units. However, the same strategies are applicable to any setting that operates a milieu and has a treatment team component (e.g., community-based programmatic residences).

BASIC NEEDS

Individuals given a diagnosis of a serious mental health condition have the same basic needs as anyone else: to belong; to participate and to be involved in meaningful pursuits; to have close, intimate relationships; and to feel productive, skilled, and capable (Baumeister & Leary, 1995; Fuligni, 2019). A pervasive experience shared by individuals on inpatient units is loneliness. In this setting, individuals are in close physical proximity to one another. But opportunities to form social bonds can be rare. Although these individuals are together, they may still feel truly alone. Inability to satisfy these basic needs impacts personal beliefs (Beck et al., 2019): self (*alone, vulnerable, defective*), others (*rejecting, controlling, demeaning*), and future (*hopeless, no likelihood that things will improve*). To protect against further hurts and disappointments, individuals build up clusters of defeatist beliefs ("I won't get what I want, so why try"; "If I don't try, I won't get disappointed") and asocial beliefs ("If I stay away from people, they can't hurt me"; "I'm better off without others"). These beliefs are then reflected in recovery-interfering behavior: individuals withdraw from other people, so they don't get hurt or disappointed, or they use passivity to avoid frustration and failure, including not talking about or taking action toward aspirations. These behaviors highlight one of the paradoxes of serious mental health challenges: the individual needs to connect, but isolates; the person desires purpose, but doesn't act. At first, it's not immediately clear why individuals engage in isolation, withdrawal, and other behaviors that leave their needs unsatisfied. But when we consider their basic beliefs about themselves, others, and their future, the picture becomes clearer.

This same formulation helps us understand other common challenges on units—for example, individuals may use aggression to fend off intrusions by other people and protect against their extreme vulnerability. While these apparent intrusions by other people are often intended to be helpful (e.g., nursing staff inviting them to attend groups or asking them to take medicine), individuals may misinterpret the actions as attempts by others to further degrade them. Why? Individuals may look for rejection to support their beliefs. An additional paradox arises: even though individuals desire to belong, their aggressive acts push people away, leading to further separation and isolation, as well as greater difficulty pursuing aspirations.

Given this understanding, a CT-R milieu approach is one that attempts to help individuals meet the need for connection. This is facilitated through frequent opportunities to activate and energize the adaptive mode. The CT-R milieu also provides opportunities in several contexts for discovering and discussing aspirations, which can help individuals connect with one another in addition to instilling greater hope for the future. The CT-R milieu can also be a catalyst for action, which can then continue in the community.

THE TREATMENT TEAM

All members of the unit treatment team play a role in creating a more collaborative, energized, and active environment. Their contributions include working together to develop an

The CT-R Inpatient Service

understanding of each individual, developing action plans for attaining aspirations with individuals, creating meaningful roles for individuals, linking unit programming to treatment targets, and guiding individuals toward more helpful and accurate beliefs. Depending on the structure of the specific hospital or organization, the team's composition and the role that each team member plays may vary. How you implement and follow through on interventions may vary as well. But the core CT-R principles remain the same.

One key function of the treatment team is to develop and share an understanding of each person on the unit. You do this with a Recovery Map (see Chapter 2), which links with the treatment plan. The Recovery Map organizes beliefs activated during the individual's positive and successful experiences, as well as those activated during more challenging times. To develop it, you gather information from all members of the team, based on their interactions with the person. Everyone has the opportunity to see individuals at their best and when challenges present. When action plans are developed, team members can decide together who will lead based on how it fits within their respective role—for example, plans regarding identifying and engaging individuals in their interests may be actioned by both a direct care worker and a specialist, such as a creative arts therapist. Specific interventions for reducing voices or uncovering the meaning of more expansive beliefs might be actioned collaboratively by a therapist and psychiatrist. Whatever the division of roles, team members can use the Recovery Map to organize ideas and communicate with one another. These individual formulations can then be translated into unit-wide programming that meets the needs of many (e.g., programs that emphasize connection, or provide opportunities for capability). This then makes the unit, as a whole, fundamentally person centered.

Based on the individual formulations, treatment team members also play a crucial role in helping individuals shift beliefs when in the adaptive mode using guided discovery (see Chapter 6). Guided discovery can occur during any unit activity, from team meetings to therapy groups or even in less structured recreational situations. When a treatment team develops individual case formulations, the specific questions asked to guide or strengthen beliefs become tailored to those that are most relevant.

Treatment teams can also help shape the overall atmosphere of the unit through intentional, collaborative decision making about how the unit is run and what type of programming is created.

THE ADAPTIVE MODE AND UNIT ATMOSPHERE

A truly exciting moment in a psychiatric inpatient unit occurs when you see individuals go into the adaptive mode. How can you tell? They are engaged and energized, participating in things they enjoy (e.g., karaoke nights, talking about their favorite sports team); discussing their interests and connected to others while working toward a mutual goal (e.g., making holiday cards); helping others on the unit.

A key mission in CT-R is to pay attention to times individuals are in the adaptive mode ("What are they like at their best?"), discover what activates the adaptive mode, and create opportunities for the individual to experience the adaptive mode more often through programming or other activities. The more times the adaptive mode is activated, the easier it is to identify and target aspirations, and the more often staff can help individuals strengthen positive beliefs and draw new conclusions about themselves. In this way, a milieu that focuses on the adaptive mode actively chips away at the influence of negative beliefs that perpetuate the challenges.

To regularly access and activate the adaptive mode, you will want to set up a stimulating environment that enables individuals to participate in activities that bring out their best self, reevaluate negative beliefs, develop new aspirations, and more. This includes opportunities to engage in pleasurable and interactive activities that involve individuals and staff partnering together.

Ideally, deciding on the specific activities will be a collaborative process where individuals and staff meet and plan together. The planning involves conversations about individuals' interests and staff sharing ideas from their own interests. The conversation can then expand to shared interests. Examples of activities might be cooking, prayer groups, video game competitions, and so on. Talking about what is good or the best part of these collective pursuits creates excitement to do them together, easing the logistical work. Planning together might involve deciding which activities are held, when, and what roles individuals and staff would like to have in those activities (e.g., setting up, leading).

Collaboration to such an extent is not always feasible, especially if the length of stay is expected to be short (e.g., acute hospitals, crisis centers). In this case, multidisciplinary staff planning can be effective. In these conversations, staff can be asked to notice, from their experience, what has been most effective at generating energy, interaction, and—frankly—really enjoyable days at work. Include those who spend the most time with individuals in these conversations, such as direct care staff, nurses, peer specialists, and others. You can ask questions such as "When are individuals at their best?" This question lends itself to person-centered and strength-based responses. When asked this question, team members often find the exceptions to the rule (e.g., "He is *always* in bed, *except* during karaoke parties when he gets to sing love songs from the 1940s"). Similarly, you can ask, "What is the unit or milieu like at its best?" This leads to discussion of more programmatic developments (e.g., when we have unitwide birthday parties, when we put music on to start the day, when we do mindfulness meditation exercises before bed). This often leads to more discussion about why these activities are helpful: it provides John a role on the unit and he has control; Terri sees herself as knowledgeable. These all inspire conversation about how the team can work together to bring about those best moments more often.

Seeking input from everyone on the team has the additional benefit of enhancing staff connectedness while actively implementing recovery programming. This connectedness comes from discussion of enjoyable elements of the job, recognizing the staff as experts in their respective areas and for their knowledge about the individuals or unit, and identifying interests, hobbies, or goals the staff can share with one another.

The following sections highlight how the different stages of the CT-R approach can be put into practice on the unit.

Accessing the Adaptive Mode

Methods for accessing and activating the adaptive mode can occur at the level of the individual or as a collective unit. Individual interventions include brief and frequent attempts at connection and seeking knowledge or advice. Milieu interventions can include interactive games to help elicit interests. The interventions highlighted here represent just a few ways you can help identify interests and access energy. Give yourself permission to be creative!

Brief, Frequent, Predictable Attempts at Connection

If you find that you and the team don't quite know yet what gets certain individuals into the adaptive mode—such as those who spend most of their time in their rooms, or who do not engage in conversation with the team—your first point of intervention is to identify interests and hooks to increase connection and counter isolation. You can do this initially through frequent low-pressure interactions. Consider the following example:

> In a team brainstorming meeting, a nurse mentions that she doesn't know a lot about Roger. She says, "Roger rarely talks to anyone. He won't come out of his room to do programming or activities on the unit. I've only seen him out when they needed to make a repair in his room, and even then he sat in a chair just outside." The psychiatrist asks whether anyone has ever successfully engaged Roger or whether they've noticed him have interactions with any other individuals on the unit. The art therapist recalls a time when Roger watched two other individuals make party decorations for a few minutes but did not remember any other interactions.

In this scenario, the team might see Roger's decoration making as an opening to get his input on something creative. The direct care staff can approach Roger and seek advice on what colors he recommends for tablecloths for an upcoming event, or to choose between two poster designs. These brief, very specific attempts at connection can uncover interests.

In other situations, you might have some sense that an individual likes music or sports, for example, but they still remain isolative. In this case, you can make brief attempts at providing the preferred activity—meeting an individual where they are, even if that's in their room under the covers. You might, for instance, play a song or get their input on who you might select as a player for your fantasy sports team.

Using this approach, you may interact with the individual for only a few minutes at a time, but the inpatient environment is one that allows for these moments to happen more often throughout the day. The more frequently these brief interactions occur, the more opportunities for positive connection and the less time the individual has to focus internally on voices, worries, or other challenges. It is helpful to spread the contact out across many different staff personnel, so that contact happens frequently, but with different people. Some units have come up with different methods of tag-teaming, such as scheduling and rotating specific times to attempt connection with the individual. Figure 13.1 is an example of what a staff activity schedule can look like.

This intervention also allows you to more quickly explore a range of possible interests and see whether you can find one that works. Topics like music, sports, food or cooking, art, television, and pop culture are all common areas of possible interest for anyone (see Chapter 3 for more ideas). By observing shifts in affect (e.g., more smiling), increased eye contact or verbal responsiveness, increased rate of speech, or easier-to-follow conversation, you can identify which area is most impactful.

Seek Advice or Knowledge

Seeking advice can be part of brief, frequent, increasingly predictable interactions. You can use short concrete questions, such as "Should we play rock or country music?" or "Should I paint my nails red or purple?" or you can ask open-ended advice questions to help you uncover

Sunday Date: ___	Monday Date: ___	Tuesday Date: ___	Wednesday Date: ___	Thursday Date: ___	Friday Date: ___	Saturday Date: ___
Hair time With: ___ Time: ___	Nails With: ___ Time: ___	Music videos With: ___ Time: ___	Makeovers With: ___ Time: ___	Singing With: ___ Time: ___	Hair time With: ___ Time: ___	Nails With: ___ Time: ___
Music videos With: ___ Time: ___	Listen to music With: ___ Time: ___	Magazines With: ___ Time: ___	Listen to music With: ___ Time: ___	Music videos With: ___ Time: ___	Listen to music With: ___ Time: ___	Listen to music With: ___ Time: ___
Exercise/dance With: ___ Time: ___	Exercise/dance With: ___ Time: ___	Knitting lessons With: ___ Time: ___	Exercise/dance With: ___ Time: ___	Exercise/dance With: ___ Time: ___	Singing With: ___ Time: ___	Exercise/dance With: ___ Time: ___
Girl talk With: ___ Time: ___	Girl talk With: ___ Time: ___	Girl talk With: ___ Time: ___	Girl talk With: ___ Time: ___	Girl talk With: ___ Time: ___	Girl talk With: ___ Time: ___	Girl talk With: ___ Time: ___
Other With: ___ Time: ___	Other With: ___ Time: ___	Other With: ___ Time: ___	Other With: ___ Time: ___	Other With: ___ Time: ___	Other With: ___ Time: ___	Other With: ___ Time: ___

Activity options

Nails	Exercise/dance
Listen to music	Watch music videos
Magazines	Singing
Makeovers	Preparing for creative arts representative role
Hair time	
Girl talk	
Knitting lessons (given by her)	

Suggested daily activity times

9:00 A.M.	2:00 P.M.
11:00 A.M.	3:00 P.M.
1:00 P.M.	6:00 P.M.
6:30 P.M.	7:00 P.M.

Staff Members

_____   _____

FIGURE 13.1. A staff activity schedule showing brief, frequent, and predictable opportunities for connection.

or discover interests, such as "What are the best recipes for a Thanksgiving dinner?" or "My daughter has a cold—do you know any tried-and-true home remedies that might help?"

Besides not requiring much energy for an individual to answer, asking for advice on a variety of topics can clue you in to the person's special areas of knowledge or experience. When you learn what topic a person responds to best, you can bring it up consistently and predictably, creating more opportunities to help boost the individual's energy and connection, and activate the adaptive mode. Beliefs you activate using this intervention include "I'm capable, helpful, knowledgeable, and useful" and "Others are interested in and care about me."

On an inpatient unit, providing advice or help to therapists, nurses, or direct care workers can also improve collaboration and partnership between individuals and the entire staff so that everyone is operating more as equals.

> **Notes on activating the adaptive mode:**
> ✓ It may be easier for people to think of things others might like than to think of what they themselves might like. This is still a helpful contribution.
> ✓ Resources on inpatient units vary. Be creative. A game of basketball, for example, can involve a paper ball and an empty trash can.

Eliciting Interests or Skills with Interactive Games

To help individuals identify interests as a group, you and other staff can create interactive games that encourage participation in a wide range of interests and activities. One example is Activity Bingo. In this game, the staff put activities that people sometimes like onto a Bingo card. They ask individuals on the unit to think of things people might like to do, and put those on the card as well (see Figure 13.2 for a sample Activity Bingo card). Activities can include things that could be done in the future (e.g., getting hair done, attending church, walking outside) or in the moment (e.g., shooting a basketball, doing exercises, sharing a favorite recipe, listening to a favorite song). Each card should include the same activities, but located in different squares.

	B	I	N	G	O
1	Describe a dream vacation	Play Tic-Tac-Toe	Take a basketball shot	Play your favorite card game	Help someone in need
2	Give someone a compliment	Tell an inspirational story	Share a favorite recipe	Do push-ups or jumping jacks	Paint nails
3	Jump rope	Share what you'd like to do in the future	Drink coffee	Throw a Frisbee with someone	Write a letter to a family member
4	Dance to your favorite song	Play video games	Talk about your favorite movie with someone	Walk a lap around the room	Have a conversation with someone
5	Sing	Get your hair done	Create music/art	Laugh with somebody	Do the electric slide

FIGURE 13.2. A sample Activity Bingo card.

In the group, you ask an individual to call out a letter and number (e.g., "B 4"). Everyone looks at the activity on their card in that specific space. Anyone who likes the activity either raises their hand or begins doing the activity, if possible. The staff write on a dry erase board or a sheet of paper how many people like each activity. When energy is high, or individuals seem to be enjoying an activity, the staff asks guiding questions, such as "How is it while you're doing this? Good, bad, or just okay?" and "If it makes you feel better or more energized, is it something you'd like to do more often?" This helps people notice the benefit of the activity in the moment.

The benefits to Activity Bingo and similar games are that these activities:

- Provide opportunities for individuals to experience energy, pleasure, socialization, and capability in the moment (learning through doing).
- Help identify interests or areas of knowledge that they might not have thought of on their own.
- Connect individuals to one another as they learn what they have in common.
- Provide a rationale for doing more activity daily.

It's likely there will be a few people on the unit with similar areas of interest. Perhaps they grew up in the same neighborhood, listened to the same music, or share a similar hobby. This is where the power of the milieu can take the initial intervention to the next level: connecting individuals with others who share their passions. Realizing that the desire to belong and connect is at the core of all people, accessing the adaptive mode not only energizes an individual but it can also facilitate opportunities for a broader social network. It helps individuals see that they can, in fact, have relationships with others, and that it is worthwhile to pursue such relationships. This neutralizes defeatist and asocial beliefs.

Energizing the Adaptive Mode: The Activity Challenge

When interests are identified, we want to expand this into opportunities to engage in them as often as possible. This is the CT-R stage of energizing the adaptive mode (see Chapter 3). You can do this with a milieuwide activity challenge and through the creation of interest-based clubs.

One fun and motivating method of energizing is to issue a challenge to individuals: "What can you do while in the hospital, and how often can you do preferred activities during the week?" This challenge sparks energy and interaction and increases how often individuals are likely to be in the adaptive mode. The following is just one example of how a unit can come together to run an activity challenge.

Keep Track of Activity

Individuals and staff carry personalized challenge cards (e.g., written on index cards), listing two to three specific activities they would like to challenge themselves to do during the week with one or more others. After engaging in their preferred activities, participants initial or sign one another's cards. The number of signatures does not represent the number of activities done, but rather the number of people someone is interacting with and doing activities with on a daily/weekly basis.

Designate Staff Challenge Champions

This is a staff member (or members) who will initiate the challenge and introduce it to the unit. This person is also a cheerleader—encouraging individuals and the staff to use their cards. For units with multiple shifts, it can be helpful to have at least one challenge champ per shift to maintain activity throughout the day.

Hold a Kickoff

Either in a group or during community meetings, individuals and the staff can come together to talk about the challenge and decide how they want it to run. The more collaborative, the better!

Start Collecting Signatures Right Away

Individuals can enjoy immediate success by earning signatures during the kickoff! Having music on in the room during the kickoff is a simple way to get cards signed and can be used as a concrete example of how the challenge works (e.g., "Does anyone have listening to music on their card? We are doing that right now! Let's sign some cards!") Other ways to start the challenge with success is to set up activity stations (e.g., with art supplies, games) and encourage people to try something out with others.

Provide Opportunities for Signatures throughout the Week

Any positive interaction can be a valuable and meaningful experience. Encourage individuals to carry their cards with them throughout the week and seek signatures from others when they engage in something they enjoy. All staff, whether participating with their own cards or not, should be aware of the challenge (it can be announced in treatment team and community meetings). The staff can remind participants to bring cards to events, such as parties or groups. If multiple participants engage in an activity together, they can seek signatures from everyone (e.g., one event, five signatures).

Add Up the Number of Signatures

Each week, initials or signatures are totaled as a group and announced to the milieu. The previous weeks' signatures are included in each new challenge count, so the number grows every time.

Use Guided Discovery and Feedback to Draw New Conclusions

While the activity challenge can be used to engage and energize a milieu, many other valuable beliefs can also be strengthened, too—for example, developing relationships is worthwhile, that they have more in common with others than they previously thought, and that they are more capable than they thought. Asking questions about what involvement in the challenge says about participants can help shift beliefs. Similarly, seeking feedback on the experience can highlight what the individual takes away from the challenge.

Examples of guiding questions include:

- "Has participating in the challenge gone better or worse than you expected?"
- "The more active you are, how do you feel? Do you have more energy or less energy?"
- "What does it say about us that we got more signatures than we expected?"
- "If this went better than we thought and we have more energy, is it worth doing these things more often? How about even outside of the hospital/residence?"

It is important to keep in mind that challenges such as these should not be used as a method of earning privileges or rewards, nor should choosing not to participate be punished. It's designed to be voluntary and fun. We've often found that participation grows as more and more activity is happening on the unit and as people see the success of others.

There are many ways to successfully run a milieu activity challenge. Some settings prefer creating unit posters over individual cards, monthly versus weekly counting, and dividing up into two teams and adding a light competition versus adding everything together as one unit. Again—be creative and flexible.

Create Interest-Based Clubs

Another method of energizing the adaptive mode and linking individual formulations to unit programming is to form social clubs—like those in the outside community—as a part of the unit's regularly scheduled programing. Clubs on a milieu are best when both staff and individuals come together to develop and run them. Some examples include gardening clubs, theater or choir clubs, fashion and beauty clubs, making a difference clubs, and exercise clubs. Individuals with those interests, or who want to help others pursue their interests, get together to engage in what they enjoy—for example, in a morning activity club, individuals might play music with one person controlling the radio, another individual leading a stretching and exercise circle, and others enjoying a cup of coffee. All are predictable ways to connect with others, build energy, and start the day with less intrusive challenges.

More general activity clubs, such as ones where individuals have open access to art, games, or music, can provide alternatives to the tradition of "quiet time" on units. Activity clubs promote interaction and reduce isolation, which can otherwise be a primary source of distressing negative and positive symptoms (see Chapters 8 and 9). They also offer opportunities for choices, which are often limited in inpatient settings.

> Recovery with restrictions: Some units have specific restrictions on activities. Clubs can still provide exciting opportunities within those confines. Use techniques such as imagery, planning for future activities, or have individuals teach and explain to staff how to help others have enjoyable experiences.

Clubs empower the staff, too, because they provide opportunities to connect with individuals as people with common interests and not just in the context of mental health challenges or treatment. Because clubs often bring about the "best" (adaptive mode) in individuals, staff members experience a real sense of success in being part of activities that help others.

Developing the Adaptive Mode: Connecting Hospital Activity to Meaningful Aspirations

When individuals are activated into the adaptive mode, it's a good time to identify and enrich aspirations for the future. Identifying and developing aspirations in an inpatient environment are important ways to increase motivation and involvement. Aspirations help link the program's work to what the individual ultimately wants. While some individuals may share goals with the treatment team, the scope of these future aims is often narrow (e.g., get discharged, attend hospital-based groups).

It's common for individuals to struggle to articulate what they want for their future at all—whether within the hospital or upon return to the community. A loss of interest in previously cherished goals contributes to this. As one individual said, "It's like a movie is playing and you hear the sound, but the screen is black—you don't know how you're going to get anywhere because you can't see a future."

To broaden an individual's view of what's possible for the future, aspirations can be built into all elements of an inpatient program. This includes the treatment team, individual therapy, and group therapy. In the next section we focus on integrating aspirations into the treatment team meetings and groups.

Draw Out Aspirations in the Treatment Team

When aspirations are at the forefront, treatment team meetings can be very empowering and meaningful for individuals. You can ask questions in the meeting that elicit and emphasize aspirations, such as:

- "When all of this is said and done and you're out of the hospital, what would you like to be doing?"
- "When we first met, you shared that it was really important for you to reconnect with your daughter and go back to school. Are those still what we're all working toward together?"
- "I know you've said going on tour as a country music artist is something you are eager to do. What would be the best part about that? What would it mean to you to do that?"
- "When you helped Mr. Smith make his way down the hallway safely, he smiled and looked like he really appreciated it. If we work together to find more ways to help others on the unit, do you think it would be a good step toward becoming a nurse?"

Additional strategies and interventions for eliciting and developing individual aspirations can be found in Chapter 4.

In each case, we focus on what is important for the individual, and the tone is collaborative. This indicates that everyone has the same goal: to use hospital or residential stays to get individuals closer to what they want. Even if aspirations seem far off, or are based on expansive beliefs, you can still discuss them in terms of what they mean for the individual. The meanings of aspirations become treatment targets.

When challenges come up—either those that led to the person's hospitalization or from an event that occurred on the unit—you can still place them in the context of aspirations. For example, when working together toward the individual's goals and a challenge arises (e.g., isolation), you can propose participation in a craft club as a way to help the individual get closer to the goal. If the challenge is not distressing to the individual or getting in the way of what they want, don't even present it as a problem.

Developing Aspirations in Groups

Aspirations are energizing and meaningful reasons for individuals to participate in activity clubs and therapy groups on the unit. Clubs can be developed as ways to achieve steps toward aspirations, such as general equivalency diploma (GED) study clubs, job preparation clubs, or clubs where people discuss how to take care of pets. The clear link between activity and aspirations often enhances access to motivation and energy.

You may find that some individuals express frustration at invitations to join therapy groups, perhaps believing "What's the point? I'm just stuck here" or "I've been there and done that!" To counter defeatist beliefs and increase motivation, it's helpful for group facilitators to incorporate individual aspirations into the mission of the group, providing a sense of purpose from the start and consistently. You might say, "So, what's the purpose of this group again? What will our work in here get us closer to?" You can ask participants to call out personal aspirations—things that will be fun, social, make them feel proud, make them feel accomplished, or be less stressed. You can also ask about the meanings of each aspiration. You can list all of these on a dry erase board or on a sheet of paper and reference them throughout the group (e.g., "We've talked a lot today about ways to de-stress. I wonder if this will get us closer to our dreams, like having a relationship or being a hard worker. What do you all think?"). Not only is this a useful way to link the program to goals, it also ends up connecting individuals to one another, as many individuals have similar aspirations or similar underlying meanings.

When people prepare for discharge from inpatient units, it can be a powerful experience for individuals to come together, imagine the future, and problem-solve together. Discharge-oriented clubs—that focus entirely on aspirations, breaking them into steps, and identifying and finding ways to be resilient against stress—are one way to achieve this. These clubs help translate activities that took place on the unit into plans for continued action upon return to the community. They also provide a safe space for individuals to connect over shared fears or stressors that naturally occur when moving toward a desired life. The CT-R approach to group therapy is detailed in Chapter 14.

Actualizing the Adaptive Mode: Positive Action

Opportunities for positive action (see Chapter 5) are an important part of a CT-R milieu. Through action, you can help individuals reactivate positive beliefs and generate new beliefs to plan for a return to the community. Some ways to provide positive action on an inpatient unit include helping others through meaningful roles, positive action scheduling, and, when possible, engaging in activities off the unit.

Help Others and Identify Meaningful Roles

It's energizing and empowering to help others. These actions can significantly shift ideas about belongingness, worthiness, capability, having control, and making a difference. The examples

The CT-R Inpatient Service

highlighted here include helping through roles on the unit milieu, helping roles in the hospital, and roles contributing to the broader community.

ROLES ON THE UNIT

Opportunities for individuals to volunteer for roles on the unit provides a sense of belonging or control in an otherwise uncontrollable environment. Having a role gives individuals and the staff a common goal of being a part of a safe, helpful, unit community. You can build roles into current events of the day, such as a community meeting, or you can create them based on a specific individual's interests—for example, community meeting president and secretary, current events representatives, weather and news reporter, club leader, movie and video-game critic, unit newsletter committee member, and peer greeters who welcome new admissions. As individuals take on unit roles, the staff can use guided discovery to consistently draw meaningful conclusions about the impact of those roles. Common beliefs you can target for those holding unit roles include:

Self: "I'm helpful, I'm capable, I can be focused, I have more control than I thought."
Others: "People appreciate me, other people respect me."
Future: "There are things I'm good at and can do at other times, too."

ROLES IN THE HOSPITAL

Beyond the specific unit, there may be roles individuals can hold in the larger hospital system—for example, they could serve in an information-sharing, advocacy capacity, or on an advisory board that communicates individuals' concerns to hospital administration. Roles like this can strengthen beliefs about individuals' ability to help others, and about their power to improve others' difficult situations—for example, while preparing for discharge, a woman on a long-term inpatient unit was designated as a unit representative. As such, she asked the head of psychiatry to extend outdoor time for other residents, which ultimately was approved. She later shared with the treatment team: "Even though I won't be able to benefit from this, I feel proud to know I helped other people have a better experience, and I think what I did will help them feel better even though they're in the hospital." She also said she believed that by volunteering or working in a care field, she could help other people after she leaves the hospital.

Other hospital roles can involve sharing talents with others, like joining unit choirs or performing arts groups. These individuals could share their own talents, or serve in supportive roles, such as making posters for events and distributing them across campus. Beliefs strengthened by these roles include the ability to gain or sustain energy through activity, beliefs about creativity and capability regarding their skills, and beliefs about their ability to work collaboratively with others and how being with other people is worthwhile.

ROLES CONTRIBUTING TO THE BROADER COMMUNITY

Unit programming that involves long-range or ongoing ways to help the community outside the hospital can access and energize the adaptive mode, link to aspirations, and be a positive action step all in one (e.g., unit clubs that make cards for veterans or sick children, holding clothing and food drives for people impacted by natural disasters, or holding drives for local animal shelters).

Of course, there are many other ways for individuals to become involved, even if a particular cause doesn't match their specific interest. A person may not be interested in animals or having a pet, yet they could use their creativity to develop posters advertising the unit's canned food drive for the local animal shelter. Projects like these bring people together, facilitate a sense of belonging, and can strengthen beliefs of capability, helpfulness, being valued by others, and being safe in interactions with others. Because they take large amounts of time or can be ongoing, activities like these also provide long-range motivation and something to look forward to on a regular basis.

Positive Action Scheduling

When meaningful activities have been identified and the individual agrees that it's valuable to engage in them more often, it's a good time to develop positive action schedules (see Chapter 3). Together with staff, the individual develops a plan to do preferred and goal-directed activities more often during the week. You can review this intervention in the treatment team meeting to see how everyone can support the individual's pursuit of action. This planning can also help increase self-initiating activity.

It's important to help individuals draw the conclusion that the positive things they enjoy in the hospital aren't restricted to life on the unit. Plans and schedules can be part of their lives outside of the hospital. You can ask individuals how they'll keep track of all they want to accomplish outside. Some choose to shift from a one-page positive action schedule to a weekly or monthly planner. Some facilities support the use of cell phones or tablets to help with future activity planning. This can be good practice for how individuals will continue their progress in the community.

Going into the Community

An excellent way to have success experiences and strengthen beliefs about one's ability to carry roles over from the unit into the community is to take community-based trips—for example, if an individual starts a clothing drive and has a chance to deliver donations to local shelters, they may feel more capable, more productive, more helpful. And they may have a stronger connection to the community they've been helping in. There are other benefits, too—for example, individuals who attend church down the street each week as a positive action step toward being more spiritual may also broaden their social network because they see that it's worthwhile to spend time with others.

A great way to maximize the success of off-unit activities is to use your understanding of the individuals' desires and skills to create a plan—for example, the team should consider:

- What beliefs are we targeting (e.g., control, capability, making a difference)?
- Where can we go to have a success experience that strengthens positive beliefs and weakens negative beliefs?

- What role can the individual play in the outing that supports their positive belief (e.g., taking orders for a food pickup, giving directions to the store)?
- What successes do we want the individual to notice during and after the outing (e.g., I can do better than I expect, I'm helpful and a good person). This helps us pick the best guided discovery question(s).

MECHANISMS FOR SUSTAINING A CT-R UNIT

Sustaining a CT-R unit involves several components to maintain the fidelity of the model, allow the treatment team to stay coordinated, and integrate new staff into the recovery-oriented system. We have developed a tool that can help you assess how well you are incorporating CT-R into these and other areas of your program. We call these the CT-R Benchmarks. The Benchmarks consist of seven domains that reflect factors related to programming, staffing, and documentation. Each domain is broken down into items, which are rated along a 4-point scale (0–3), with a "3" representing the CT-R ideal. The CT-R ideal is aspirational and can provide a sense for where a program might like to be eventually. A full version of this self-assessment tool is found in Appendix H. To highlight just a couple of ways inpatient settings can meet CT-R Benchmarks and support sustainability of CT-R practices, we next describe the benefit of regular team brainstorming meetings, use of CT-R-guided documentation in team and clinical meetings, and identification of CT-R champions.

Team Brainstorming Meetings

Outside of the context of formal treatment team meetings with individuals, the treatment team can meet regularly to review individual Recovery Maps and discuss how each member has followed through on their action plans to execute specific interventions. This meeting can be referred to in many ways—for example, clinical roundtable or team huddle. An efficient way to do this is to focus on individuals expected to be seen in a treatment team meeting that week. Reviewing the Recovery Map in this way reminds team members about gaps in understanding (e.g., not knowing someone's aspirations) and provides a specific area of focus for the upcoming meeting.

Besides focusing on specific individuals, clinical round-tables provide an opportunity to discuss CT-R and interventions more broadly—for example, several individuals who used to be on a unit were interested in fashion and they started a club. But now there are individuals on the unit who are more interested in cooking. The team can discuss how the unit can adjust to meet new interests and aspirations as the census changes. Review of guided discovery techniques during clinical round-tables may help ensure that the staff are paying attention to modifying beliefs. In sum, team brainstorming meetings can provide an opportunity for internal consultation, developing or updating formulations, and reviewing programming.

CT-R-Informed Documentation

CT-R can be maintained if it's integrated into the documentation of the unit. Recovery Maps can be used as one form of documentation. They provide a concise guide to understanding individuals, as well as relevant interventions. Treatment plans and progress notes can also link challenges to recovery targets and beliefs, and to respective strategies for change. Other documents that can incorporate CT-R are nursing rounds sheets, which typically annotate individual behaviors throughout the shift—every 15, 30, or 60 minutes—and often include sections for making note of challenges. Existing rounds sheets can be modified to also note positive behaviors and interactions, and whether the individual is engaged in opportunities offered by the unit (e.g., fulfilling a unit role). These documents focus staff attention on recovery-promoting behaviors and can prompt staff to encourage individuals to participate in such things more often.

CT-R Champions

When a unit successfully adopts CT-R, staff members become experts in understanding individuals, connecting with them, eliciting interests and aspirations, and creating opportunities for action. It's helpful to identify champions for the unit whose role is to understand the CT-R approach in depth and how it looks on the unit. Champions can be from any discipline, or from several disciplines. Champions can also serve as internal trainers for new staff, or for the reorientation of seasoned staff to the approach, refreshing their enthusiasm and keeping skills sharp. Champions might be involved in developing staff orientation materials specific to CT-R, or in presenting case studies or successful interventions to administrators. Champions are leaders on the unit who provide suggestions when challenges arise and help guide individuals to draw impactful conclusions.

ADDITIONAL CONSIDERATIONS

When Challenges Come Up, Turn to Formulation and Aspirations

A CT-R-oriented milieu can neutralize negative beliefs that contribute to many challenges—however, challenges, such as isolation, attending to voices, aggression, and others, will likely present. When this happens, the treatment team should review their understanding of the individual (looking at the Recovery Map) and consider what beliefs may have been activated when the challenge was occurring. The team can also do a chain analysis with the individual to better understand what happens in these times (see Chapter 6). Was there a rejection? Loss of control? The team may subsequently plan increased interventions, such as increasing connection and interaction for individuals whose negative symptoms are more challenging, or who believe they cannot do anything to control their voices. Seeking advice and help from individuals who may feel powerless—and are therefore destroying property—may be another intervention. Specific interventions for challenges are detailed in Chapters 7–11. The motivation for tackling challenges is greater when it impacts progress toward what an individual wants for the future.

When challenges need to be addressed in the treatment team meetings, the perspective is that they are keeping the individual from attaining their aspirations. Does the challenge get them closer to or further from achieving their meaningful aspirations? If further, you can ask, "Would it be worth us working together to find ways to not have this get in your way so much?" This helps make potentially useful interventions and skills worth trying (e.g., progressive muscle relaxation, refocusing exercises).

You Don't Need Interventions Tailored to Every Single Person

Though individual formulations can inform programming, they do so on a broader level that brings people together over similar desires, or provides opportunities for many individuals to have roles, even if their goals are unique. Keeping this in mind, you do not need to have 20 unique clubs or groups for 20 different individuals—rather, you will want to find many opportunities for people to come together, work together, and help one another.

Milieu Programs Can Evolve as New People Arrive

As the composition of a unit changes—new people transitioning in, others transitioning out—it is likely that interests and desires will change. Be flexible. If an exercise club or acting club was a big hit at one time, but now no one really holds that interest, it may be time to change things. One way to do this is through regular conversation with individuals and staff seeking feedback on current programming and requesting assistance in keeping it fresh. This is another opportunity for collaboration and roles.

Adapting for Different Lengths of Stay

When an inpatient setting has a short length of stay (a few days to a couple weeks), you may not have sufficient time to fully develop and revamp Recovery Maps or formulations. Similarly, it may not be practical to develop positive action-focused programming for achieving aspirations. In this circumstance, the most important areas of focus are identifying interests and aspirations. What gets someone in the adaptive mode? Can you help them notice this and plan for doing more of these activities either upon discharge to the community or at the next treatment

---

WORDS OF WISDOM

BOX 13.1. A Milieu More Than the Sum of Its Parts

Milieus teem with possibility, whether inpatient, residential, or in a community agency or program. These congregating spaces can be dominated by beliefs that isolate and create a group that is *together alone*. However, staff action can transform the milieu from this resting state into its full active potential. A dynamic therapeutic atmosphere that doesn't look at all like therapy creates mutual positive attitudes, positive affect, and positive action.

This is a network of belonging, purpose, respect, and equality. Activities tap into the interests and values of the individuals. Roles allow them to participate and experience their best selves. Positive attitudes, enthusiasm, and positive action all interact with one another, simultaneously strengthening the adaptive mode of staff and individuals alike.

The ultimate aim is the establishment of a beneficial community atmosphere in which the whole is more than the sum of the parts. The staff become powerful partners, meeting individuals where they are, accessing adaptive modes, imbuing daily living with purpose, and collaboratively developing resiliency in the face of life's inevitable stresses.

Individuals are transformed from feeling defeated to flourishing, from chronic institutionalization to life in the community. There is a successful integration of adaptive beliefs and confidence that enables individuals to thrive.

location? Likewise, if you can identify a meaningful aspiration and develop a rich recovery image, this is incredibly useful in enhancing access to motivation postdischarge.

In short-stay settings, work with individuals on plans to easily recall their strengths and desires; they can then refer to whatever the next step may be—for example, you might say, "Now that we have a clear idea of what you hope for in your life, how can we remember this when the stressful stuff comes up? Should we write it down? How can we best remember the steps?" If the individual in a short-stay setting is able to address a challenge head-on, you can link the use of a clinical intervention to aspirations. For instance, you can use the short stay to identify an aspiration, teach a voice-control technique, and then say, "When things become stressful or the voices feel uncontrollable, how can you remember that using this skill helps you be in control and gets you closer to your dream of being an entrepreneur?"

SUMMARY

- Application of CT-R to an inpatient unit involves integrating the core elements of CT-R into all aspects of clinical care, including treatment team, groups, and on the milieu.
- The emphasis is on creating *connection* between staff and individuals and among the individuals themselves, a sense of *control* over their environment and desires, and *consistency* in opportunities for positive action and progression toward aspirations.

A CT-R unit:
- Understands what individuals and the unit are like when functioning at their best.
- Views individuals' interests and aspirations as being similar to the staff's, which invites interaction and connection.
- Is active and engaging. It activates the adaptive mode by identifying and energizing interests, skills, and areas of knowledge.
- Emphasizes the importance of aspirations, putting them at the forefront of treatment teams, clubs, and groups.
- Provides opportunities for collaboration with staff and others, including ways to be in a helping role, contributing to the unit community and the community outside of the hospital.
- Encourages positive action steps toward aspirations and planning ahead for the future outside of the hospital.
- Strengthens beliefs about energy, capability, self-worth, helpfulness, how worthwhile it is to interact with others, and how there is hope for the future.
- Sustains the approach through coordinated teams, recovery-oriented documentation, and selection of champions to encourage consistency and fidelity to the model.

CHAPTER 14
CT-R Group Therapy

The group at the clinic has been getting together for 2 months now. On this particular day, Daniel comes in especially tired and mentions to the facilitator that he doesn't even know how he made it in. As other people arrive, they all seem to notice that Daniel is really out of sorts. He doesn't respond when they ask him what's wrong, though he does appear to be whispering under his breath.

The facilitator asks others about their energy level, and several agree that it's not very high. She then invites Erica, another group member, to help lead a light stretching exercise for the group, which they'd done a few weeks before, to see whether they can get their energy up. The facilitator asks Daniel, "Should we listen to something slow or more upbeat during the stretching?" Daniel says, "Upbeat." Another individual turns on a radio station playing pop music, and Erica leads the stretching. Some people, including Daniel, start off in their chairs doing the moves, while others stand. The facilitator begins asking different people whether they have stretches they'd like to show the group. When she asks Daniel, he gets up and teaches a leg stretch. The group continues in this way for about 5 minutes.

As she's wrapping it up, the facilitator notices everyone seems to have more energy—and that Daniel is smiling while thanking Erica for getting them started. The facilitator asks everyone about their energy again, and they agree—it's better! They agree that it was worth doing. And they all agree that they now feel more ready to keep going with the group session.

Group therapy and the group process are powerful vehicles for change. Groups present opportunities for connection, belonging, problem solving, taking action toward goals, and new experiences that empower and inspire movement toward aspirations (Yalom, 1963). You can use the recovery-oriented cognitive therapy approach to create new groups. You can also infuse it into existing groups that you facilitate. This chapter presents the phases of the CT-R group process, including the overall structure of a CT-R (or CT-R-informed) group session, and concludes with specific considerations for successfully realizing CT-R in group therapy.

CT-R GROUP PHASES

There is a natural progression that you can expect to see in a course of CT-R group therapy. This set of phases maps on to the basic elements of the CT-R approach. There is no designated number of sessions for each phase to allow you to be flexible as the needs of the group members become evident. Sometimes, you will move stepwise through each phase, but sometimes you will need to reenergize, reassess aspirations, or address new challenges.

Accessing and Energizing Phase

To start, you want to welcome individuals into the group, build connection among members, find common ground, and develop a group identity. This building of cohesion also involves setting the expectation that the group sessions will be active and build energy. At its core, group CT-R is an opportunity for participants to gain a sense of belonging and purposeful action together.

You will be most effective by having conversations that activate the adaptive mode (see Chapter 3). Energized discussion about interests, such as the best pizza and favorite toppings, listening to music together, or exercising, are connecting experiences that group members may not routinely experience in their day-to-day lives. You can also play games, such as trying to keep a balloon in the air, playing Activity Bingo (see Chapter 13) or Name That Tune, as well as others to create energy and teamwork.

You also want to collaboratively develop a group mission. A mission is unifying and can serve as a brief reminder of why everyone is there. If you're creating a new group, you might say, "I'm hoping our new group can be really fun but also get us moving toward the things we really care about. What do you all think?" For existing groups, you might say, "We're been doing anger management together for a little while. Let's see how it fits into what we want in life. What's the mission of our time together?"

A more interactive approach to developing a mission can include the facilitator putting empowering and resilience-oriented words and pictures on a dry erase board or on a sheet of paper, and inviting individuals to point to or write the ones that hold a lot of meaning to them. Together, the group can then use the different words or pictures to create a mission statement. It can take a few sessions to develop the mission.

Examples of CT-R group missions include "Getting out and staying out: Smoothing the path to recovery" (an inpatient group) and "Empowerment group: Taking it to the streets and taking action toward our desires!" (a community-based group).

Developing Phase

Now, you want to identify, elicit, and develop group members' aspirations. Share and discuss aspirations and their meanings (e.g., What would be good about them?), and then draw attention to shared meanings that underlie everyone's aspirations. We find time and again that individuals may have different dreams for the future, but that there are themes that may be similar—for example, one person might want to work and someone else might want to volunteer, but the meaning of both might be having a sense of purpose or a desire to provide for others.

One group member might want to return to school, while another wants to join a community book club, or work with their brother to learn plumbing. Although these aspirations may seem distinct, the connecting thread might be a desire to expand their minds, to feel accomplished, or to have a way of connecting to others.

Similarly, individuals might desire a romantic partner, to spend more time with a parent, or to join Bible study; connection and meaningful relationships may be the common thread. Finally, individuals might share desires to manage their own money, have their own place, or have their own businesses; independence and capability might be the common meaning.

You can spend several sessions identifying and elaborating on as many group members' long-range goals as possible.

You elicit and enrich aspirations in the same way described in Chapter 4. However, for the group, you want to bring individuals into the conversation, even if it is not their own aspiration—for example, when someone identifies an aspiration, you first ask them what the best part would be. Then, you can ask the group, "What do you all think? Does anyone else want that? What are some other good things about that?" Group members can help enrich, as well: "What other details might you want to know about their aspiration?"

Inviting people to think about others' aspirations can be inspiring. People who may have otherwise had difficulty identifying an aspiration for themselves may discover a passion or remember a desire. You may find that when some individuals are asked about the best part or the meaning of their aspiration, they share challenges instead (e.g., "Well, I don't know if I can keep a job, and what if my income goes down?"). You can use the group to help rekindle the excitement. You might say, "That's interesting. In thinking about the best part of working you came up with a few reasons it might be tough. Can anyone else think what might be the best part of working for Sophia? What might be good about it?" In response, the other individuals often give supportive and encouraging responses, such as "She's so social, she'd probably help a lot of people" and "You could make more money to help your son." The group members begin to play a role in helping one another build hope for the future.

Refer back to member's aspirations and meanings in each session—for instance, you might say, "So, we're still working together on getting you two back to work; you three into new relationships, and you two moving toward opening your clothing and ice cream business. Right?" This is how the aspirations support continuity and provide the basis for moving forward.

> Actualizing the adaptive mode in groups:
>
> ✓ Break down aspirations into intermediate and immediate action steps.
> ✓ Create a group project linked to shared meanings under aspirations.
> ✓ Plan for action between group sessions.
> ✓ Collaborate with group members to problem-solve challenges.
> ✓ Act out problem-solving strategies.

Actualizing Phase

Once the group mission is established and meaningful aspirations are elicited, you want to develop ways to take action toward aspirations or their meanings. You break aspirations down into steps, try some steps out together, and plan for action between groups.

Breaking Aspirations into Small Steps

The group members need to see recovery goals as attainable. Therefore, you need to break aspirations down into intermediate and immediate action steps (see Chapter 5). The advantage of doing this in a group setting is that many people are better at seeing solutions for others than for themselves. Group members often provide good suggestions for how to break one another's goals down into smaller steps. This is also an opportunity to help others, which is beneficial in and of itself.

Conclusions that can be drawn as group members help one another include "What does it say that everyone came together to help you make plans to get back to work? Other people sometimes care a lot about us, don't they?" and "What does it say about you that you helped Thomas think of steps he hadn't considered before? Would you say you're a pretty good problem-solver?"

Actualizing Steps as a Group Project

You can also actualize by creating a collective project that links to some of the shared meanings underlying members' aspirations. Examples might be developing a group cookbook (linked to an aspiration of being a better parent, and tied to some group members' interests and skills around cooking), drawing pictures or making cards for organizations that care for homeless veterans or sick children (linked to an aspiration of helping others and using people's creative interests), or organizing a clothing drive for the community shelter (linked to an aspiration of giving back to the community).

Working on these projects together provides opportunities to experience energy and connection regularly (accessing and energizing the adaptive mode), serves as direct links to aspirations (developing the adaptive mode), and is a way to achieve meaning related to aspirations right in the moment (actualizing the adaptive mode). The projects are prime opportunities for strengthening beliefs about purpose, self-worth, and the ability to work well with others (strengthening the adaptive mode). The work is efficient because everyone is simultaneously benefitting from the collective action.

Problem Solving

You will find it straightforward to identify possible challenges as individuals consider steps toward aspirations or begin taking action—for example, a group member made a plan to listen to music with their sister, but they were too worried about what their sister would think (anxiety); or a person wanted to join the local book club but instead spent the day in bed listening to voices; or perhaps they did not get a job interview and went home and used substances. You want to collaborate with group members to identify and problem-solve some of these challenges of everyday living.

Don't open with the problem. Rather, you first want to review and generate energy around aspirations. This puts hope and purpose front and center—the reason why it is ultimately worth overcoming the challenges. After reviewing aspirations, you can ask the group to pick a specific aspiration and break it down into steps. Then you can ask, "What might be some things that could make it difficult to achieve this?" It is best if the specific challenges are selected by the individuals.

In some groups, you may have members who are willing to talk about times when things did not work out well for them. If this is the case, you can move directly to problem solving together. You might find, at times, that asking about challenges can have the opposite effect. It can bring about negative beliefs and contribute to shutting down, expansive beliefs, or agitation among the group members. To provide a balance, you can ask advice for a problem you or someone else might have, or try role-playing and acting.

Solving a problem for others takes some of the pressure off of the group members who may feel especially vulnerable. You can ask questions such as "What might happen if I really wanted to take this action step but I just felt too tired?" or "My sister gets really nervous when she thinks about trying to meet someone new. Do you have any ideas of what she can do when she feels anxious?" You might also ask, "Is there anything you've done that's helped if you've ever felt this way?"

As group members generate ideas, you express appreciation for their helpfulness and ask whether you can write them down. Ideally, you can write them on a dry erase board or on a sheet of paper that everyone can see. You can then move from solving someone else's challenges to their own. You can ask the group, "Has anyone here ever experienced this?" You might then try one of the group's suggestions in session, such as deep breathing.

Finally, suggest using these strategies in the future: "Would it be worth us trying some of these strategies we came up with outside of group, too? Maybe as our action plan?" At the conclusion of the conversation, you can use guided discovery to strengthen beliefs about individuals' ability to be helpful, smart, and reap the benefits of working together.

Role playing or acting out different problem-solving strategies (Beck, 2020) is another way to help group members fully participate and collectively benefit. It can be a fun way to think through many options. One approach is as follows:

1. Identify a challenge to focus on and invite everyone to give suggestions on how to help.
2. Encourage all possible responses: "There are no wrong answers—we all have many choices we can make. Some might get us closer to our aspirations than others, but that's what we're going to figure out as we act them out!"
3. List the suggestions in a place where everyone can see them.
4. Invite individuals to decide who would like to play the role of director—the director says, "Action!" and "Cut!" as others act out the scene.
5. Invite individuals to play the role of someone with a challenge or who wants to take an action step toward their aspiration. (It does not have to be one they themselves experience or desire.) Someone else can play the person they will interact with (e.g., a family member, potential partner, potential boss).
6. Test all of the suggestions and get the whole group's reactions about what they noticed, what worked well, and what was less helpful.
7. As a group, everyone can then identify some of the best strategies and an action plan can be developed.

Activities such as these encourage creativity, and also help people evaluate decisions without being shamed.

Consider an individual who brings up the challenge of fearing that if they get a job, other people might use them for their money, and they might give in. Suggestions might include to give away the money, fight, talk about why you can't help out right now, and suggest other ways you can help out without giving money. Acting out each option (or imagining it, such as in the case of fighting) can help people evaluate the pros and cons of each choice. Then the options can be weighed against the aspirations: "Which choice or choices might make it easier to reach your aspiration of feeling independent and capable of caring for yourself? Which might make it harder?

We have seen this type of "act it out" group produce a lot of excitement and group cohesion, as well as good ideas for handling some of life's toughest challenges (Tang et al., 2020). We have also seen such groups facilitated effectively by the individuals themselves.

Planning for Action between Sessions

A final approach to actualizing is to plan action between group sessions and check on progress. In an inpatient setting, this might involve participation in an activity challenge (see Chapter 13) or joining another milieu or club program. In the community, this may involve positive action scheduling (see Chapters 3 and 5). Group members can help one another develop action plans, celebrate successes as people make progress, and help one another problem-solve if they run into challenges.

Strengthening Phase

Strengthening the adaptive mode can happen at any phase of a CT-R group. The guided discovery techniques discussed in Chapter 6 are just as effective in groups as they are individually or on a milieu. You want to promote future action and to strengthen adaptive beliefs and beliefs about group members' abilities to feel resilient in the face of challenges or setbacks. Using guided discovery in a group can be especially effective because other individuals may provide empowering comments about how resilient the person is—for example, while doing a group activity you might point out "Did you notice Paula's reaction to your poster? What does that say about you that you made her smile like that?" and "Paula, what was it like to have Chris help you like that? Sounds like you're both really helpful and a good team. Did either of you expect that?"

Similarly, as people are successful at action steps toward aspirations or come up with problem-solving strategies in the group, you can ask the group, "What do you guys think it says about Dave that he started his resumé?" Questions that might be useful in other phases include "Was it worth us doing this to get our blood pumping and get some energy?" and "Does it seem worth going over our mission a bunch so we can always keep our eyes on the prize?"

CT-R GROUP SESSION STRUCTURE

The structure of a CT-R or CT-R-informed group, as shown in Figure 14.1, provides a guide for what to plan as a facilitator. Use the same formula as you move through the phases of the approach. The structure includes the following components: accessing the adaptive mode, a bridge between group meetings, review of aspirations, problem solving, and developing action plans for between sessions.

Opening: Accessing the Adaptive Mode

To open a group session, you can check on the energy level or mood of the group members, and then engage in conversations or actions that facilitate connection to one another and bring group

Group Phases	Group Structure
Phase 1: Accessing and Energizing Building connection, group identity, and cohesion	**Opening: Accessing the Adaptive Mode** Focus on energy, connection, getting people into the adaptive mode
Phase 2: Developing Identifying, eliciting, and developing aspirations	**Bridge: Shared Mission** Why are we here and why do we keep coming back?
Phase 3: Actualizing Identifying and participating in meaningful action related to aspirations	**Aspirations: Elicited and Developed** Can guide the mission and be the reason why challenges are addressed
Phase 4: Problem Solving Addressing challenges as they arise	**Challenges: Problem Solving in Context of Aspirations** May be a theme of the group or may come up only as it applies to achieving the aspirations
Phase 5: Strengthening Building Resiliency	**Action Plan** Based on what we did in group, what might we do during the week or before the next group?

FIGURE 14.1. CT-R group therapy structure and phases for new or existing groups.

members into the adaptive mode—for example, you may ask members to rate their energy level as low, medium, or high, or on a scale from 1 to 10, where 1 = *No energy*, 5 = *Some energy but not a lot*, and 10 = *Extraordinarily energized*. You might then ask about topics such as agency outings, special events for holidays, or local events (e.g., fairs, parades), sporting events, and so on. For example:

FACILITATOR: Are people getting ready for the holidays?

EDWARD: Yeah.

FACILITATOR: How many other people are getting ready? [*people raise hands*] What's your favorite part of the season?

PAT: I like seeing the kids enjoying the decorations. Seeing people excited.

KEVIN: I like the food.

GROUP: Me too!

Activity examples include music, throwing a ball around the room, or stretching, such as in this chapter's opening vignette. Spend enough time in this portion of the group to increase the group's energy sufficiently for proceeding to the next step. You can also help people notice that talking with others about enjoyable topics or doing a fun activity feels better and gives them some power. You can use strengthening and guided discovery interventions to help them notice the effects of these opening exercises. This part of the group often only takes a few minutes. If energy remains low, however, you can shift your approach (e.g., from conversation to action) or suggest that the mission of the group for that session focus on building some momentum to get through the rest of their day.

Bridge: Shared Mission

The next step in the group is a conversation that serves as a bridge connecting the last session to the current one. The first part of the bridge asks individuals to share why it is that the group gets together—the group's mission. You can also review action plans from the previous session and see how everyone did. When a new individual joins the group, the bridge is an opportunity for the more seasoned members to serve in an expert role and explain the mission so as to get new members up to speed.

Aspirations: Elicited and Developed

Early in the group process, it is very important to elicit and enrich aspirations. Once you have a sense for group members' aspirations and their valued meanings, you will want to briefly review and reference them in each session. Early on in the group's course, you will want to do this step before introducing the bridge, as aspirations can guide the development of a mission. By recalling the aspirations each session, you continue to build the excitement and create reasons for the potentially hard work of addressing challenges.

Challenges: Problem Solving in the Context of Aspirations

Once energy is sufficient, the mission is highlighted, and the aspirations are confirmed, you can begin to plan action and address challenges that may impede progress toward aspirations. Challenges may be the theme of the group (e.g., anger management) or they may come up in a CT-R-specific group after aspirations have been broken into steps. In either case, it is in this part of the session that you will either introduce skills or invite individuals to help one another problem-solve. This takes most of the session's time, particularly after you have moved out of the aspiration development phase.

Action Plan

At the end of each group, you will want to collaborate with the group members to develop an action plan. Based on what was discussed in the group, what might the individuals do during the week before the next session? You want to elicit summaries from individuals about what they got out of the group. You can also share your own takeaways (e.g., "What I'm hearing you say is we learned today that you gain more from doing things with others than alone. Is that right?" and "Since listening to music with the group gave you so much happiness and connection, could each of us try that this week? Can you think of at least one person to listen to music with? What song would you want to try?").

At the end of the session you can also elicit feedback on its activities, assessing what was most useful, least useful, and what the group members would like to do similarly or differently in future groups.

Interest-based clubs (see Chapter 12) can follow a similar structure—for example, community service clubs can have a shared mission and can still be linked to individual aspirations. Similarly, individuals can develop action plans around future engagement in preferred activities and positive beliefs about the adaptive mode can be strengthened. Existing groups, such as those focused on drug and alcohol treatment, legal issues, or stress management, can apply this structure to maintain motivation for addressing these specific challenges. Figure 14.1 illustrates the group phases and structure.

ADDITIONAL CONSIDERATIONS

When Individuals Have Low Energy or Low Participation

Develop a formulation to understand what might be limiting group participation. When individuals have low energy or attend but don't participate in the group, possible active beliefs include "I just don't have the energy"; "What's the point?"; "I'm not worth it"; "I can't relate to other people"; or "Other people don't care; they can't understand me anyway."

Strategies that activate the adaptive mode (see Chapter 3) are helpful here. Spend time finding energizing hooks for individuals, and possibly ones that many enjoy. When asking questions, present them in closed-ended ways (e.g., yes/no questions, offer choices).

In an inpatient setting, you might start with accessing techniques right in the person's room. You can also hold group programs on the milieu if low energy is a more global challenge. Another effective approach is to provide opportunities for individuals to have roles in the group: ask for advice about the opening activity, invite someone to be the timekeeper so that the group starts and ends on time, ask for help setting up the room to start. Roles can increase energy, increase equality to you, and can be low pressure while still contributing.

The focus on aspirations is also helpful here. If individuals get excited by their aspirations, and others share or support their interests, it counters beliefs of being alone or misunderstood. It strengthens beliefs that they may have more in common with people than they thought.

When Challenges Carry over from Outside the Group

Sometimes people have a rough day—or many. Irritation and frustration can carry over from the day's events into the group, making it difficult to proceed as planned. We might understand this as an individual's attempt at communicating their experiences and having their voices heard. It could also be related to beliefs that their situation cannot improve, and nothing will get better.

In these situations, you want to take approaches that provide as much connection, choice, and control as possible. Connection can be in the form of being nonjudgmental and empathic: "I hear you saying how difficult things are. I imagine I would be angry, too, if I were you!" or "I imagine that when tough things happen, it can be hard to feel safe. What do you think?" Choice and control can be in the form of providing meaningful, helpful roles. This can also help refocus attention.

Maintaining Attention

Maintaining attention in a group can sometimes be a challenge for the members. People may be struggling with negative symptoms, distracting voices, or the sedating effects of certain medications. The energizing, aspiration-focused, and action-oriented components of each group session can combat some of these challenges. Additional suggestions include hopping around the room to elicit ideas and seek participation, rather than going one-by-one around the room. You can also incorporate nonverbal attention strategies, such as throwing a ball around to one another, even during conversation. If the group as a whole seems to have reduced energy and attention, it can be helpful to stay in—or return to—the *accessing the adaptive mode* step of the group for the duration of the session. This can provide valuable experiences that individuals can generate their own energy and that, as a group, you are all in it together to help one another overcome this challenge.

Transitions and Changes in Group Composition

Changes in group membership can present interesting challenges and opportunities. In an open-attendance group, new group members can be welcomed when more experienced members serve in helpful roles, such as explaining the mission or describing the session structure. Many group members may share this role. Group members may also discontinue attendance. This may be because of discharge or stepping down from services. In this case, celebrate leaving members and their accomplishments. Celebrations can be great times to reiterate strengthened beliefs and lessons learned. It can also be an opportunity for the parting member to share messages of inspiration or hope to other members. An important conclusion to draw is that,

---

WORDS OF WISDOM

BOX 14.1. Affiliation and Spreading Activation of Purpose

Doing things together brings out the best in everyone at the same time. Participating with others and identifying with the group activates interpersonal connections and desire for affiliation. The goals of the group may transcend the individual's own personal values and goals, allowing the members to do something bigger than any one of them can do individually. Generosity, empathy, and compassion are particularly powerful social processes that emerge in the spirit of collaboration, be it decorating the unit or residence, cooking a meal together, putting on a play, running a clothing drive, or cleaning up the neighborhood.

Think of the group as a network. Individuals fuse together, forming a team with a group identity. Members have different roles in achieving the overall group mission, creating a dynamic flow from group to individual and back. Everyone can achieve the specific meaning of their aspirations together, precisely because the group allows for individualized roles in actualizing the group mission.

Motivation and optimism are contagious, spreading across the group members electrically. The group project can be something to get up for, an activity that makes each day special, and a safe place to experience affiliation, collaboration, appreciation, and purpose. These qualities are connected with one another, within each person and across persons. Enthusiasm grows and reflects between members dynamically. This mutual reinforcement of positive emotion and success can impact each member's sense of being worthwhile, capable, belonging, and mattering. It can also help members dream bigger dreams and live bigger lives. Since they have exceeded expectations in the group or club, who knows what they might be capable of?

even though leaving members may not attend the group, they remain connected because of all they've done together—that is something that does not go away.

Individuals might also leave abruptly due to experiencing considerable challenges or other reasons. You can acknowledge the person's absence and share with the group that you hope they will be able to join again in the future or work hard to achieve their aspirations. This reflects your hopeful desires for all group members, and further demonstrates how connection can continue even if the person is not physically present.

SUMMARY

- The strategy for change in a group context is the same as in individual therapy. The facilitator collaborates with individuals to connect and build trust with others, to increase energy, to identify and enrich aspirations, to plan action toward aspirations, and to strengthen beliefs around success and capability.
- CT-R groups help individuals connect with one another around the shared meanings of their aspirations.
- With one another's aspirations in mind, a CT-R group supports problem solving and developing action steps together. People feel less alone when describing challenges, providing further opportunities to strengthen resiliency beliefs.
- The best groups are experiential—giving opportunities for individuals to experience energy, take action steps toward aspirations, or practice problem-solving strategies. Success in the moment provides opportunities for strengthening positive beliefs and countering those that drive challenges.

CHAPTER 15
Families as Facilitators of Empowerment

Much of the approach described in this book plays to the strengths of families. They often have a lot of information about their relative. They can inform about passionate interests, hidden strengths, possible aspirations, and positive beliefs to strengthen, as well as about challenges and negative beliefs to weaken. Families are at their best when doing meaningful activities together, sharing a meal, playing a game, telling stories, or taking a trip. Being part of a family satisfies an elemental sense of belonging to a group. There are many opportunities for roles within the family, too, that make it stronger and more successful, promoting every member's happiness.

In short, the family is an ideal partner in helping to promote the empowerment of individuals with serious mental health challenges (Klapheck, Lincoln, & Bock, 2014). In this chapter, we focus on how you can collaborate with the family to produce betterment for all. We acknowledge the difficulty that can be involved, but also believe in the benefits of successful partnerships.

FOCUS THE FAMILY ON BELIEFS

You can be helpful to the family by providing a new way to understand their relative in terms of underlying beliefs. We start with and emphasize the positive beliefs and *at-their-best* moments. Families can be useful by providing stories that might inform or confirm the person's passions and the beliefs the person holds. The person that the family has always known is still there. With the right approach, the family can see more of this side of their relative. Family can encourage action that amplifies positive beliefs that are the opposite of the negative ones that govern the challenges. The relative wants to be a good person, a helping person, to belong, to make the world a better place, to love and be loved.

Families can be involved in adding to the relative's Recovery Map and can also take important information from your formulation. Share your understanding from the Recovery Map that captures the whole person. This helps the family be better partners with their relative to pursue a fuller, desired life. Work with the family on how to bring out the individual's strengths and interests, and what these may mean about them. You can also help the family take action steps that are less likely to evoke vulnerabilities.

> CT-R steps for families:
>
> ✓ Ask for the family's help in understanding their relative's *at-their-best* moments.
> ✓ Learn about times the family is or was at its best.
> ✓ Encourage the family to support big aspirations and their meanings.
> ✓ Help the family to understand situations and beliefs that can bring about challenges.
> ✓ Draw conclusions about the individual's and their family's successes.
> ✓ Strengthen positive beliefs through action and problem solving as a team.

FACILITATE FAMILY EMPOWERMENT

Adaptive Mode and the Best Self

The first step in working with families is to introduce them to the concept of the adaptive mode and get them thinking of the individuals' at-their-best moments. You can ask, "What is he like at his best?"; "What was she doing before all the challenges came up?"; or "Can you think of times that are the exceptions to the rule—he's yelling a lot at his voices, but are there times he *isn't* and what is happening at those times?" Next, ask what their relative might think during these at-their-best moments. Do they see themselves as connected? Capable? A good person? Ask how their relative might feel. Happy? Content? Proud? These are all conjectures for the Recovery Map.

You can discuss with the family strategies for accessing their relative's adaptive mode. Help the family to select activities that will be mutually beneficial and appeal strongly to their relative. Consider interests, skills, and passions. Can the family seek the person's advice? Can the family restart activities they used to love doing? Doing together is best. Being creative is a plus.

Energizing the Adaptive Mode—Family at Its Best

A good way to help the family begin to assist in building up their relative's adaptive mode is to pose the question "When is the family at *its* best? What types of activities are you doing together?" At these times there is likely to be a sense of interconnectedness. Everyone is pitching in, much like a team. It is this spirit that cultivates the right activity to energize the adaptive mode of the relative. Do what is good for everyone and the right activities will be there.

Part of the family moving toward being at its best is giving everyone a role, which means giving the relative a productive, helping purpose within the family. Often individuals given a mental health diagnosis are offered a lot of help. They can grow weary of receiving help. This might even strengthen beliefs they have about being defective. Instead, offer the relative a role that supports the family. Have the family look for shared interests: meals together, listening to music, dancing, walks, going to services, watching sporting events, going to live arts events, supporting the kids or grandkids. This will lead naturally to more activity together; their relative might begin to entertain future aspirations. The possibilities are endless. The key is to help the family do these things predictably and often.

Help the family to notice how good these at-their-best activities feel. Suggest they comment on how good it feels and ask everyone, including the relative, how it feels to them. Draw conclusions with families in the same way we do with their relative. What does it say about the family that they are doing good things for one another? Helping one another? Connecting better with one another? What more like this could they be doing?

Aspirations—Dreaming Big Together

Given their history together, the family may well have ideas about aspirations their relative might want to pursue, or know what their relative wanted prior to the onset of the challenges. The family can be enthusiastic supporters of aspirations. Make sure to encourage the family's support of big dreams and draw their attention to the role of aspirations as a counterbalance to the powerful beliefs that amplify challenges.

Family can especially help their relative savor the idea in the aspiration by asking, "What would be the best part?" and "What would it feel like?" They can be ready for the relative to talk about helping make the world a better place, feeling like they matter, contributing. The family can ask more questions to get at the dream: "Paint me a picture?"; "What will your day look like?"; "Who will you be doing things with?": "How will you feel doing those kinds of things?"; and "What will it say about you?"

Guiding families to have these conversations with their relative emphasizes connection and partnership and helps them avoid power struggles about whether or not the aspirations are attainable, because the meanings are real and achievable.

Here's an example of how a dialogue with an individual and his brother could go:

PROVIDER: Thank you for coming in today. I think we had a really great start! Some of those plans you made sound exciting! Which ones do you think your brother would be the most interested in?

INDIVIDUAL: Oh, the guitar. We used to play music together as kids.

BROTHER: What about the guitar?

INDIVIDUAL: Oh, I want to get back to playing. I also want to play at church on Sundays eventually and maybe teach. . . .

BROTHER: Are you kidding me? Me on drums again and you on guitar? That would be awesome. Don't think the pastor could take that again.

INDIVIDUAL: I don't think he'd stand for any of our goofing off.

BROTHER: Maybe . . . maybe not [*laughing*]. Also, teaching? You're going to show my daughter some stuff, right?

INDIVIDUAL: [*hesitantly*] I guess so . . . really?

BROTHER: Who else would I want teaching my girl?

Ultimately, the dreaming together is powerful. It strengthens the family members' bonds with one another. They feel closer. And the relative sees the dream as more achievable. The family at its best can promote everyone in their highly valued missions.

Families as Facilitators of Empowerment

Positive Action Toward Aspirations—Family Getting Even Better

Once the relative's aspiration has been developed, the family can be a great place to plan activities that have the same underlying meaning. They can also collaborate on activities that move their relative closer to achieving the aspiration. This is a continuation of the family at its best. This will work best if it is mutual, and everyone feels a part of the team and helping goes in all directions.

Successes can be celebrated as they accrue. Problems can be solved together as they crop up. It will be important for the family to foster a spirit of collaboration, planning activities together, and making sure the relative maintains a sense of control throughout by being offered choices. The family can collaborate to help their relative extend beyond a particular comfort zone (e.g., applying for jobs, going to school, dating, having an apartment). For instance, as an individual starts a job, his sister might commiserate with the frustrations of waking up and getting ready: getting up, packing lunch, figuring out transportation, remembering to take breaks. She might share some of her tricks and see what he thinks of them, both of them sharing notes later about how well these worked.

Frequency and predictability of family activities works well, but surprises add an occasional spice. Mission work should not crowd out fun. Working out, cooking, going to services, watching shows together—along with weekly pursuit of aspirations—all exemplify the family at its best getting better. We have seen great success for family members who use a combined positive action schedule (see Chapters 3 and 5) to plan activities they will do together. (You can modify Figure 13.1 for this purpose.)

Because challenges tend to come up in the course of taking all this action, it can sometimes be useful for families to understand in terms of beliefs. Questions they might have are:

- Why doesn't she have friends anymore?
- Why does he sleep all day?
- Why doesn't he know that what he hears isn't real?
- Why does he believe he owns the whole state?
- Why does she hurt herself?

Though no one wants their loved one to hold such defeating beliefs, it can be helpful to know that the person sees themselves as a failure, other people as treacherous, and the future as nonexistent or that they see themselves as vulnerable and incompetent, and others as rejecting (Beck et al., 2019).

Understanding these challenges in terms of beliefs can be empowering for the family, helping empathize better with how their relative must feel, and giving them a chance to come up with ways for their relative to have more experiences to counter such negative expectations and worldviews.

To help them consider which beliefs might be most relevant to the challenges, ask the family about what the person might be thinking most of the time when not in this adaptive mode. You can ask, "Why might it be that anyone might withdraw from others?" You can float possible beliefs, such as "What's the point of trying? I am going to fail anyway"; "Something is wrong with me"; and "I will do it when I have the energy." It can help the family see how their relative might experience a strong pull toward inactivity. Accessing the adaptive mode combats this demoralized state.

Building Resilience

Family can have the greatest role in helping their relative to persevere—thrive even—when things don't work out. Doing more and going for aspirations entails risks. With risks come setbacks, as well as victories. Stress is tougher on some days than others. Living one's purpose involves all of this. The relative might change course. They might experience dead ends, rejections, and disappointments. When life is tough and more challenging, the family can aid their relative. Resiliency is the ability to handle life's challenges, expressed in the phrase "I got this."

The relative has most likely experienced a period in which they did not feel strong or capable. They may have believed "I can't handle this; I am just going to fail." They may have given up each time things got a little hard: "Why try? I can't succeed." Now that they are in the adaptive mode building their desired life, those old ideas may still crop up.

The family can help their relative see things more accurately and flexibly. What appear to be big setbacks can be brought down to the right size. Things not working out is just a part of life and not a catastrophe. Types of conclusions the relative can draw include "It did not turn out the way I thought it would, but it was still worth it" and "I may not have gotten it the first time, but I will if I keep trying."

Having the relative help other family members solve daily problems can be especially effective. This activity has a lot of meaning, and the solutions that are hit upon can be transferred to the relative themselves: "Why don't we both try this solution?" This can set up the whole family as a group of problem solvers who can anticipate ways to manage future challenges for everyone.

ADDITIONAL CONSIDERATIONS

How to Help Families Promote Empowerment When Challenges Arise

Whatever challenges the relative tends to experience, the feeling of disconnection is likely to be at the core. At its essence, family embodies powerful connections; perhaps the strongest ones we know are being a mother, father, brother, sister, son, or daughter. These connections can be brought to bear, often with some creativity, when the relative has a flare-up of mental health challenges. With the right set of actions, family can reaccess their relative's adaptive mode. You can help the family do this.

Negative Symptoms

Since the negative symptoms are sometimes misunderstood as laziness or a character flaw, you can make sure the family has a sense of what to look for in their relative's inaction and how to understand what they see in terms of beliefs. When the family sees a reduction or elimination of activity, socializing, and pleasure, their relative is feeling demoralized and disconnected. Beliefs they might hold include "Failing partway is the same as failing all the way" (limited access to motivation), "Nobody likes me" (limited socializing), and "I can't enjoy anything" (limited pleasure).

The family can provide opportunities to counter inactivity with positive action that appeals to the relative and can bring out their best self. The family can help turn the tide and move the relative toward more purpose. The relative can draw conclusions about themselves, others, and the future—for example:

- Doing an appealing or pleasurable activity together (going for a walk, playing a game, cooking) increases energy and can lead to useful beliefs, such as "The more I do that I enjoy, the better I feel" and "Once I get going, I always feel better."
- Contributing to the family in some way (fixing a cell phone or data assistant, such as Alexa) leads to success and having a role; possible positive beliefs include "It went better than I thought it would"; "It was hard at first, but I am glad I did it"; and "I can make meaningful contributions."

Delusions

These beliefs can be quite divisive for family. Their relative can exist in modes that are either expansive or safety seeking, both of which can be very concerning to the family. Because these beliefs can be hard to comprehend and cause much worry, you can help the family understand better what they are seeing. The beliefs grow out of disconnection. Their relative highly values these hard-to-understand beliefs. This is why challenging the truthfulness of these beliefs can be counterproductive, further disconnecting and isolating. In some cases, challenging the delusion strengthens the beliefs.

You can help the family see that the beliefs represent the basic needs for value, control, autonomy, and safety. If their relative has grandiose beliefs, these compensate for lack of importance, of success, of respect. If their relative has paranoid beliefs, these reflect a sense of being vulnerable and incapable and highly valuing safety and control.

The successful approach is to meet the need of a delusion rather than address the belief directly. Families are good at providing interactions that embody connection. Helping their relative have a valuable role within the family and in the community can go a long way toward helping the person feel important and capable. It can also give the person a sense of control and show them that others are helpful and value them.

Hallucinations

Voices and other hallucinations can also be hard for the family to understand. They can be tempted to tell the person that the voices are not real, that it is all in their relative's head. You can help the family see that this approach can also be invalidating. The person's experience is a very real one, much like any perceptual experience we have. It is important to call the experience what the relative calls it (e.g., headaches, stress, pressure, spirits).

Help the family to understand the experience better. Since hallucinations commonly occur for many people, you can show the family that the problem comes when focusing on the hallucination impedes their relative's ability to connect with others and make personally meaningful contributions. If it is voices, help the family see that what is said comes from beliefs their relative has about themselves ("I'm a bad person") and others ("They hate me"). If they listen to voices a lot, it is because they believe the voices are credible or that the voices have control and are more powerful than the individual themselves. The family can also recognize times when the voices and other hallucinations might become worse; the relative will seem stressed, isolated, or lonely.

The strategy with hallucinations is to help the person refocus back to the things in life that matter to them. Family activities can be great opportunities to help the person feel connected, in control, and doing important things. If the relative knows specific refocusing techniques, such as the Look-Point-Name game (see Chapter 9), family members can do it with their relative, enhancing connection and success. If the person likes to refocus by singing along to music, sing with the family. In each of these cases, you can enable the family to help their relative see the impact of the refocusing activity:

FAMILY MEMBER: We just sang together; what happened to the things that make it hard to focus?

RELATIVE: They went down.

FAMILY MEMBER: Seemed like it! Can we do this again sometime?

RELATIVE: Totally!

FAMILY MEMBER: We are in this together to control that stuff the best we can!

Family can ultimately be a place where the individual participates in many activities and has several roles that help them feel confident and strong. The person can have such roles in the community, as well. Together these are terrific opportunities to focus away from hallucinations and ultimately to draw different beliefs about their own capability and merit; at the same time the person comes to see that the hallucinations are not all that interesting and they do not have time for them.

When the Person Has No Family

Life can be unfair. It can be cruel. Some individuals find themselves with no family. This usually entails considerable suffering and loss, no matter why it is that the family is no longer available to them. Many still passionately yearn for their family. What do you do when the person doesn't have one?

First, you can empathize, appreciating how much less connected the person might feel, perceiving themselves to be alone in the world. You can then turn these painful emotions to a kind of gold. Ask the person, "What is the best part about the idea of family?" Explore what the person misses most or would most want from family. Is it possible to get these feelings and experiences with new people? Perhaps one can create a new family—be that friends, a family of their own, or some other way. This is an empowering approach to loss. The person may not be able to be with the ones they want to love and have love them. But they can love and develop familial-like relationships with the ones they are with. The same approach can be taken when family is unsupportive or is minimally involved.

Family Is Skeptical about Mental Health Providers

There are enumerable reasons that can lead families to not trust you at the outset—for example, these might arise from cultural factors, or personal history (Kuipers, Leff, & Lam, 2002). You need not see this as personal. A lot is going on for them. They may feel responsible for what is happening. The health care system can be hard to navigate. They may have gotten their hopes up only to have them dashed. They may have felt let down by people in your role in the past. They also may have a preferred way of understanding why their relative is struggling, which has been a source of disagreement in the past with mental health providers.

An advantage that you have is the active approach you are taking with their relative. You can trade on this. Skepticism is healthy. You can respect it. It is surely well earned. What you are hoping to do with the family is for them to go along with the process for a while and see what happens. They can judge for themselves. Try beginning with "Can we start with what your relative is like at-their-best?" Collaborating on aspirations and goals for the whole family can be a conduit to mutual understanding, connection, trust, and hope for everyone.

WORDS OF WISDOM

BOX 15.1. FOCUSING THE FAMILY

Over the past 70 years the explanation for schizophrenia has swung back and forth between external factors, such as a schizophrenogenic mother (Fromm-Reichmann, 1948) and expressed emotion, on the one side, and internal factors, such as high heritability and brain dysfunction (Henriksen, Nordgaard, & Jansson, 2017) on the other. Both pose liabilities for families—guilt over past actions that cannot be undone compared to hopelessness at the inability of correcting biological misfortune.

Families can be empowered with the knowledge that their relative holds beliefs about self, others, and the future that get expressed in a variety of challenges: difficulties accessing motivation, focusing attention, and sustaining effort; complete withdrawal from others; profound inactivity; and internal focus on voices or beliefs that are hard to understand. With these beliefs in mind, the family can get back to doing what they do best—meaningful and fun activities together, bolstering one another's dreams, and helping one another through hard times and setbacks.

It can start with having fun and pursuing mutual interests. This could be a good meal, an outing, going into nature, watching or playing sports, or working on cars. The family can set up desired goals for everyone. Working as a group, it is possible to generate positive ideas for everyone to move toward their aspirations. All can have roles in one another's successes, compounding cohesion and the positive family identity. What may seem insoluble can be addressed by drawing on collective experiences to problem-solve and overcome adversity.

The family identity can be based on resilience and strength. They can say, "We are Smiths; we are tough; and we help one another."

The combination of mutual success and group strength produces positive attitudes about self, others, and the future—belonging, capability, resilience, and so on—which run counter to the negative beliefs that feed challenges. Being connected to a meaningful identity—being a Smith—diffuses the disconnection that so often is the source of so much unhappiness.

SUMMARY

- Families can be ideal partners for facilitating recovery because of their unique perspective on an individual's at-their-best moments and the family's at-its-best moments.
- Roles in the family that extend beyond "caretaker" and "patient" and that support a more natural, dynamic unit can be a significant source of empowerment for all—moving families beyond the power struggles that can arise around treatment, diagnosis, and the challenges.
- Because negative beliefs about connection often underlie challenges, the family can be a strong source of connection, pursuit of mutual aspirations, and has an important role in building up resilience beliefs and providing encouragement when challenges arise.
- Frequent, planned action that realizes collective meanings realizes the family at its best.
- Families, providers, and the individuals themselves can partner together to employ and test-drive interventions to overcome challenges as they arise.

APPENDICES

APPENDIX A	CT-R Terminology	233
APPENDIX B	Blank Recovery Map	234
APPENDIX C	Recovery Map How-To Guide	235
APPENDIX D	Suggestions for Activities to Access the Adaptive Mode	237
APPENDIX E	Blank Activity Schedule	238
APPENDIX F	Blank Chart for Breaking Aspirations into Steps	239
APPENDIX G	Interventions for Individuals Experiencing Negative Symptoms	240
APPENDIX H	CT-R Benchmarks	241

APPENDIX A — CT-R Terminology

Here is how we define some of the commonly used terms in this text:

Action plan: A step toward an individual's aspiration or step toward handling a specific challenge in the context of an aspiration; this replaces the term "homework."

Activity: Individual or group-oriented programs; opportunities for interaction and the pursuit of interests and/or aspirations.

Adaptive mode: When individuals are at-their-best or feel most like themselves; when energy, focus, and connection are apparent; this is when there is greatest potential to access positive beliefs. Accessing the adaptive mode is a formulation-based approach to what is often referred to as engagement.

Aspirations: An individual's personal desires for the future; the meaning individuals seek for themselves in the future.

Challenges: A catchall term for problems, symptoms, or obstacles; challenges are anything that impedes progress toward aspirations.

Empowerment: Strength in the face of stress or challenges; developing resiliency beliefs; interventions that help individuals achieve this strength and resiliency.

Expansive or grand beliefs: Replaces the term "grandiose"; reflects big ideas about the self or world that may be difficult for others to understand and that reflect a deeper meaning than what may appear on the surface.

Individual: A person who has been given a diagnosis of a serious mental health condition or who is a participant in mental health services; we do not refer to individuals as "patients" in this text.

Milieu: Any environment where many people are together in a shared space; can be a dayroom, dining room, waiting room, creative arts space, or any other community space.

Negative beliefs: Beliefs that underlie many challenges and can impede movement toward aspirations.

"Patient" mode: Used to describe the opposite of the adaptive mode. This is when challenges are most prominent; when connection and interaction are based on perceived psychopathology; the adaptive mode is dormant. "Patient" is used in quotes as to not endorse the concept of patienthood as an identity.

Positive beliefs: Adaptive beliefs about the self, others, the future, and the world that reflect strengths, skills, capabilities, and belonging.

Recovery: Living the meaningful life of one's choosing.

Resiliency beliefs: Beliefs about the ability to overcome challenges or to continue in the pursuit of aspirations despite challenges or stressors; beliefs about the ability to bounce back after challenges.

Serious mental health conditions: A term referring to any diagnosis an individual may be given (whether or not they agree or accept the diagnosis), including schizophrenia and schizoaffective disorder; the term also acknowledges the significance of some challenges impacted by mental health conditions, such as aggressive behavior and nonsuicidal self-injury.

From *Recovery-Oriented Cognitive Therapy for Serious Mental Health Conditions* by Aaron T. Beck, Paul Grant, Ellen Inverso, Aaron P. Brinen, and Dimitri Perivoliotis. Copyright © 2021 The Guilford Press. Permission to photocopy this material is granted to purchasers of this book for personal use or use with clients (see copyright page for details). Purchasers can download additional copies of this material (see the box at the end of the table of contents).

APPENDIX B — Blank Recovery Map

Recovery Map	
ACCESSING AND ENERGIZING THE ADAPTIVE MODE	
Interests/Ways to Engage:	**Beliefs Activated While in Adaptive Mode:**
ASPIRATIONS	
Goals:	**Meaning of Accomplishing Identified Goal:**
CHALLENGES	
Current Behaviors/Challenges:	**Beliefs Underlying Challenges:**
POSITIVE ACTION AND EMPOWERMENT	
Current Strategies and Interventions:	**Beliefs/Aspirations/Meanings/Challenges Targeted:**

From *Recovery-Oriented Cognitive Therapy for Serious Mental Health Conditions* by Aaron T. Beck, Paul Grant, Ellen Inverso, Aaron P. Brinen, and Dimitri Perivoliotis. Copyright © 2021 The Guilford Press. Permission to photocopy this material is granted to purchasers of this book for personal use or use with clients (see copyright page for details). Purchasers can download additional copies of this material (see the box at the end of the table of contents).

APPENDIX C: Recovery Map How-To Guide

Recovery Map	
Accessing and Energizing the Adaptive Mode **Recovery Component—Connection**	
Interests/Ways to Engage: What does a person look like at-their-best? • Shared interests • What can they teach you or help you with? Develop understanding of when things are going well or what they were doing when they were at-their-best. Let the individual guide you. Look for a brightening of affect, eye contact, focus, etc.	**Beliefs Activated While in Adaptive Mode:** What positive beliefs are activated when in the adaptive mode? How does a person see themselves? Others? The future? How does the person feel while they are in the adaptive mode? Initially you may have to hypothesize, but as you get to know the individual, make sure you test and confirm your hypotheses (e.g., "What does it say about you that you taught me this?").
Aspirations—Developing the Adaptive Mode **Recovery Component—Hope**	
Goals: If everything was how they want it to be, what would they be doing? Getting? All responses accepted without judgment. Use questions to distinguish between steps (e.g., discharge) and aspirations (longer range, bigger meaning).	**Meaning of Accomplishing Identified Goal:** What would be the best part about the that [aspiration]? How might they see themselves or others if they achieved their aspiration? How would they feel? Meanings are the most important aspect of distant, expansive, or high-risk aspirations. Meanings can be actioned every day, even if aspirations change over time.
Challenges	
Current Behaviors/Challenges: Challenges that are getting in the way of working toward aspirations. Why are they still here in current level of care (symptoms, behaviors, experiences)?	**Beliefs Underlying Challenge:** What beliefs might a person hold about self, others, or the future that contributes to the challenge occurring? What feeling(s) might they be experiencing?

(continued)

From *Recovery-Oriented Cognitive Therapy for Serious Mental Health Conditions* by Aaron T. Beck, Paul Grant, Ellen Inverso, Aaron P. Brinen, and Dimitri Perivoliotis. Copyright © 2021 The Guilford Press. Permission to photocopy this material is granted to purchasers of this book for personal use or use with clients (see copyright page for details). Purchasers can download additional copies of this material (see the box at the end of the table of contents).

Recovery Map How-To Guide *(page 2 of 2)*

Positive Action and Empowerment—Actualizing and Strengthening Adaptive Mode
Recovery Component—Purpose and Resilience

Current Strategies and Interventions:	Beliefs/Aspirations/Meanings/Challenges Targeted:

Strategy: Transforming starting belief into more accurate and helpful belief; gaining information on the adaptive mode or aspirations.
 	
Interventions: Methods used to achieve the strategy.
 	
How can we increase positive beliefs, work toward an aspiration and its meaning, or target a challenge and the negative belief?
 	
Examples:
 	
1. **Access adaptive mode/reduce isolation.**
   a. Identify hook by asking for advice.
   b. Brief, frequent, predictable interaction time.
2. **Increase control.**
   a. Provide leadership role.
   b. Develop skills or strategies for managing hallucinations (e.g., music).
3. **Increase connection.**
   a. Invite individual to teach others.
   b. Develop/involve in a club or group activity/project.
4. **Increase consistency.**
   a. Daily activity planning.
5. **Develop/enrich existing aspirations.**
   a. Future-focused discussion/thoughts.
   b. Identify valued goals.
   c. Develop recovery image (e.g., What would their future home look like?).
6. **Discover meaning of goals/aspirations.**
   a. What would be the best part about that?
   b. How would it feel to be doing that?
	Carried down from above sections in this column.
	
	Provides the clinical rationale and target for the strategies and interventions used.
	
	Examples:
	
	1. **"I am safe"** (belief)/**increase connection and safety** (meaning)/**reduce isolation** (challenge).
	2. **"I have control over my life"/leave hospital/independence/hallucinations.**
	3. **"Others want to be around me and care about my interests"/having close relationships/connection/aggressive behaviors.**
	4. **"My days have purpose and meaning"/volunteering/feeling helpful/delusions.**
	5. **"My future is hopeful," "I am working toward something meaningful," or "Others believe in me"/purpose.**

APPENDIX D Suggestions for Activities to Access the Adaptive Mode

Connected

- Listen to a song together, discuss music or sing.
- Play cards or a game.
- Create art together.
- Take a walk.
- Watch clips of interests (sports, dancing, movies, animals).
- Cook or discuss food.
- Talk about or play sports (play catch; use arms as a paper ball basketball hoop).
- Read together (passage from religious text, poem, literature).

During or afterward, say: "I really enjoyed spending time together, how about you?"

Helpful

- Take on a helping role at the facility (help with a group/community meeting/club, take notes at a meeting, clean/set up for something, update people about the news).
- Decorate the unit.
- Write cards for organizations (e.g., VA, children's hospitals).
- Organize a charity project on the unit (clothing drive, items for an animal shelter).

During or afterward, say: "You're a really helpful person, aren't you?"

Capable

- Ask for advice about something (fashion, food).
- Have them teach you how to do something they are skilled in.
- Do an activity or talk about an individual's unique knowledge pocket (previous trade or job, playing music or singing, cooking).
- Unit talent show/open mic night/art show.

During or afterward, say: "What does it say about you that you know so much about that?"

Energized

Brief but predictable interactions about something simple that doesn't require a lot of verbal participation:

- Listen to a song.
- Play cards or a game.
- Watch a video clip.
- Do something artistic.
- Exercise or stretch.
- Read together.

During or afterward, say: "I have a lot more energy after doing that, how about you?"

**Bolded items can be done without access to technology.

From *Recovery-Oriented Cognitive Therapy for Serious Mental Health Conditions* by Aaron T. Beck, Paul Grant, Ellen Inverso, Aaron P. Brinen, and Dimitri Perivoliotis. Copyright © 2021 The Guilford Press. Permission to photocopy this material is granted to purchasers of this book for personal use or use with clients (see copyright page for details). Purchasers can download additional copies of this material (see the box at the end of the table of contents).

APPENDIX E — Blank Activity Schedule

Instructions. If the individual's aspirations are not known, schedule activities to increase energy and connection. Write each activity under a day that the individual selects. Aspirations (when clear) go in the space indicated by blank lines below the chart, and then meanings go in the space below that. Next, add activities under the person's chosen day that relate to getting closer to these aspirations and meanings, increasing lived purpose daily. *Remember: Build schedules gradually and collaboratively.* See Chapters 3 and 5 for elaborated instructions.

CT-R Weekly Activity Schedule

Sunday	Monday	Tuesday	Wednesday	Thursday	Friday	Saturday

Aspirations:

_____

_____

Meanings:

_____

_____

From *Recovery-Oriented Cognitive Therapy for Serious Mental Health Conditions* by Aaron T. Beck, Paul Grant, Ellen Inverso, Aaron P. Brinen, and Dimitri Perivoliotis. Copyright © 2021 The Guilford Press. Permission to photocopy this material is granted to purchasers of this book for personal use or use with clients (see copyright page for details). Purchasers can download additional copies of this material (see the box at the end of the table of contents).

APPENDIX F — Blank Chart for Breaking Aspirations into Steps

Meanings of Aspiration

ASPIRATION

STEPS TO ASPIRATION

Instructions: Prior to using this chart, confirm the individual's aspiration and reflect any meanings you recall, or elicit new ones. This chart should be worked on only when the individual is in the adaptive mode.

Write, draw, or add a picture representing a person's aspiration at the top of the "steps" side of the figure on the right. Enter what the individual says are the best parts of their aspiration—including meanings, positive beliefs, or values—in the box labeled "Meanings of Aspiration" on the left side. Next, ask the individual what they or anyone working toward that aspiration would need to do to get there. Responses do not need to be provided in a particular order—rather, organize each answer by asking the individual where it goes on the stepwise chart, with earlier steps going toward the bottom, intermediate steps in the middle, and so on. You can always revise the order as the individual comes up with more ideas. Feel free to float ideas of steps to them. For more instruction and examples, see Chapter 5; Figure 5.1 contains a completed Aspirations and Steps chart.

From *Recovery-Oriented Cognitive Therapy for Serious Mental Health Conditions* by Aaron T. Beck, Paul Grant, Ellen Inverso, Aaron P. Brinen, and Dimitri Perivoliotis. Copyright © 2021 The Guilford Press. Permission to photocopy this material is granted to purchasers of this book for personal use or use with clients (see copyright page for details). Purchasers can download additional copies of this material (see the box at the end of the table of contents).

APPENDIX G — Interventions for Individuals Experiencing Negative Symptoms

Purpose: Connect over interests/activities that increase sense of pleasure and ability to access energy

Introduction: "Let's listen to a song together! Should we pick this artist or that artist?"

Brief, predictable interactions

Meet individual where they are.

Start with forced-choice questions (e.g., "Should we listen to rock or pop?").

Prioritize activities over talking

(e.g., listening to a song, watching a video, playing cards, taking a walk)

Draw attention to positive beliefs during and after.

Energy

"I feel more energized after that, how about you?"

Pleasure

"I really enjoyed doing that, how about you?"

Success

"Did that go better or worse than expected? Is it worth doing it again?"

If attempts at conversation or connection are rejected:
- Keep it low pressure.
- Ask for advice.
- Try different interests and activities.

Example: "No problem, later on I'll come by and maybe we can look up recipes together!"

From *Recovery-Oriented Cognitive Therapy for Serious Mental Health Conditions* by Aaron T. Beck, Paul Grant, Ellen Inverso, Aaron P. Brinen, and Dimitri Perivoliotis. Copyright © 2021 The Guilford Press. Permission to photocopy this material is granted to purchasers of this book for personal use or use with clients (see copyright page for details). Purchasers can download additional copies of this material (see the box at the end of the table of contents).

APPENDIX H CT-R Benchmarks

RECOVERY-ORIENTED COGNITIVE THERAPY (CT-R) BENCHMARKS FIDELITY SCALE

1. What is this?
   - A self-assessment tool to measure the degree to which your program/site realizes the CT-R approach.
2. What is the purpose?
   - Demonstrates how CT-R principles can translate into day-to-day work by describing components of a program that is consistent with the CT-R model.
   - Helps sites reflect on the ways in which CT-R informs their practice, gauges the strengths of the site, and identifies areas that need improvement in relation to the CT-R model.
   - Guides action plans to strengthen programming.
   - Regular use of this tool will aid in sustainability of the CT-R model at your site.
3. Who should complete this?
   - We recommend that this self-assessment be completed together by staff from multiple disciplines who are familiar with the day-to-day happenings at a site. This may include psychologists, nursing staff, social workers, peer support specialists, recreational therapists, psychiatrists, and others.
4. When should it be completed?
   - We recommend that this be readministered at least once per year. In the first year of CT-R implementation, however, we suggest that staff should revisit the action plan section of the tool more frequently to track progress and make adjustments to action plans if needed (i.e., every 3–4 months).

Instructions

- This scale is broken into seven different domains and each domain has three to six items.
- Read the description of the domain and the definition of relevant terms for each domain.
- Determine the score for each item that most accurately describes the usual happenings at your site. Of note, a "3" is considered aspirational and many sites will not achieve this score in the early stages of implementation.
- At the end of each domain, record your scores for each item and sum those items to get the domain score.
- Identify the areas of strength and opportunities for growth within that domain based on the item scores.
- Complete this process for all seven domains.
- Turn to the summary page:
  - Copy domain scores onto the summary page.
  - Based on these scores identify two to three areas that would benefit from improvement relative to CT-R.
  - Develop an action plan and timeline for these areas. Of note, it may make sense to focus on one area first before addressing the other areas.

(continued)

From *Recovery-Oriented Cognitive Therapy for Serious Mental Health Conditions* by Aaron T. Beck, Paul Grant, Ellen Inverso, Aaron P. Brinen, and Dimitri Perivoliotis. Copyright © 2021 The Guilford Press. Permission to photocopy this material is granted to purchasers of this book for personal use or use with clients (see copyright page for details). Purchasers can download additional copies of this material (see the box at the end of the table of contents).

CT-R Benchmarks *(page 2 of 16)*

I. Milieu Factors

An ideal CT-R milieu is a lively atmosphere filled with activity and connection. There are ample opportunities for individuals to engage with others in activities that are connected to their interests and the things that they value in their lives (e.g., music, reading, sports, spirituality, exercise, family). An active milieu provides multiple opportunities for individuals to draw conclusions about their capability, strength, and connection with others.

Terms

Activity: Individual or group-oriented programs; opportunities for interaction and the pursuit of interests and/or aspirations.

Aspirations: An individual's personal desires for the future; the meaning individuals seek for themselves in the future.

Milieu: Any environment where many people are together in a shared space.

---

1. **CT-R Milieu Programming Frequency**
   - 0: There is very little activity at the site (i.e., less than 10% of shift waking hours).
   - 1: There are occasional activities available at the site (i.e., more than 10% but less than 30% of waking hours).
   - 2: There are frequent activities at the site (i.e., more than 30% but less than 50% of waking hours).
   - 3: The milieu is very active during the day (i.e., more than 50% of waking hours).

2. **Individual and Staff Interaction Level**
   - 0: There is no interaction between staff and individuals during activities.
   - 1: There is minimal connection/interaction between staff and individuals during activities.
   - 2: There is some interaction between staff and individuals, as evidenced by some opportunities for shared conversation and activity.
   - 3: There is significant engagement between staff and individuals during activities.

3. **Connection to Interests and Aspirations**
   - 0: Activities are not connected to the individuals' interests and aspirations. There is no system in place to learn about individuals' interests/aspirations and modify programming accordingly.
   - 1: Activities are occasionally connected to individuals' interests and aspirations (i.e., less than 30% of the time). There is a feedback system to modify programming accordingly, but it is used inconsistently.
   - 2: Activities are often connected to individuals' interests and aspirations (i.e., approximately 50% of the time). There is a feedback system to modify programming as necessary, but it may not always be used.
   - 3: Activities are frequently connected to individuals' interests and aspirations (i.e., at least 75% of the time). There is a consistent feedback system to modify programming as necessary

(continued)

CT-R Benchmarks *(page 3 of 16)*

4. Opportunities for Roles
- 0: There are no opportunities for individuals to have roles or leadership positions in the milieu programs.
- 1: There are minimal opportunities for individuals to have roles or leadership positions in the milieu programs.
- 2: There are some opportunities for individuals to have roles or leadership positions in the milieu programs.
- 3: There are opportunities for roles or leadership positions in the milieu programs for almost every individual.

5. Drawing Conclusions
- 0: There are no attempts to draw conclusions during the milieu activities about successes or individuals' abilities and strengths.
- 1: There are minimal attempts to draw conclusions during the milieu activities about successes or individuals' abilities and strengths.
- 2: There are some attempts to draw conclusions during the milieu activities about successes or individuals' abilities and strengths.
- 3: There are frequent attempts to draw conclusions during the milieu activities about successes or individuals' abilities and strengths.

Scoring

1. **CT-R Milieu Programming Frequency:** _____
2. **Individual and Staff Interaction Level:** _____
3. **Connection to Interests and Aspirations:** _____
4. **Opportunities for Roles:** _____
5. **Drawing Conclusions:** _____

Total Milieu Factors Score [1 + 2 + 3 + 4 + 5]: _____

Areas of Strength:

Opportunities for Growth:

(continued)

CT-R Benchmarks *(page 4 of 16)*

II. Community Involvement

Ideally, a CT-R program provides individuals with many chances to connect to the things that matter to them in the community, regardless of level of care—for example, individuals may have the opportunity to participate in community activities (e.g., attending exercise classes, volunteering, taking classes). In facilities where individuals are not able to go into the community, they may engage in activities on the unit that are directly related to their community aspirations (e.g., cooking group, book club, spirituality group). Engaging in meaningful activities or taking steps toward one's aspirations fosters hope, purpose, and builds confidence.

Terms

Aspirations: An individual's personal desires for the future; the meaning individuals seek for themselves in the future.

---

1. **Frequency of Community Involvement**
   - 0: There is no community involvement:
     - At a site where community outings are possible, no community outings occur.
     - At a site where community outings are *not* possible (e.g., locked forensic setting), activities that take place in the milieu are not linked in any meaningful way to future community involvement.
   - 1: There is minimal community involvement, either through community outings or on-site activities linked to the larger community (i.e., less than 15% of activities).
   - 2: There is some community involvement, either through community outings or on-site activities linked to the larger community (i.e., less than 50% of activities).
   - 3: There is frequent and predictable community involvement, either through community outings or on-site activities linked to the larger community (i.e., more than 50% of activities).

2. **Connection to Interests and Aspirations**
   - 0: Community involvement activities are not connected to individuals' interests and aspirations. There is no system in place to learn about individuals' interests/aspirations and modify programming accordingly.
   - 1: Community involvement activities are occasionally connected to individuals' interests and aspirations (i.e., less than 30% of the time). There is a feedback system to modify programming accordingly, but it is used inconsistently.
   - 2: Community involvement activities are often connected to individuals' interests and aspirations (i.e., approximately 50% of the time). There is a feedback system to modify programming as necessary, but it may not always be used.
   - 3: Community involvement activities are frequently connected to individuals' interests and aspirations (i.e., at least 75% of the time). There is a consistent feedback system to modify programming as necessary.

(continued)

CT-R Benchmarks *(page 5 of 16)*

3. **Opportunities for Roles**
   - 0: There are no opportunities for individuals to have roles or leadership positions in the community involvement activities.
   - 1: There are minimal opportunities for individuals to have roles or leadership positions in the community involvement activities.
   - 2: There are some opportunities for individuals to have roles or leadership positions in the community involvement activities.
   - 3: There are multiple opportunities for individuals to have roles or leadership positions in the community involvement activities.

4. **Drawing Conclusions**
   - 0: There are no attempts to draw conclusions during the community involvement activities about successes or individuals' abilities and strengths.
   - 1: There are minimal attempts to draw conclusions during the community involvement activities about successes or individuals' abilities and strengths.
   - 2: There are some attempts to draw conclusions during the community involvement activities about successes or individuals' abilities and strengths.
   - 3: There are frequent attempts to draw conclusions during the community involvement activities about successes or individuals' abilities and strengths.

Scoring

1. **Frequency of Community Involvement:** _____
2. **Connected to Interests and Aspirations:** _____
3. **Opportunities for Roles:** _____
4. **Drawing Conclusions:** _____

Total Community Involvement Score [1 + 2 + 3 + 4]: _____

Areas of Strength:

Opportunities for Growth:

(continued)

CT-R Benchmarks *(page 6 of 16)*

III. Treatment Planning

Treatment planning occurs as a collaboration between treatment providers and individuals. The plan for treatment is anchored by an individual's aspirations. In the context of aspirations, treatment providers and individuals work together to identify meaningful steps toward these aspirations and manage challenges that may impact an individual's ability to move toward their aspirations. Treatment team meetings or treatment plan reviews offer the opportunity to celebrate successes (big or small), draw meaningful conclusions, and foster beliefs related to resiliency.

Terms

Action plan: A step toward an individual's aspiration or step toward handling a specific challenge in the context of an aspiration.

Activating the adaptive mode: Use of methods that increase energy, focus, and connection.

Aspirations: An individual's personal desires for the future; the meaning individuals seek for themselves in the future.

Treatment team: A group consisting of an individual and all providers involved in the individual's treatment.

Treatment team meeting: A meeting where the treatment team comes together to develop and review treatment plans.

---

1. **Including Individuals in the Treatment Team Meeting**
    - 0: Treatment team or provider does not involve individuals in treatment planning.
    - 1: Treatment team or provider invites individuals to participate in treatment planning some of the time (i.e., more than 30% of the time).
    - 2: Significant attempts are made to invite individuals to participate in treatment planning (i.e., more than 50% of the time).
    - 3: Individuals are almost always invited to participate in treatment planning.

2. **Activating the Adaptive Mode during the Treatment Team Meeting**
    - 0: No attempts at activating the adaptive mode are made at the beginning of treatment planning meetings.
    - 1: Occasional, but inconsistent, attempts at activating the adaptive mode are made at the beginning of treatment planning meetings.
    - 2: Some consistent attempts at activating the adaptive mode are made at the beginning of treatment planning meetings.
    - 3: Meetings to discuss/develop the treatment plan almost always begin with opportunities to activate the adaptive mode.

3. **Use of Aspirations to Frame Treatment Plan**
    - 0: Individuals' aspirations are not accounted for in treatment plans and treatment providers make no attempts to identify aspirations.
    - 1: Individuals' aspirations are occasionally incorporated into the treatment planning process, when known. If not known, treatment providers occasionally attempt to collaborate with individuals to identify aspirations (i.e., less than 30% of the time).

(continued)

CT-R Benchmarks *(page 7 of 16)*

   2: Individuals' aspirations are often incorporated into the treatment planning process, when known. If not known, treatment providers often attempt to collaborate with individuals to identify aspirations (i.e., less than 50% of the time).

   3: If aspirations are known, the team will revisit and explore during the meeting (i.e., more than 75% of the time). The team frequently supports individuals in identifying aspirations if unknown.

4. **Collaboration in Treatment Planning**

   0: Individuals are not part of developing their treatment plan.

   1: Treatment plan (i.e., meeting agenda, treatment goals, action plans) is dictated by the team rather than individuals.

   2: Individuals provide feedback about current treatment, but treatment goals and action plans are still generated and dictated by the treatment team.

   3: Individuals are actively engaged in the development of the treatment plan (collaborating on goals and action plans).

5. **Drawing Conclusions**

   0: There are no attempts made to draw conclusions about successes connected to the treatment plan and/or individuals' abilities and strengths.

   1: There are minimal attempts made to draw conclusions about successes connected to the treatment plan and/or individuals' abilities and strengths.

   2: There are some attempts made to draw conclusions about successes connected to the treatment plan and/or individuals' abilities and strengths.

   3: There are frequent attempts made to draw conclusions about successes connected to the treatment plan and/or individuals' abilities and strengths.

Scoring

1. **Including Individuals in the Treatment Team Meeting:** _____
2. **Activating the Adaptive Mode during the Treatment Team Meeting:** _____
3. **Use of Aspirations to Frame Treatment Plan:** _____
4. **Collaboration in Treatment Planning:** _____
5. **Drawing Conclusions:** _____

   Total Treatment Planning Score [1 + 2 + 3 + 4 + 5]: _____

Areas of Strength:

Opportunities for Growth:

(continued)

CT-R Benchmarks *(page 8 of 16)*

IV. Transition Planning

Ideally, individuals and treatment providers begin to discuss transitions to different levels of care as soon as possible. Individuals are actively involved in these discussions and decisions. Individuals and treatment providers collaborate together to ensure that transitions are aligned with the individual's aspirations—for example, if an individual is interested in pursuing more schooling, their educational goals should be a relevant part of the transition planning. There are opportunities to identify meaningful plans for action and connection after the transition occurs. Staff and the individual work together to foster resiliency in the context of potential challenges related to transitions.

> **Terms**
>
> *Aspirations:* An individual's personal desires for their future; the meaning individuals seek for themselves in the future.
>
> *Transition steps:* Actions that staff and individuals can engage in at their current level of care that are related to the transition process (e.g., garden club at current residence, visiting next level of care, finding the community garden near the next level of care).

1. **Individuals' Participation in Transition Planning**
   0: Individuals are never involved in transition planning.
   1: Individuals are kept informed of transition plans but are not invited to participate in decisions.
   2: Individuals are kept informed of transition plans and are occasionally invited to participate in decisions.
   3: Individuals are actively and collaboratively involved in transition planning.

2. **Connecting Transitions/Discharges to Aspirations**
   0: Aspirations are not incorporated into transition plans.
   1: Individuals' aspirations are occasionally incorporated into the transition plan (i.e., less than 30% of the time).
   2: Individuals' aspirations are often incorporated into the transition plan (i.e., approximately 50% of the time).
   3: Individuals' aspirations are frequently discussed and connected to the transition plan (i.e., at least 75% of the time).

3. **Planning for Next Steps**
   0: The staff do not collaborate with individuals to plan for next steps in the transition process.
   1: The staff occasionally collaborate with individuals to identify next steps in the transition process (i.e., less than 30% of the time).
   2: The staff often collaborate with individuals to identify next steps in the transition process (i.e., approximately 50% of the time).
   3: The staff consistently and frequently collaborate with individuals to identify next steps in the transition process (i.e., at least 75% of the time).

(continued)

CT-R Benchmarks *(page 9 of 16)*

4. Building Resiliency Relative to Transitions

0: There are no attempts made to draw conclusions about being able to manage potential transition-related opportunities and challenges using prior successes and/or individuals' abilities and strengths.

1: There are minimal attempts to draw conclusions about being able to manage potential transition-related opportunities and challenges using prior successes and/or individuals' abilities and strengths.

2: There are some attempts made to draw conclusions about being able to manage potential transition-related opportunities and challenges using prior successes and/or individuals' abilities and strengths.

3: There are frequent attempts made to draw conclusions about being able to manage potential transition-related opportunities and challenges using prior successes and/or individuals' abilities and strengths.

Scoring

1. **Individuals' Participation in Transition Planning:** _____
2. **Connecting Transitions/Discharges to Aspirations:** _____
3. **Planning for Next Steps:** _____
4. **Building Resiliency Relative to Transitions:** _____

Total Transition Planning Score [1 + 2 + 3 + 4]: _____

Areas of Strength:

Opportunities for Growth:

V. CT-R Formulation

A CT-R formulation is the anchor for rich understandings and developing meaningful and effective action plans. Ideally, sites will develop, review, and revise formulations regularly as they evolve as individuals become empowered and pursue their aspirations. Sites also develop and implement interventions based on each individual's formulation and have a method for communicating both formulations and intervention strategies to team members.

(continued)

CT-R Benchmarks

> **Terms**
>
> *Adaptive mode:* When individuals are at-their-best or feel most like themselves.
>
> *Aspirations:* An individual's personal desires for the future; the meaning individuals seek for themselves in the future.
>
> *Formulation:* How we use the cognitive model to understand an individual's positive beliefs, aspirations, and challenges.

1. **Documented CT-R Formulations**
   - 0: CT-R formulations have not been created.
   - 1: CT-R formulations are complete for some individuals (i.e., less than 30% of individuals).
   - 2: CT-R formulations have been created for many individuals (i.e., approximately 50% of individuals).
   - 3: CT-R formulations are completed for all individuals, and there is a plan in place to complete them as new individuals begin to participate in services.

2. **Completeness of CT-R Formulations**
   - 0: CT-R formulations have not been completed.
   - 1: Formulations that have been developed may be missing significant components (i.e., only challenges are identified).
   - 2: Formulations are all complete but may lack sufficient detail (e.g., meaning of aspirations, adaptive beliefs).
   - 3: Formulations are clearly individualized and detailed.

3. **Strategies and Interventions**
   - 0: Strategies and interventions do not connect to strengthening adaptive beliefs and action toward the meaning of aspirations.
   - 1: Strategies and interventions occasionally connect to strengthening adaptive beliefs and action toward the meaning of aspirations (i.e., less than 30% of the time).
   - 2: Strategies and interventions sometimes connect to strengthening adaptive beliefs and action toward the meaning of aspirations (i.e., approximately 50% of the time).
   - 3: Strategy and interventions are clearly and consistently connected to strengthening adaptive beliefs and action toward the meaning of aspirations (i.e., at least 75% of the time).

4. **Team-Based Development of CT-R Formulations**
   - 0: CT-R formulations have not been developed.
   - 1: CT-R formulations may be created with only limited input from team members.
   - 2: CT-R formulations may be created with input from some team members but not in all disciplines.
   - 3: CT-R formulations have been created with feedback and input from team members from multiple disciplines.

5. **Communication of CT-R Formulations**
   - 0: There is no plan in place to share/communicate CT-R formulations and action plans with team members.
   - 1: CT-R formulations and action plans are inconsistently shared/communicated with team members (i.e., less than 30% of the time).

(continued)

CT-R Benchmarks *(page 11 of 16)*

2: CT-R formulations and action plans are sometimes shared/communicated with team members (i.e., approximately 50% of the time).

3: CT-R formulations and action plans are frequently shared/communicated with team members (i.e., at least 75% of the time).

6. **Staff Knowledge of CT-R Formulation/Action Plans**

    0: Team members are not aware of the CT-R formulations and/or action plans for the individuals with whom they work.

    1: Team members are infrequently aware of the CT-R formulations and/or action plans for the individuals with whom they work (i.e., less than 30% of individuals).

    2: Team members are somewhat aware of the CT-R formulations and/or action plans for the individuals with whom they work (i.e., approximately 50% of individuals).

    3: Team members are familiar with the components of the CT-R formulation and/or action plans for all individuals with whom they work directly.

Scoring

1. **Documented CT-R Formulations:** _____
2. **Completeness of CT-R Formulations:** _____
3. **Strategies and Interventions:** _____
4. **Team-Based Development of CT-R Formulations:** _____
5. **Communication of CT-R Formulations:** _____
6. **Staff Knowledge of CT-R Formulation/Action Plans:** _____

Total CT-R Formulation Score [1 + 2 + 3 + 4 + 5 + 6]: _____

Areas of Strength:

Opportunities for Growth:

(continued)

CT-R Benchmarks *(page 12 of 16)*

VI. Outcomes

CT-R sites have a plan in place to assess outcomes for individuals who are receiving services. These assessments include a focus on aspiration attainment, participation in individually meaningful activities, and satisfaction with the program. Programs have plans in place to make programmatic or individualized changes based on outcomes.

> **Terms**
>
> *Aspirations:* An individual's personal desires for the future; the meaning individuals seek for themselves in the future.

1. **Outcomes Assessment**
   - 0: No outcomes are collected.
   - 1: Outcomes are assessed inconsistently (i.e., less than 30% of the time).
   - 2: Outcomes are sometimes assessed (i.e., approximately 50% of the time).
   - 3: Outcomes are frequently assessed (i.e., at least 75% of the time).

2. **Types of Outcomes Assessed**
   - 0: No outcomes are assessed.
   - 1: Outcome assessments focus on symptom severity rather than participation in individually meaningful activities, aspiration attainment, and satisfaction with the program.
   - 2: Outcome assessments sometimes focus on participation in individually meaningful activities, aspiration attainment, and satisfaction with the program.
   - 3: Outcome assessments almost always address participation in individually meaningful activities, aspiration attainment, and satisfaction with the program.

3. **Use of Outcomes**
   - 0: There is no plan in place to make programmatic or individualized changes based on outcomes.
   - 1: Outcomes are inconsistently used to make programmatic or individualized changes (i.e., less than 30% of the time).
   - 2: Outcomes are sometimes used to make programmatic or individualized changes (i.e., approximately 50% of the time).
   - 3: Outcomes are consistently used to make programmatic or individualized changes.

> **Scoring**
>
> 1. **Outcomes Assessment:** _____
> 2. **Types of Outcomes Assessed:** _____
> 3. **Use of Outcomes:** _____
>
> **Total Outcomes Score [1 + 2 + 3]:** _____

(continued)

CT-R Benchmarks *(page 13 of 16)*

Areas of Strength:

Opportunities for Growth:

VII. Staff Factors

Ideally, a strong CT-R program has a robust training program in place to support new staff as they learn CT-R. Of note, this can provide staff who are well versed in CT-R with opportunities for leadership and mentoring roles. Additionally, programs support ongoing improvement of staff CT-R skills by assessing their skills, conducting advanced or refresher trainings, and holding regular consultations.

> **Terms**
>
> *Consultation:* Meetings where staff or team members come together to discuss CT-R theory, interventions, challenges, and possibly individual formulations.

1. Assessment of Staff CT-R Skills
- 0: Staff CT-R skills are not assessed.
- 1: Staff CT-R skills are inconsistently assessed. Feedback is inconsistent and there are no clear plans for improving skills.
- 2: CT-R skills are assessed on a regular basis. Feedback is provided but there are inconsistent plans for improving skills.
- 3: CT-R skills are assessed on a regular basis. Feedback is provided consistently and clear/collaborative plans are consistently developed to improve CT-R skills within a given period of time.

2. Training and Integration of New Staff
- 0: New staff are not introduced to the CT-R model and there is no training plan in place.
- 1: Initial CT-R training is inconsistently provided to new staff (i.e., less than 30% of staff).
- 2: Initial CT-R training is sometimes provided to new staff (i.e., approximately 50% of staff).
- 3: Initial CT-R training is provided to the majority of new staff from all disciplines (i.e., at least 75% of staff).

(continued)

CT-R Benchmarks *(page 14 of 16)*

3. **Ongoing CT-R Training for Staff**
   - 0: There is no ongoing training program in place to support staff in improving CT-R skills.
   - 1: Infrequent advanced or refresher CT-R trainings are offered.
   - 2: Advanced or refresher CT-R trainings are offered but may not be part of a consistent ongoing training plan.
   - 3: The facility has a consistent ongoing training program to support staff in improving their CT-R skills.

4. **Internal CT-R Consultation**
   - 0: Staff do not have regularly scheduled CT-R consultations.
   - 1: Staff occasionally meet for CT-R consultation (i.e., less than one meeting per month).
   - 2: Staff have regularly scheduled CT-R consultations (i.e., at least twice a month).
   - 3: Staff have regularly scheduled CT-R consultations (i.e., at least twice a month) with team members from multiple disciplines.

5. **Action Plan/Feedback System from Trainings or Consultations**
   - 0: There is no system in place to follow up on plans from trainings or consultations.
   - 1: Plans made in trainings or consultations inconsistently receive follow-up (i.e., less than 30% of the time) and there is no consistent feedback strategy regarding the success of these plans.
   - 2: Plans made in trainings or consultations sometimes receive follow-up (i.e., approximately 50% of the time). Feedback regarding the success of these plans is communicated inconsistently.
   - 3: Staff have a plan in place to ensure consistent follow-up on interventions, share feedback on the identified interventions during consultation, and identify new strategies as necessary.

Scoring

1. **Assessment of Staff CT-R Skills:** _____
2. **Training and Integration of New Staff:** _____
3. **Ongoing CT-R Training for Staff:** _____
4. **Internal CT-R Consultation:** _____
5. **Action Plan/Feedback System from Trainings or Consultations:** _____

Total Staff Factors Score [1 + 2 + 3 + 4 + 5]: _____

Areas of Strength:

(continued)

CT-R Benchmarks *(page 15 of 16)*

Opportunities for Growth:

CT-R FIDELITY SCALE SUMMARY SHEET

Domain	Domain score	Items	Item score
I. Milieu factors		1. CT-R milieu programming frequency	
		2. Individual/staff interaction level	
		3. Connection to interests and aspirations	
		4. Opportunities for roles	
		5. Drawing conclusions	
II. Community involvement		1. Frequency of community involvement	
		2. Connected to interests and aspirations	
		3. Opportunities for roles	
		4. Drawing conclusions	
III. Treatment planning		1. Including individuals in treatment team meeting	
		2. Activating the adaptive mode during treatment team meeting	
		3. Use of aspirations to frame treatment plan	
		4. Collaboration in treatment planning	
		5. Drawing conclusions	
IV. Transition planning		1. Individuals' participation in transition planning	
		2. Connecting transitions/discharges to aspirations	
		3. Planning for next steps	
		4. Building resiliency relative to transitions	
V. CT-R formulation		1. Documented CT-R formulations	
		2. Completeness of CT-R formulations	
		3. Strategies and interventions	
		4. Team-based development of CT-R formulations	

(continued)

CT-R Benchmarks

Domain	Domain score	Items	Item score
V. CT-R formulation *(continued)*		5. Communication of CT-R formulations	
		6. Staff knowledge of CT-R formulation/action plans	
VI. Outcomes		1. Outcomes assessment	
		2. Types of outcomes assessed	
		3. Use of outcomes	
VII. Staff factors		1. Assessment of staff CT-R skills	
		2. Training and integration of new staff	
		3. Ongoing CT-R training for staff	
		4. Internal CT-R consultation	
		5. Action plan/feedback system from trainings or consultations	

CT-R FIDELITY SCALE PLANS FOR IMPROVEMENT

Action Plan 1:

Domain/item addressed:

Timeline:

Plan for improvement:

Action Plan 2:

Domain/item addressed:

Timeline:

Plan for improvement:

Action Plan 3:

Domain/item addressed:

Timeline:

Plan for improvement:

Completed by: _____

Resources

RECOVERY-ORIENTED COGNITIVE THERAPY

Book

Visit *beckinstitute.org/CTR-resources* for:

- Handouts from this book
- Videos that show what the strategies and interventions look like
- New multimedia materials
- CT-R telehealth materials

Connect

Visit *www.beckinstitute.org/CTR* for:

- Information about training opportunities
- Joining the CT-R community

GENERAL COGNITIVE-BEHAVIORAL THERAPY

Training Programs

Beck Institute for Cognitive Behavior Therapy is a nonprofit organization in suburban Philadelphia. It offers a variety of on-site, off-site, and online training programs in CBT and CT-R for individuals and organizations worldwide, along with supervision and consultation programs: *https://beckinstitute.org*.

Additional Resources

- Worksheet packet
- Client booklets

- Books, CDs, and DVDs by Aaron T. Beck, MD, and Judith S. Beck, PhD
- Videos with Aaron T. Beck
- COVID-19 resource bank: *https://beckinstitute.org/covid-19-resources*

BECK CBT Certification

- Information about the Beck CBT Certification program and certified clinicians directory—*https://beckinstitute.org/certification*.

Connect with Beck Institute

- Monthly newsletter with CBT tips, news, and announcements
- Blog with articles from Beck Institute leadership and faculty
- Links to Beck Institute's social accounts

References

American Psychiatric Association. (2013). *Diagnostic and statistical manual of mental disorders* (5th ed.). Arlington, VA: Author.

Andreasen, N. C. (1984). *The broken brain: The biological revolution in psychiatry.* New York: Harper & Row.

Andreasen, N. C., & Grove, W. M. (1986). Thought, language and communication in schizophrenia: Diagnosis and prognosis. *Schizophrenia Bulletin, 12*, 348–358.

Anthony, W. A. (1980). *Principles of psychiatric rehabilitation.* Baltimore: University Park Press.

Arieti, S. (1974). *The interpretation of schizophrenia.* New York: Basic Books.

Baumeister, R. F., & Leary, M. R. (1995). The need to belong: Desire for interpersonal attachments as a fundamental human motivation. *Psychological Bulletin, 117*(3), 497–529.

Beavan, V., Read, J., & Cartwright, C. (2011). The prevalence of voice-hearers in the general population: A literature review. *Journal of Mental Health, 20*(3), 281–292.

Beck, A. T. (1963). Thinking and depression: I. Idiosyncratic content and cognitive distortions. *Archives of General Psychiatry, 9*(4), 324–333.

Beck, A. T. (1996). Beyond belief: A theory of modes, personality, and psychopathology. In P. M. Salkovskis (Ed.), *Frontiers of cognitive therapy* (pp. 1–25). New York: Guilford Press.

Beck, A. T. (1999). *Prisoners of hate: The cognitive basis of anger, hostility, and violence.* New York: HarperCollins.

Beck, A. T. (2019a). My journey through psychopathology, beginning and ending with schizophrenia. *Psychiatric Services, 70*(11), 1061–1063.

Beck, A. T. (2019b). A 60-year evolution of cognitive theory and therapy. *Perspectives on Psychological Science, 14*(1), 16–20.

Beck, A. T., Davis, D. D., & Freeman, A. (2014). *Cognitive therapy of personality disorders* (3rd ed.). New York: Guilford Press.

Beck, A. T., Finkel, M., & Beck, J. S. (2020). The theory of modes: Applications to schizophrenia and other psychological conditions. *Cognitive Therapy and Research.*

Beck, A. T., Himelstein, R., Bredemeier, K., Silverstein, S. M., & Grant, P. (2018). What accounts for poor functioning in people with schizophrenia: A re-evaluation of the contributions of neurocognitive v. attitudinal and motivational factors. *Psychological Medicine, 48*(16), 2776–2785.

Beck, A. T., Himelstein, R., & Grant, P. M. (2019). In and out of schizophrenia: Activation and deactivation of the negative and positive schemas. *Schizophrenia Research, 203*, 55–61.

Beck, A. T., Rector, N. R., Stolar, N. M., & Grant, P. M. (2009). *Schizophrenia: Cognitive theory, research and therapy.* New York: Guilford Press.

Beck, A. T., Rush, A. J., Shaw, B. F., & Emery, G. (1979). *Cognitive therapy of depression.* New York: Guilford Press.

Beck, A. T., Wright, F. D., Newman, C. F., & Liese, B. S. (1993). *Cognitive therapy of substance abuse.* New York: Guilford Press.

Beck, J. S. (2020). *Cognitive behavior therapy: Basics and beyond* (3rd ed.). New York: Guilford Press.

Bellack, A. S., Mueser, K. T., Gingerich, S., & Agresta, J. (2013). *Social skills training for schizophrenia: A step-by-step guide* (2nd ed.). New York: Guilford Press.

Bentall, R. P., Corcoran, R., Howard, R., Blackwood, N., & Kinderman, P. (2001). Persecutory delusions: A review and theoretical integration. *Clinical Psychology Review, 21*(8), 1143–1192.

Birtel, M. D., Wood, L., & Kempa, N. J. (2017). Stigma and social support in substance abuse: Implications for mental health and well-being. *Psychiatry Research, 252,* 1–8.

Blanchard, J. J., & Cohen, A. S. (2006). The structure of negative symptoms within schizophrenia: Implications for assessment. *Schizophrenia Bulletin, 32*(2), 238–245.

Bleuler, E. (1950). *Dementia praecox or the group of schizophrenias.* New York: International Universities Press.

Broadway, E. D., & Covington, D. W. (2018). *A comprehensive crisis system: Ending unnecessary emergency room admissions and jail bookings associated with mental illness.* Alexandria, VA: National Association of State Mental Health Program Directors.

Callard, A. (2018). *Aspiration: The agency of becoming.* New York: Oxford University Press.

Campellone, T. R., Sanchez, A. H., & Kring, A. M. (2016). Defeatist performance beliefs, negative symptoms, and functional outcome in schizophrenia: A meta-analytic review. *Schizophrenia Bulletin, 42*(6), 1343–1352.

Center for Substance Abuse Treatment. (2014). Understanding the impact of trauma. In *Trauma-informed care in behavioral health services.* Rockville, MD: Substance Abuse and Mental Health Services Administration.

Chadwick, P. (2014). Mindfulness for psychosis. *British Journal of Psychiatry, 204,* 333–334.

Chadwick, P., Birchwood, M., & Trower, P. (1996). *Cognitive therapy for delusions, voices and paranoia.* Chichester, UK: Wiley.

Chamberlin, J. (1990). The ex-patients' movement: Where we've been and where we're going. *Journal of Mind and Behavior, 11,* 323–336.

Chang, N. A., Grant, P. M., Luther, L., & Beck, A. T. (2014). Effects of a recovery-oriented cognitive therapy training program on inpatient staff attitudes and incidents of seclusion and restraint. *Community Mental Health Journal, 50*(4), 415–421.

Clay, K., Raugh, I., Chapman, H., Bartolomeo, L., Visser, K., Grant, P. M., . . . Strauss, G. P. (2019). *Defeatist performance beliefs are associated with negative symptoms, cognition, and global functioning in individuals at clinical high-risk for psychosis.* Paper presented at the annual meeting of the Society for Research in Psychopathology, Buffalo, NY.

Cohen, A. N., Hamilton, A. B., Saks, E. R., Glover, D. L., Glynn, S. M., Brekke, J. S., & Marder, S. R. (2017). How occupationally high-achieving individuals with a diagnosis of schizophrenia manage their symptoms. *Psychiatric Services, 68*(4), 324–329.

Cohen, B. D., & Camhi, J. (1967). Schizophrenic performance in a word-communication task. *Journal of Abnormal Psychology, 72*(3), 240–246.

Crow T. J. (1980). Molecular pathology of schizophrenia: More than one disease process? *British Medical Journal, 280,* 66–68.

Curson, D. A., Pantelis, C., Ward, J., & Barnes, T. R. (1992). Institutionalism and schizophrenia 30 years on: Clinical poverty and the social environment in three British mental hospitals in 1960 compared with a fourth in 1990. *British Journal of Psychiatry, 160,* 230–241.

Davidson, L., Harding, C., Spaniol, L., Rowe, M., Tondora, J., O'Connell, M. J., & Lawless, M. S. (2008). *A practical guide to recovery-oriented practice: Tools for transforming mental health care.* Oxford, UK: Oxford University Press.

Davidson, L., Rakfeldt, J., & Strauss, J. (2011). *The roots of the recovery movement in psychiatry: Lessons learned.* Hoboken, NJ: Wiley.

de Bont, P. A., van den Berg, D. P., van der Vleugel, B. M., de Roos, C., Mulder, C. L., Becker, E. S., . . . van Minnen, A. (2013). A multi-site single blind clinical study to compare the effects of prolonged exposure, eye movement desensitization and reprocessing and waiting list on patients with a current diagnosis of psychosis and comorbid post traumatic stress disorder: Study protocol for the randomized controlled trial treating trauma in psychosis. *Trials, 14,* 151.

De Hert, M., Correll, C. U., Bobes, J., Cetkovich-Bakmas, M., Cohen, D., Asai, I., . . . Leucht, S. (2011). Physical illness in patients with severe mental disorders: I. Prevalence, impact of medications and disparities in health care. *World Psychiatry, 10*(1), 52–77.

Delespaul, P., deVries, M., & van Os, J. (2002). Determinants of occurrence and recovery from hallucinations in daily life. *Social Psychiatry and Psychiatric Epidemiology, 37*(3), 97–104.

Dixon, L. B., Holoshitz, Y., & Nossel, I. (2016). Treatment engagement of individuals experiencing mental illness: Review and update. *World Psychiatry, 15*(1), 13–20.

Frankl, V. (1946). *Man's search for meaning.* Boston: Beacon Press.

Freeman, D. (2007). Suspicious minds: The psychology of persecutory delusions. *Clinical Psychology Review, 27*(4), 425–457.

Freeman, D., & Garety, P. (2014). Advances in understanding and treating persecutory delusions: A review. *Social Psychiatry and Psychiatric Epidemiology, 49*(8), 1179–1189.

Fromm-Reichmann, F. (1948). Notes on the development of treatment of schizophrenics by psychoanalytic psychotherapy. *Psychiatry, 11*(3), 263–273.

Fuligni, A. J. (2019). The need to contribute during adolescence. *Perspectives in Psychological Science, 14*(3), 331–343.

Galderisi, S., Mucci, A., Buchanan, R. W., & Arango, C. (2018). Negative symptoms of schizophrenia: New developments and unanswered research questions. *Lancet Psychiatry, 5*(8), 664–677.

Grant, P. M. (2019a, September). *Recovery-oriented cognitive therapy (CT-R) approaches for individuals with serious mental health conditions.* Paper presented at the International Initiative for Mental Health Leadership and International Initiative for Disability Leadership, Washington, DC.

Grant, P. M. (2019b). *Recovery-oriented cognitive therapy: A theory-driven, evidence-based, transformative practice to promote flourishing for individuals with serious mental health conditions that is applicable across mental health systems.* Alexandria, VA: National Association of State Mental Health Program Directors.

Grant, P. M., & Beck, A. T. (2009a). Defeatist beliefs as a mediator of cognitive impairment, negative symptoms, and functioning in schizophrenia. *Schizophrenia Bulletin, 35*(4), 798–806.

Grant, P. M., & Beck, A. T. (2009b). Evaluation sensitivity as a moderator of communication disorder in schizophrenia. *Psychological Medicine, 39*(7), 1211–1219.

Grant, P. M., & Beck, A. T. (2010). Asocial beliefs as predictors of asocial behavior in schizophrenia. *Psychiatry Research, 177*(1–2), 65–70.

Grant, P. M., & Best, M. W. (2019, July). *It is always sunny in Philadelphia: The adaptive mode and positive beliefs as a new paradigm for understanding recovery and empowerment for individuals with serious mental health challenges.* Paper presented at the annual meeting of the International CBT for Psychosis, Philadelphia, PA.

Grant, P. M., Best, M. W., & Beck, A. T. (2019). The meaning of group differences in cognitive performance. *World Psychiatry, 18*(2), 163–164.

Grant, P. M., Bredemeier, K., & Beck, A. T. (2017). Six-month follow-up of recovery-oriented cognitive therapy for low-functioning individuals with schizophrenia. *Psychiatric Services, 68*(10), 997–1002.

Grant, P. M., Huh, G. A., Perivoliotis, D., Stolar, N. M., & Beck, A. T. (2012). Randomized trial to evaluate the efficacy of cognitive therapy for low-functioning patients with schizophrenia. *Archives of General Psychiatry, 69*(2), 121–127.

Grant, P. M., & Inverso, E. (in press). Recovery-oriented cognitive therapy: Using the cognitive triad to map and achieve best selves in the face of tough challenges. *Cognitive Therapy and Research*.

Grant, P. M., Perivoliotis, D., Luther, L., Bredemeier, K., & Beck, A. T. (2018). Rapid improvement in beliefs, mood, and performance following an experimental success experience in an analogue test of recovery-oriented cognitive therapy. *Psychological Medicine, 48*(2), 261–268.

Hackmann, A., Bennett-Levy, J., & Holmes, E. A. (2011). *Oxford guide to imagery in cognitive therapy.* Oxford, UK: Oxford University Press.

Harding, K. (2019). *The rabbit effect: Live longer, happier, and healthier with the groundbreaking science of kindness.* New York: Atria Books.

Henriksen, M. G., Nordgaard, J., & Jansson, L. B. (2017). Genetics of schizophrenia: Overview of methods, findings and limitations. *Frontiers in Human Neuroscience, 11*, 1–9.

Honig, A., Romme, M. A., Ensink, B. J., Escher, S. D., Pennings, M. H., & deVries, M. W. (1998). Auditory hallucinations: A comparison between patients and nonpatients. *Journal of Nervous and Mental Disease, 186*(10), 646–651.

Hooley, J. M., & Franklin, J. C. (2017). Why do people hurt themselves?: A new conceptual model of nonsuicidal self-injury. *Clinical Psychological Science, 6*(3), 428–451.

Jacobson, E. (1938). *Progressive relaxation.* Chicago: University of Chicago Press.

Jay, M. (2016). *This way madness lies.* London: Thames & Hudson.

Kiran, C., & Chaudhury, S. (2009). Understanding delusions. *Industrial Psychiatry Journal, 18*(1), 3–18.

Klapheck, K., Lincoln, T. M., & Bock, T. (2014). Meaning of psychoses as perceived by patients, their relatives and clinicians. *Psychiatry Research, 215*(3), 760–765.

Knowles, R., McCarthy-Jones, S., & Rowse, G. (2011). Grandiose delusions: A review and theoretical integration of cognitive and affective perspectives. *Clinical Psychology Review, 31*(4), 684–696.

Koh, A. W. L., Lee, S. C., & Lim, S. W. H. (2018) The learning benefits of teaching: A retrieval practice hypothesis. *Applied Cognitive Psychology, 32*, 401–410.

Kraepelin, E. (1971). *Dementia praecox and paraphrenia.* Huntington, NY: Krieger.

Kreyenbuhl, J., Nossel, I. R., & Dixon, L. B. (2009). Disengagement from mental health treatment among individuals with schizophrenia and strategies for facilitating connections to care: A review of the literature. *Schizophrenia Bulletin, 35*(4), 696–703.

Kuipers, E., Leff, J., & Lam, D. (2002). *Family work for schizophrenia.* London: RCPsych.

Le, T. P., Najolia, G. M., Minor, K. S., & Cohen, A. S. (2017). The effect of limited cognitive resources on communication disturbances in serious mental illness. *Psychiatry Research, 248*, 98–104.

Lee, E. E., Liu, J., Tu, X., Palmer, B. W., Eyler, L. T., & Jeste, D. V. (2018). A widening longevity gap between people with schizophrenia and general population: A literature review and call for action. *Schizophrenia Research, 196*, 9–13.

Liberman, R. P. (2008). *Recovery from disability: Manual of psychiatric rehabilitation.* Washington, DC: American Psychiatric Publishing.

Lieberman, J. A., Stroup, T. S., Perkins, D. O., & Dixon, L. B. (Eds.). (2020). *The American Psychiatric Association Publishing textbook of schizophrenia* (2nd ed.). Washington, DC: American Psychiatric Publishing.

Lutterman, T., Shaw, R., Fisher, W., & Manderscheid, R. (2017). *Trend in psychiatric inpatient capacity, United States and each state, 1970 to 2014.* Alexandria, VA: National Association of State Mental Health Program Directors.

Maslow, A. H. (1954). *Motivation and personality.* New York: Harper & Row.

McKenna, P. J., & Oh, T. M. (2005). *Schizophrenic speech: Making sense of bathroots and ponds that fall in doorways.* New York: Cambridge University Press.

Mervis, J. E., Lysaker, P. H., Fiszdon, J. M., Bell, M. D., Chue, A. E., Pauls, C., . . . Choi, J. (2016). Addressing defeatist beliefs in work rehabilitation. *Journal of Mental Health, 25*(4), 366–371.

Mote, J., Grant, P. M., & Silverstein, S. M. (2018). Treatment implications of situational variability in cognitive and negative symptoms of schizophrenia. *Psychiatric Services, 69*(10), 1095–1097.

Murthy, V. H. (2020). *Together: The healing power of human connection in a sometimes lonely world.* New York: HarperCollins.

Nock, M. K. (2009). *Understanding nonsuicidal self-injury: Origins, assessment, and treatment.* Washington, DC: American Psychological Association.

Olmstead v. LC, 527 581 (Supreme Court 1999).

Oshima, I., Mino, Y., & Inomata, Y. (2003). Institutionalisation and schizophrenia in Japan: Social environments and negative symptoms: Nationwide survey of in-patients. *British Journal of Psychiatry, 183,* 50–56.

Oshima, I., Mino, Y., & Inomata, Y. (2005). Effects of environmental deprivation on negative symptoms of schizophrenia: A nationwide survey in Japan's psychiatric hospitals. *Psychiatry Research, 136*(2–3), 163–171.

Patel, R., Jayatilleke, N., Broadbent, M., Chang, C.-K., Foskett, N., Gorrell, G., . . . Stewart, R. (2015). Negative symptoms in schizophrenia: A study in a large clinical sample of patients using a novel automated method. *BMJ Open, 5*(9), e007619.

Perivoliotis, D., Morrison, A. P., Grant, P. M., French, P., & Beck, A. T. (2009). Negative performance beliefs and negative symptoms in individuals at ultra-high risk of psychosis: A preliminary study. *Psychopathology, 42*(6), 375–379.

Pinals, D. A., & Fuller, D. A. (2017). *Beyond beds: The vital role of a full continuum of psychiatric care.* Alexandria, VA: National Association of State Mental Health Program Directors.

Posey, T. B., & Losch, M. E. (1984). Auditory hallucinations of hearing voices in 375 normal subjects' imagination. *Cognition and Personality, 3*(2), 99–113.

Powers, A. R., III, Kelley, M. S., & Corlett, P. R. (2017). Varieties of voice-hearing: Psychics and the psychosis continuum. *Schizophrenia Bulletin, 43*(1), 84–98.

President's New Freedom Commission on Mental Health. (2003). Achieving the promise: Transforming mental health care in America (Final Report: Pub SMA-03-3832). Rockville, MD: U.S. Department of Health and Human Services. Retrieved from *www.sprc.org/sites/default/files/migrate/library/freedomcomm.pdf.*

Reddy, F., Reavis, E., Polon, N., Morales, J., & Green, M. (2017). The cognitive costs of social exclusion in schizophrenia. *Schizophrenia Bulletin, 43*(Suppl. 1), S54.

Resick, P. A., Monson, C. M., & Chard, K. M. (2017). *Cognitive processing therapy for PTSD: A comprehensive manual.* New York: Guilford Press.

Rogers, C. (1951). *Client-centered therapy: Its current practice, implications and theory.* London: Constable.

Romme, M. A., & Escher, A. D. (1989). Hearing voices. *Schizophrenia Bulletin, 15*(2), 209–216.

Romme, M. A., Honig, A., Noorthoorn, E. O., & Escher, A. D. (1992). Coping with hearing voices: An emancipatory approach. *British Journal of Psychiatry, 161,* 99–103.

Ruiz, I., Raugh, I., Chapman, H., Gonzalez, C., Grant, P. M., Beck, A. T., & Strauss, G. P. (2019). *Defeatist performance beliefs predict negative symptoms in daily life for people with schizophrenia: Evidence from ecological momentary assessment and geolocation.* Paper presented at the Society for Research in Psychopathology, Buffalo, NY.

Sacks, O. (2012). *Hallucinations.* Hampshire, UK: Pan Macmillan.

Saha, S., Chant, D., & McGrath, J. (2007). A systematic review of mortality in schizophrenia: Is the differential mortality gap worsening over time? *Archives of General Psychiatry, 64*(10), 1123–1131.

Satcher, D. (2000). Mental health: A report of the surgeon general—executive summary. *Professional Psychology: Research and Practice, 31*(1), 5–13.

Savill, M., Banks, C., Khanom, H., & Priebe, S. (2015). Do negative symptoms of schizophrenia change over time?: A meta-analysis of longitudinal data. *Psychological Medicine, 45*(8), 1613–1627.

Tandon, R., Nasrallah, H. A., & Keshavan, M. S. (2009). Schizophrenia, "just the facts" 4: Clinical features and conceptualization. *Schizophrenia Research, 110*(1–3), 1–23.

Tang, S. X., Seelaus, K. H., Moore, T. M., Taylor, J., Moog, C., O'Connor, D., . . . Gur, R. C. (2020). Theatre improvisation training to promote social cognition: A novel recovery-oriented intervention for youths at clinical risk for psychosis. *Early Intervention in Psychiatry, 14*(2), 163–171.

Thomas, E. C., Luther, L., Zullo, L., Beck, A. T., & Grant, P. M. (2017). From neurocognition to community participation in serious mental illness: The intermediary role of dysfunctional attitudes and motivation. *Psychological Medicine, 47*(5), 822–836.

van den Berg, D. P., & van der Gaag, M. (2012). Treating trauma in psychosis with EMDR: A pilot study. *Journal of Behavior Therapy and Experimental Psychiatry, 43*(1), 664–671.

Varvogli, L., & Darviri, C. (2011). Stress management techniques: Evidence-based procedures that reduce stress and promote health. *Health Science Journal, 5*(2), 74–89.

Vilhauer, R. P. (2017). Stigma and need for care in individuals who hear voices. *International Journal of Social Psychiatry, 63*(1), 5–13.

Wing, J. K., & Brown, G. W. (1970). *Institutionalism and schizophrenia: A comparative study of three mental hospitals 1960–1968*. Cambridge, UK: Cambridge University Press.

Wolpe, J. (1990). *The practice of behavior therapy*. New York: Pergamon Press.

Yalom, I. D. (1963). *Inpatient group psychotherapy*. New York: Basic Books.

Zarlock, S. P. (1966). Social expectation, language, and schizophrenia. *Journal of Humanistic Psychology, 6*(1), 68–74.

Index

Note. Page numbers followed by an *f* or a *t* indicate a figure or a table.

Accessing and energizing the adaptive mode
   aggression and, 164–165
   communication challenges and, 146–149, 146*f*, 154
   considerations in, 53, 55–57
   CT-R interactions and, 12, 12*f*
   decision tree to follow in navigating, 33–43, 34*f*, 36*f*, 38*f*, 40*f*, 42*f*
   delusions and, 119–120, 120*f*, 125–127, 125*f*, 126*f*
   developing ideas and guesses about beliefs and activities that may excite, 30–33, 32*t*
   family empowerment and, 223–224
   group CT-R and, 212, 217*f*
   guiding for positive and resilience beliefs and, 94–95
   hallucinations and, 136–139, 138*f*
   individual CT-R and, 180–182, 182*f*, 188, 190*f*
   inpatient CT-R and, 196–202, 198*f*, 199*f*, 210
   negative symptoms and, 107–109, 108*f*, 109*f*, 115
   objective of, 30
   overview, 1*f*, 8–9, 8*f*, 16, 29–30, 30*f*, 57
   Recovery Map and, 18, 19–20, 21*f*, 53, 54*f*
   self-injury and, 161
   strengthening positive beliefs and, 43–47, 43*t*, 44*f*, 45*f*
   substance use and, 170–171
   at-their-best moments and, 31
   trauma and, 157–158
   See also Adaptive mode; Connection; Core features of CT-R; Energizing the adaptive mode; Recovery Map
Action plan
   CT-R Benchmarks, 249–251
   CT-R interactions and, 12, 12*f*
   empowerment cards and, 98
   group CT-R and, 213–216, 217*f*, 218–219, 221
   increasing positive action towards aspirations and, 80
   individual CT-R and, 184–185, 190–191, 190*f*
   inpatient CT-R and, 195
   negative symptoms and, 110
   overview, 233
   See also Actualizing the adaptive mode; Planning; Positive action scheduling; Recovery Map; Steps
Activities
   common activities to consider, 32*t*
   communication challenges and, 146, 147–149
   compared to rewards, 55
   delusions and, 119–120, 132
   developing ideas and guesses about, 31–33, 32*t*
   energizing the adaptive mode and, 48–49, 48*f*, 57
   family empowerment and, 228, 229
   high-risk interests or response and, 41–43, 42*f*
   individual CT-R and, 180
   inpatient CT-R and, 200–202
   negative symptoms and, 109–110, 110*f*
   overview, 233
   Recovery Map and, 19–20, 21*f*
   remembering positive and resilience beliefs and, 98
   self-injury and, 161
   suggestions for, 237
   See also Accessing and energizing the adaptive mode; Activity scheduling
Activity Bingo game, 199–200, 199*f*
Activity challenge, 200–202
Activity scheduling
   energizing the adaptive mode and, 48, 48*f*, 50, 57
   example of, 51*f*
   form for, 238
   inpatient CT-R and, 197, 198*f*
   See also Activities; Positive action scheduling

Actualizing the adaptive mode
  aggression and, 166–168, 167f, 168f
  communication challenges and, 150, 150f
  considerations in, 84, 86
  CT-R interactions and, 12, 12f
  delusions and, 121–122, 128, 128f
  evaluating progress and drawing conclusions from positive action, 83–84
  example of, 79, 84
  group CT-R and, 213–216, 217f
  hallucinations and, 139
  individual CT-R and, 183–186, 187f
  inpatient CT-R and, 204–207
  negative symptoms and, 110
  overview, 1f, 8–9, 8f, 10, 16, 79, 79f, 87
  self-injury and, 162
  substance use and, 171–173, 172f
  trauma and, 158–159
  See also Adaptive mode; Aspirations; Core features of CT-R; Empowerment; Positive action
Adaptive mode
  accessing and energizing, 9
  actualize core feature of CT-R and, 10
  aspirations and, 57
  CT-R interactions and, 12, 12f
  defining aspirations and, 60
  delusions and, 132
  develop core feature of CT-R and, 9–10
  family empowerment and, 223–226
  individual CT-R and, 180
  inpatient CT-R and, 195–196
  negative symptoms and, 107–109, 108f, 109f, 115
  overview, 7, 8–11, 8f, 16, 57, 233
  Recovery Map and, 18
  strengthening, 10–11
  strengthening positive beliefs and, 43–47, 43t, 44f, 45f
  See also Accessing and energizing the adaptive mode; Actualizing the adaptive mode; Developing the adaptive mode; Modes; Strengthening the adaptive mode
Advice, 32–33, 41, 197, 199
Aggressive behavior
  accessing and energizing the adaptive mode and, 164–165
  actualizing the adaptive mode and, 166–168, 167f, 168f
  considerations in, 173–176, 174f
  developing the adaptive mode and, 165–166
  overview, 163–164, 163f, 176
  Recovery Map and, 22
  strengthening the adaptive mode and, 168
  See also Challenges; Trauma
Alcohol use. *See* Substance use
Alogia, 143. *See also* Communication challenges
Anxiety, 124
Aspirations
  adaptive mode as the gateway, 57
  aggression and, 165–166
  challenges and, 84, 86
  changing through the course treatment, 76
  chart for breaking into steps, 239
  communication challenges and, 149–150, 154
  considerations in, 75–77
  CT-R interactions and, 12, 12f
  decision trees and, 61, 62f, 69, 69f, 71, 72f
  defining, 59–60, 59f, 60f, 73f
  delusions and, 120–121, 120f, 121f, 127–128, 128f
  discovering the meaning of, 71–72, 72f, 73f
  distinguishing from other targets, 61, 62f, 63–67, 68t
  eliciting and enriching, 9–10, 61, 62f, 68, 68f, 69–71, 69f, 73–74, 73f, 74f
  family empowerment and, 224–226, 230
  group CT-R and, 204, 212–213, 217f, 218, 221
  guiding for positive and resilience beliefs and, 95
  hallucinations and, 139, 142
  increasing positive action towards, 80–83, 82f
  individual CT-R and, 182–183, 183f, 184, 190, 190f
  inpatient CT-R and, 193, 195–196, 203–207, 208, 210
  multiple aspirations, 76
  negative symptoms and, 109–110, 110f, 115
  overview, 78, 87, 233
  positive action scheduling for, 82–83
  Recovery Map and, 18, 21–22, 22f, 28
  self-injury and, 162
  substance use and, 171–172
  transforming goal targets into aspirations and, 68t
  trauma and, 158, 176
  See also Actualizing the adaptive mode; Developing the adaptive mode; Goals; Recovery Map
Assessments, 14, 193–194
Attention difficulties, 14, 153, 219–220
At-their-best moments, 7, 30–31. *See also* Adaptive mode
Auditory hallucinations. *See* Hallucinations

B

Beliefs
  aggression and, 164
  with both grandiose and paranoid features, 131
  challenges and, 22–23, 23f
  communication challenges and, 154
  discovering the meaning of aspirations and, 71–72, 72f, 73f
  eliciting, 89–93
  family empowerment and, 222–223, 225–226, 228, 229, 230
  grandiose beliefs, 116–122, 118f, 120f, 121f, 122f, 123f
  hallucinations and, 134–135, 135f, 142
  individual CT-R and, 180
  inpatient CT-R and, 193, 206–207
  negative symptoms and, 106–107, 110–111, 112–113, 112f, 115

paranoid beliefs and the safety mode, 123–129, 125*f*, 126*f*, 128*f*, 130*f*
Recovery Map and, 18, 19–20, 21*f*, 22–23, 23*f*
self-injury and, 160
strengthening, 52, 52*f*, 55, 57, 101
substance use and, 169
trauma and, 158, 176
See also Delusions; Negative beliefs; Positive beliefs
Beliefs Activated while in Adaptive Mode section of the Recovery Map, 19–20, 21*f. See also* Recovery Map
Biases, 112–113
Big dreams or desires, 76–77. *See also* Aspirations
Brain functioning, 14
Bridge between sessions, 188, 190, 190*f*, 218. *See also* Individual CT-R
Brief interactions, 35, 39, 41, 197, 198*f. See also* CT-R interactions

C

Capability
communication challenges and, 154
family empowerment and, 228
guiding for positive and resilience beliefs and, 93*t*
inpatient CT-R and, 194
remembering positive and resilience beliefs and, 97–99, 99*f*
suggestions for activities, 237
teaching others and, 97
Caretaker roles, 230
Case formulation. *See* Formulation
Chain analysis, 91–93, 167–168, 167*f*, 168*f*
Challenges
achieving aspirations and, 84, 86
CT-R interactions and, 12, 12*f*
empowerment cards and, 99
family empowerment and, 225–228, 230
group CT-R and, 217*f*, 218
individual CT-R and, 190, 190*f*
inpatient CT-R and, 203–204, 208–209
overview, 11, 103, 233
Recovery Map and, 18, 22–23, 23*f*
removal of in eliciting aspirations, 62*f*, 63, 64–65, 68*t*
scheduling activity and, 50
trauma and, 157–159
See also Aggressive behavior; Communication challenges; Delusions; Empowerment; Hallucinations; Negative symptoms; Positive symptoms; Recovery Map; Self-injury; Substance use
Closed-ended questioning, 46–47. *See also* Questioning
Clubs, 202, 204, 209, 210. *See also* Interests
Cognitive model, 7–8, 13, 16, 28, 257–258
Cognitive triad, 28
Collaboration
actualizing the adaptive mode and, 159
aspirations and, 75

challenges related to trauma and, 175
communication challenges and, 150
CT-R interactions and, 12, 12*f*
delusions and, 132
eliciting beliefs and, 91
family empowerment and, 230
group CT-R and, 212, 221
increasing positive action towards aspirations and, 82
individual CT-R and, 191
inpatient CT-R and, 194–195, 196, 210
overview, 8
Recovery Map and, 27, 28
strengthening the adaptive mode and, 10–11
Collusion, 131
Communication challenges
accessing and energizing the adaptive mode and, 37–39, 38*f*, 146–149, 146*f*
actualizing the adaptive mode and, 150, 150*f*
aspirations and meaning and, 149–150
considerations in, 151–154
overview, 143–145, 145*f*, 154
Recovery Map and, 22
strengthening the adaptive mode and, 151, 152*f*
See also Challenges
Community
CT-R Benchmarks, 244–245, 255
inpatient CT-R and, 205–206
recovery-oriented care and, 5–6, 5*f*, 6*f*
See also Life, prioritizing; Relationships; Social network
Compliments, 99–100
Conclusions
challenges related to trauma and, 176
communication challenges and, 154
delusions and, 132
group CT-R and, 214
hallucinations and, 142
individual CT-R and, 180
inpatient CT-R and, 201–202
overview, 10–11
positive action and, 52, 52*f*, 57, 83–84
strengthening positive beliefs and, 45–47
See also Strengthening the adaptive mode
Connection
accessing and energizing the adaptive mode and, 57
aggression and, 164–165
communication challenges and, 145, 150, 152–153, 154
CT-R approach and, 4
defining aspirations and, 60
delusions and, 120
family empowerment and, 230
group CT-R and, 219, 220–221
guiding for positive and resilience beliefs and, 93*t*
individual CT-R and, 180
inpatient CT-R and, 194–195, 196, 197, 198*f*, 200–202
negative symptoms and, 106, 107, 115

Connection (cont.)
  overview, 8–9, 8f
  recovery-oriented care and, 6
  seeking advice, 32–33
  self-injury and, 161, 162
  shared interests and, 32
  substance use and, 170–171
  suggestions for activities, 237
  teaching others and, 97
  trauma and, 156, 157
  See also Accessing and energizing the adaptive mode; Disconnection; Relationships; Therapeutic relationship
Consistency, 115
Control
  accessing and energizing the adaptive mode and, 39
  activities and, 55
  guiding for positive and resilience beliefs and, 93t
  hallucinations and, 142
  self injury and, 160, 161
  trauma and, 156, 157–158
Core features of CT-R, 1f, 16. *See also* Accessing and energizing the adaptive mode; Actualizing the adaptive mode; Developing the adaptive mode; Strengthening the adaptive mode
Corrections facilities, 55–56, 75–76
Crisis situations, 175
CT-R approach. *See* Recovery-oriented cognitive therapy (CT-R) overview
CT-R Benchmarks, 193–194, 241–256
CT-R interactions
  brief interactions, 35
  control and safety and, 39, 41
  inpatient CT-R and, 197, 198f
  overview, 16
  Recovery Map and, 28
  structure of, 12, 12f
Curiosity, therapist, 56, 154, 165–166

D

Daily life, 12, 12f, 49, 90, 173
Dangerous or risky goals, 62f, 63, 66–67, 68t. *See also* Aspirations; Goals; High-risk interests or response
Dating, 5–6, 5f, 6f. *See also* Life, prioritizing; Relationships
Deescalation of crisis situations, 175
Defeatist beliefs, 13, 80. *See also* Negative beliefs
Delusions
  accessing and energizing the adaptive mode and, 119–120, 120f, 125–127, 125f, 126f
  actualizing the adaptive mode and, 121–122, 128, 128f
  aspirations and meaning and, 120–121, 121f
  with both grandiose and paranoid features, 131
  considerations in, 129–131
  family empowerment and, 227
  grandiose beliefs, 116–122, 118f, 120f, 121f, 122f, 123f
  overview, 132
  paranoid beliefs and the safety mode, 123–129, 125f, 126f, 128f, 130f
  strengthening the adaptive mode and, 122, 122f, 123f, 129, 130f
  See also Beliefs; Challenges
Developing the adaptive mode
  aggression and, 165–166
  considerations in, 75–77
  CT-R interactions and, 12, 12f
  defining aspirations and, 59–60, 59f, 60f
  discovering the meaning of aspirations and, 71–72, 72f, 73f
  distinguishing aspirations from other targets and, 61, 62f, 63–67, 68t
  eliciting aspirations and, 61, 62f
  enriching aspirations and, 69–71, 69f
  example of, 58, 68, 68f
  group CT-R and, 212–213, 217f
  individual CT-R and, 182–183, 183f
  inpatient CT-R and, 203–204
  overview, 1f, 8–10, 8f, 16, 59, 78
  self-injury and, 162
  trauma and, 158
  See also Adaptive mode; Aspirations; Core features of CT-R
Diagnosis, 5–6, 5f, 6f
Direct verbal approach, 33–34, 34f
Disconnection, 106, 107, 113, 161. *See also* Connection
Distant goals, 62f, 63, 66, 68t. *See also* Aspirations; Goals
Distraction, 142
Documentation, 24, 207–208
Drawing conclusions. *See* Conclusions
Dreams, 109–110, 110f. *See also* Aspirations
Drug use. *See* Substance use

E

Emotions, 71, 134–135, 135f, 153, 154
Empathy, 154, 219, 228
Empowerment
  aspirations and, 75
  challenges and, 65, 103, 145
  communication challenges and, 145
  delusions and, 122, 122f
  empowerment cards, 98–99, 99f
  families and, 223–226
  hallucinations and, 135–140, 136f, 138f, 142
  individual CT-R and, 183–186, 187f
  motivation and, 14
  negative symptoms and, 107–111, 108f, 109f, 110f, 115
  overview, 11, 233
  Recovery Map and, 19, 23–24, 24f
  removal of a challenge and, 65
  responding to stressors and, 99

strengthening positive beliefs and, 45f
See also Accessing and energizing the adaptive mode; Actualizing the adaptive mode; Challenges; Positive action; Recovery Map
Energizing the adaptive mode
    communication challenges and, 146f, 147–149
    delusions and, 119–120, 120f
    example of, 53
    family empowerment and, 223–224
    group CT-R and, 212, 214
    inpatient CT-R and, 200–202
    overview, 9, 47–52, 48f, 51f, 52f, 53, 54f
    self-injury and, 161
    substance use and, 170–171
    trauma and, 157–158
    See also Accessing and energizing the adaptive mode; Energy; Recovery Map
Energy
    communication challenges and, 147
    eliciting aspirations and, 61
    evaluating progress and drawing conclusions from positive action and, 84
    group CT-R and, 214, 219, 221
    guiding for positive and resilience beliefs and, 93t
    increasing positive action towards aspirations and, 80
    inpatient CT-R and, 193, 200
    negative symptoms and, 106, 107
    suggestions for activities, 237
    See also Energizing the adaptive mode
Expansive mode
    grandiose beliefs, 116–122, 118f, 120f, 121f, 122f, 123f, 129
    overview, 132, 233

F

Families
    beliefs and, 222–223
    considerations in, 226–229
    empowerment cards and, 223–226
    family empowerment and, 223–226
    lack of family, 228
    overview, 222, 230
    See also Setting for treatment
Fast progress, 114
Feelings, 71, 134–135, 135f, 153, 154
Feelings as hallucinations. *See* Hallucinations
Flexibility, 89
Forensic facilities, 55–56, 75–76
Formal thought disorder, 143. *See also* Communication challenges
Formulation
    CT-R Benchmarks, 249–251, 255–256
    inpatient CT-R and, 195, 208, 209–210
    Recovery Map and, 28
    See also Recovery Map
Future, dreams for. *See* Aspirations

G

Games, 199–200, 199f, 212
Genuineness, 56
Goals
    distinguishing aspirations from other targets and, 62f, 63–67, 68f
    eliciting aspirations and, 62f, 63
    individual CT-R and, 182–183, 183f, 184
    overview, 60
    Recovery Map and, 21–22, 22f
    transforming goal targets into aspirations and, 68t
    See also Aspirations
Grand desires, 62f, 63, 65–66, 68t. *See also* Aspirations; Goals
Grandiose beliefs
    actualizing the adaptive mode and, 121–122
    considerations in, 129–131
    overview, 116–122, 118f, 120f, 121f, 122f, 123f, 132, 233
    See also Beliefs; Delusions
Grounding skills, 162. *See also* Refocusing process
Group CT-R
    accessing and energizing the adaptive mode and, 212, 216–218, 217f
    actualizing the adaptive mode and, 213–216, 217f
    aspirations and, 204, 217f, 218
    challenges and, 217f, 218
    considerations in, 219–221
    developing the adaptive mode and, 212–213, 217f
    inpatient CT-R and, 210
    overview, 211, 221
    phases of CT-R group therapy, 212–216
    session structure and, 216–219, 217f
    strengthening the adaptive mode and, 216, 217f
    See also Setting for treatment
Guarded individuals, 39–41, 40f
Guessing, 90–91. *See also* Questioning
Guiding and guided discovery questions
    considerations in, 99–101
    group CT-R and, 215, 216
    guiding for positive and resilience beliefs and, 93–97, 93t
    inpatient CT-R and, 201–202, 207
    meeting people where they are with, 100–101
    See also Questioning

H

Hallucinations
    accessing and energizing the adaptive mode and, 136–139, 138f
    actualizing the adaptive mode and, 139
    aspirations and meaning and, 139
    considerations in, 140, 142
    family empowerment and, 227–228
    overview, 133–135, 135f, 136f, 142

Hallucinations (cont.)
　　strengthening the adaptive mode and, 139–140, 141f
　　See also Challenges
Health outcomes, 11
Helping role
　　accessing and energizing the adaptive mode and, 32–33, 41
　　group CT-R and, 220–221
　　inpatient CT-R and, 197, 199, 204–206
　　suggestions for activities, 237
Highly restrictive settings, 55–56, 75–76
High-risk interests or response, 41–43, 42f. See also Dangerous or risky goals
Hope
　　big dreams or desires and, 76–77
　　defining aspirations and, 59–60, 59f, 60f
　　increasing positive action towards aspirations and, 80
　　overview, 8–9, 8f
　　trauma and, 158

I

Imagery, 69–71, 69f, 73f, 139
Individual CT-R
　　accessing and energizing the adaptive mode and, 180–182, 182f, 188
　　actualizing the adaptive mode and, 183–186, 187f
　　considerations in, 188–192, 190f
　　developing the adaptive mode and, 182–183, 183f
　　ending therapy, 187–188, 189f, 191
　　overview, 189f, 192
　　See also Setting for treatment
Individuals, 233
Inpatient CT-R
　　accessing and energizing the adaptive mode and, 196–202, 198f, 199f
　　actualizing the adaptive mode and, 204–207
　　basic needs and, 194
　　considerations in, 208–210
　　CT-R Benchmarks, 241–256
　　developing the adaptive mode and, 203–204
　　group CT-R and, 219
　　overview, 193–194, 210
　　sustaining a CT-R unit, 207–208
　　See also Setting for treatment
Interactions, CT-R. See Brief interactions; CT-R interactions
Interactive games, 199–200, 199f
Interests
　　developing ideas and guesses about, 31–33, 32t
　　high-risk interests or response and, 41–43, 42f
　　inpatient CT-R and, 197, 198f, 199–200, 199f, 202, 204
　　Recovery Map and, 28
　　shared interests, 32
Interests/Way to Engage section of the Recovery Map, 19–20, 21f. See also Recovery Map
Interventions, 19, 28, 113, 176

Isolated individuals
　　accessing and energizing the adaptive mode and, 35–37, 36f
　　communication challenges and, 145
　　inpatient CT-R and, 197, 198f
　　negative symptoms and, 106, 113

L

Life, prioritizing, 5–6, 5f, 6f, 61, 106
Life expectancy, 11
Look-Point-Name game, 137–139, 228
Low-resource settings, 55–56, 75–76

M

Mapping recovery. See Recovery Map
Meaning
　　aspirations and, 21–22, 22f, 71–72, 72f, 73f
　　communication challenges and, 149–150
　　CT-R interactions and, 12, 12f
　　delusions and, 120–121, 121f, 127–128, 128f, 132
　　hallucinations and, 139
　　individual CT-R and, 184
　　inpatient CT-R and, 194
　　negative symptoms and, 114
　　positive action and, 81–82, 83–84
　　Recovery Map and, 18
　　substance use and, 171–172
Meaningful roles
　　inpatient CT-R and, 204–206, 207
　　negative symptoms and, 106
　　overview, 8
　　recovery-oriented care and, 5–6, 5f, 6f
　　See also Life, prioritizing; Purpose
Media, 35, 37
Memory difficulties, 14, 50, 97–99, 153
Mental flexibility, 61
Mental illness, 5–6, 5f, 6f, 156–157, 233
Milieu treatment, 193–194, 233, 242–243, 255. See also Inpatient CT-R
Mind–body skills, 162
Mindfulness, 140
Modes, 7, 16. See also Adaptive mode; Expansive mode; Patient mode; Safety mode
Mood, 84, 112–113, 154
Motivation
　　aspirations and, 87
　　empowerment and, 14, 98
　　group CT-R and, 220
　　inpatient CT-R and, 203
　　negative symptoms and, 107
　　positive action scheduling for aspirations and, 82–83
Multidisciplinary team, 75. See also Collaboration; Treatment team
Mutual activities. See Activities

N

Negative beliefs
  challenges related to trauma and, 176
  communication challenges and, 154
  family empowerment and, 230
  increasing positive action towards aspirations and, 80
  inpatient CT-R and, 206–207
  negative symptoms and, 112–113, 115
  overview, 233
  research and evidence to support the use of CT-R and, 13–14
  See also Beliefs
Negative symptoms
  accessing and energizing the adaptive mode and, 107–109, 108f, 109f
  actualizing the adaptive mode and, 110
  aspirations and, 109–110, 110f
  considerations in, 111–115
  family empowerment and, 226–227
  interventions for, 240
  overview, 105–107, 115
  Recovery Map and, 22
  See also Challenges
  strengthening the adaptive mode and, 110–111, 112f
New Freedom Commission on Mental Health (2003), 5
Noticing in the moment, 90

O

Observations, 90
Olfactory hallucinations. *See* Hallucinations
Olmstead v. L. C. (1999), 4–5
Open-ended questioning, 46–47. *See also* Questioning
Optimism, 112–113, 220
Outcomes, 13–16, 252–253, 256
Outpatient individual therapy settings. *See* Individual CT-R

P

Paranoid beliefs
  aggression and, 167–168, 167f, 168f
  considerations in, 129–131
  overview, 123–129, 125f, 126f, 128f, 130f, 132
  See also Beliefs; Delusions
Patient mode
  challenges and, 22
  family empowerment and, 230
  individual CT-R and, 180
  overview, 7–8, 233
Pie technique, 171–172, 172f
Planning
  communication challenges and, 153
  defining aspirations and, 60
  evaluating progress and drawing conclusions from positive action and, 84
  increasing positive action towards aspirations and, 80–81
  negative symptoms and, 110
  See also Action plan
Pleasurable activities. *See* Activities
Positive action
  accessing and energizing the adaptive mode and, 57
  aggression and, 176
  delusions and, 122, 122f, 123f
  energizing the adaptive mode and, 48
  evaluating progress and drawing conclusions from, 83–84
  example of, 84
  family empowerment and, 225–226
  guiding for positive and resilience beliefs and, 95–97
  hallucinations and, 135, 136f, 142
  increasing positive action towards aspirations, 80–83, 82f
  individual CT-R and, 183–186, 187f
  inpatient CT-R and, 210
  overview, 10
  Recovery Map and, 19, 23–24, 24f, 28
  self-injury and, 176
  strengthening positive beliefs and, 45f
  substance use and, 172–173, 176
  See also Action plan; Actualizing the adaptive mode; Empowerment; Positive action scheduling; Recovery Map
Positive Action and Empowerment section of the Recovery Map, 19. *See also* Empowerment; Positive action; Recovery Map
Positive action scheduling
  accessing and energizing the adaptive mode and, 57
  for aspirations, 82–83
  energizing the adaptive mode and, 48, 48f, 50
  example of, 51f
  inpatient CT-R and, 206–207
  remembering positive and resilience beliefs and, 98
  strengthening positive beliefs and, 52, 52f
  See also Activity scheduling; Positive action
Positive beliefs
  aggression and, 168
  communication challenges and, 154
  considerations in, 99–101
  eliciting, 89–93
  guiding for, 93–97, 93t, 99–101
  individual CT-R and, 180
  inpatient CT-R and, 206–207
  negative symptoms and, 111
  overview, 16, 233
  Recovery Map and, 19, 28
  remembering, 97–99, 99f

Positive beliefs *(cont.)*
   research and evidence to support the use of CT-R and, 13
   strengthening, 43–47, 43t, 44f, 45f, 52, 52f, 55, 57, 88–89, 101
   See also Beliefs; Strengthening the adaptive mode
Positive emotion, 71, 134–135, 135f, 153, 154
Positive symptoms, 22. *See also* Challenges
Posttraumatic stress disorder (PTSD), 155. *See also* Trauma
Power, 158
Predictability, 157–158, 165
Problem solving
   defining aspirations and, 60
   group CT-R and, 214–216, 217f, 218, 221
   poor performance on tests and tasks and, 14
   self-injury and, 162
Program outcomes, 15–16, 193–194, 207–208, 241–256
Progress, rate of, 113–114
Progress evaluation, 83–84
Provider roles, 175
Public health, 11
Purpose
   CT-R interactions and, 12, 12f
   group CT-R and, 220
   inpatient CT-R and, 194
   negative symptoms and, 106, 110
   overview, 8–9, 8f, 61
   recovery-oriented care and, 5–6, 5f, 6f
   self-injury and, 162
   See also Meaningful roles

Q

Quality of life, 5–6, 5f, 6f, 11, 61
Questioning
   aspirations and, 73f
   eliciting aspirations and, 61, 62f
   eliciting beliefs and, 90–91
   group CT-R and, 215, 216
   guiding for positive and resilience beliefs and, 93–97, 93t
   identifying steps and, 80–81
   inpatient CT-R and, 201–202
   meeting people where they are, 100–101
   rather than complimenting, 99–100
   strengthening positive beliefs and, 46–47
   transforming goal targets into aspirations and, 68t
   See also Closed-ended questioning; Open-ended questioning

R

Recovery, 4–6, 5f, 6f, 15, 233
Recovery check, 188, 190, 190f. *See also* Individual CT-R
Recovery Map
   accessing and energizing the adaptive mode and, 9, 53, 54f
   actualize core feature of CT-R and, 10
   aspirations and, 68, 68f, 74, 74f
   benefits of, 18
   challenges and, 11
   communication challenges and, 145, 145f, 146, 146f, 150, 150f, 151, 152f
   deciding when to use, 27–28
   delusions and, 118f, 119, 120, 120f, 121, 121f, 122f, 123f, 125, 125f, 126, 126f, 128, 128f
   develop core feature of CT-R and, 10
   as documentation, 24, 207–208
   example of a completed Recovery Map, 26f
   families and, 223
   filling out, 18–24, 21f, 22f, 23f, 24f
   form for, 234
   hallucinations and, 135, 135f
   individual CT-R and, 182, 182f, 183, 183f, 189f, 191
   inpatient CT-R and, 195, 207–208, 209–210
   negative symptoms and, 108, 108f, 109–110, 109f, 110f, 112f
   over the course of treatment, 24–25
   overview, 9, 16, 17–18, 28
   positive action and, 84, 85f
   Recovery Map How-To Guide, 235–236
   shared Recovery Maps, 27
   strengthening positive beliefs and, 44–45, 44f, 45f
   strengthening the adaptive mode and, 11
   substance use and, 170
   sustaining a CT-R unit and, 207
   treatment planning and, 25
   See also Accessing and energizing the adaptive mode; Action plan; Aspirations; Challenges; Empowerment; Positive action
Recovery-oriented care, 5–6, 5f, 6f
Recovery-oriented cognitive therapy (CT-R) overview
   core features of, 1f
   CT-R Benchmarks, 241–256
   overview, 3–4, 8–11, 8f, 16
   research and evidence to support, 13–16
   resources for, 257–258
Refocusing process
   challenges related to trauma and, 176
   family empowerment and, 228
   hallucinations and, 135–140, 136f, 138f, 142
   self-injury and, 162
Rejecting individuals, 39–41, 40f
Rejection beliefs, 160, 164. *See also* Beliefs
Relapse, 174, 174f
Relationships
   communication challenges and, 150
   defining aspirations and, 60
   inpatient CT-R and, 194–195
   negative symptoms and, 106
   recovery-oriented care and, 5–6, 5f, 6f
   See also Community; Connection; Dating; Life, prioritizing; Social network; Therapeutic relationship

Index

Relaxation, 140, 153, 162
Removal of a challenge, 62f, 63, 64–65, 68t. *See also* Aspirations; Challenges
Repeated experiences, 47
Repetition, 55, 101, 115, 119–120
Resilience
 aspirations and, 75
 communication challenges and, 145, 151, 152f
 delusions and, 122, 122f, 123f, 129, 130f
 eliciting positive beliefs and, 89–93
 empowering, 10–11
 family empowerment and, 226, 229
 group CT-R and, 217f
 guiding for positive and resilience beliefs and, 93–97, 93t, 100–101
 negative symptoms and, 110–111, 112f
 overview, 8–9, 8f, 11, 233
 remembering positive and resilience beliefs and, 97–99, 99f
 repetition in strengthening beliefs and, 55
 responding to stressors and, 100
 substance use and, 173
 See also Strengthening the adaptive mode
Risky behaviors. *See* Aggressive behavior; Self-injury; Substance use; Trauma
Risky goals. *See* Dangerous or risky goals
Roles. *See* Helping role; Meaningful roles

S

Safety
 accessing and energizing the adaptive mode and, 39
 aggression and, 175
 dangerous aspirations and, 67
 defining aspirations and, 60
 negative symptoms and, 106
 paranoid beliefs and the safety mode and, 123–129, 125f, 126f, 128f, 130f, 132
 trauma and, 156, 158, 176
Safety mode, 124
School, 5–6, 5f, 6f. *See also* Life, prioritizing
Seeing things that aren't there. *See* Hallucinations
Self-assessment, program, 15–16, 193–194, 207–208, 241–256
Self-concept, 156
Self-injury
 accessing and energizing the adaptive mode and, 161
 actualizing the adaptive mode and, 162
 considerations in, 173–176, 174f
 developing the adaptive mode and, 162
 overview, 159–161, 160f, 176
 Recovery Map and, 22
 strengthening the adaptive mode and, 162–163
 See also Challenges; Trauma
Sensory experiences, 69f, 70
Serious mental health conditions. *See* Mental illness

Setting for treatment, 55–56, 75–76, 179. *See also* Families; Group CT-R; Individual CT-R; Inpatient CT-R
Slow progress, 113–114
Smells as hallucinations. *See* Hallucinations
Social network, 5–6, 5f, 6f, 202, 204. *See also* Community; Life, prioritizing; Relationships
Speech that is hard to follow. *See* Communication challenges
Spirituality, 5–6, 5f, 6f. *See also* Life, prioritizing
Staff. *See* Treatment team
STEER process, 167–168, 167f, 168f
Steps
 chart for breaking aspirations into, 239
 evaluating progress and, 83–84
 group CT-R and, 213–216, 221
 identifying steps and, 82f
 increasing positive action towards aspirations and, 80–82, 82f
 overview, 62f, 63–64, 87
 transforming goal targets into aspirations and, 68t
 See also Actualizing the adaptive mode; Aspirations; Goals
Stigma, 142, 168–169
Strategy, 19, 28
Strengthening the adaptive mode
 aggression and, 168
 communication challenges and, 151, 152f
 considerations in, 99–101
 CT-R interactions and, 12, 12f
 delusions and, 122, 122f, 123f, 129, 130f
 eliciting beliefs and, 89–93
 example of, 88
 group CT-R and, 216, 217f
 guiding for positive and resilience beliefs and, 93–97, 93t
 hallucinations and, 139–140, 141f
 negative symptoms and, 110–111, 112f
 overview, 1f, 8–9, 8f, 10–11, 16, 88–89, 89f, 101
 remembering positive and resilience beliefs and, 97–99, 99f
 self-injury and, 162–163
 substance use and, 173
 See also Adaptive mode; Beliefs; Conclusions; Core features of CT-R; Positive beliefs; Resilience
Stressors, 100, 145, 154
Substance use
 accessing and energizing the adaptive mode and, 41–43, 42f, 170–171
 actualizing the adaptive mode and, 171–173, 172f
 considerations in, 173–176, 174f
 overview, 168–169, 176
 Recovery Map and, 22
 strengthening the adaptive mode and, 173
 See also Challenges; Trauma
Symptoms. *See* Aggressive behavior; Anxiety; Delusions; Formal thought disorder; Hallucinations; Negative symptoms; Self-injury; Substance use; Trauma

T

Targets
- distinguishing aspirations from, 61, 62f, 63–67, 68t
- Recovery Map and, 19, 28
- transforming goal targets into aspirations and, 68t

Teaching others, 97
Technology, 50
Termination, 187–188, 189f, 191, 192
Therapeutic relationship
- accessing and energizing the adaptive mode and, 56
- aggression and, 164–165
- communication challenges and, 151–153, 154
- defining aspirations and, 60
- delusions and, 120, 129–131
- eliciting beliefs and, 91–93
- individual CT-R and, 191
- *See also* Connection; Relationships; Trust

Therapist factors, 56
Transition planning, 248–249, 255
Trauma
- accessing and energizing the adaptive mode and, 157–158
- actualizing the adaptive mode and, 158–159
- considerations in, 173–176, 174f
- developing the adaptive mode and, 158
- individual CT-R and, 186
- overview, 155–157, 176
- *See also* Aggressive behavior; Self-injury; Substance use

Treatment, 5–6, 5f, 6f, 14
Treatment planning, 25, 246–247, 255
Treatment team
- CT-R Benchmarks, 253–255, 256
- inpatient CT-R and, 194–195, 201, 203–204, 208, 210
- multidisciplinary teams, 70
- sustaining a CT-R unit, 207–208
- *See also* Collaboration

Treatment-oriented goals, 62f, 63, 64, 68t. *See also* Aspirations; Goals
Trust
- aspirations and, 60, 61
- CT-R approach and, 4
- delusions and, 120
- families and, 229
- individual CT-R and, 186, 191
- negative symptoms and, 106, 107
- trauma and, 157
- *See also* Therapeutic relationship

V

Value of activities, 46. *See also* Activities
Visual aids, 153
Visual hallucinations. *See* Hallucinations
Voices, hearing. *See* Hallucinations

W

Withdrawn individuals, 35–37, 36f, 219. *See also* Negative symptoms
Work, 5–6, 5f, 6f. *See also* Life, prioritizing
Worth, 156, 160, 176